SIXTH EDITION

The Voice and Voice Therapy

Daniel R. Boone

University of Arizona

Stephen C. McFarlane

University of Nevada Medical School

Allyn and Bacon

Boston ■ London ■ Toronto ■ Sydney ■ Tokyo ■ Singapore

To two of our heroes,
G. Paul Moore, Ph.D.
and Robert W. Blakeley, Ph.D.

Executive Editor: Stephen D. Dragin
Editorial Assistant: Bridget McSweeney
Marketing Managers: Ellen Dolberg and Brad Parkins
Editorial Production Service: Chestnut Hill Enterprises
Manufacturing Buyer: David Repetto
Cover Administrator: Linda Knowles

Copyright © 2000 by Allyn & Bacon
A Pearson Education Company
160 Gould Street
Needham Heights, MA 02494
Copyright 1994, 1988, 1983, 1977, 1971 by Prentice Hall

Internet: www.abacon.com

Between the time Website information is gathered and published, some sites may have closed. Also, the transcription of URLs can result in typographical errors. The publisher would appreciate notification where these occur so that they may be corrected in subsequent editions.

Library of Congress Cataloging-in-Publication Data

Boone, Daniel R.
    The voice and voice therapy / Daniel R. Boone, Stephen C.
  McFarlane. — 6th ed.
      p.   cm.
    Includes bibliographical references and index.
    ISBN 0-205-30843-0 (alk. paper)
    1. Voice disorders. 2. Larynx—Diseases. I. McFarlane, Stephen C.
  II. Title.
    [DNLM: 1. Voice Disorders—diagnosis. 2. Speech, Alaryngeal.
  3. Voice—physiology. 4. Voice Disorders—etiology. 5. Voice
  Disorders—therapy. 6. Voice Training. WV 500 B724v 1999]
RF540.B8S   1999
616.85'5—dc21
DNLM/DLC
for Library of Congress   99-22921
                                                  CIP

Printed in the United States of America

10 9 8 7 6 5   04 03

CONTENTS

PREFACE

The study of the normal voice and voice disorders and their management has caught on. When the first edition of *The Voice and Voice Therapy* was written in the late 1960s, there were few publications, books or journal articles, about clinical voice disorders. Today, the management of voice disorders may be found in the journals and texts of speech–language pathologists, otolaryngologists, voice and drama teachers, vocal coaches, singing teachers, self-improvement consultants, and other specialists who give priority to the need for a healthy voice. Although this sixth edition of *The Voice and Voice Therapy* keeps its introductory emphasis for the student in speech–language pathology, we have attempted to maintain a clear perspective on the normal voice, its disorders, and their management and/or voice therapy for most professional readers interested in voice.

We are indebted to former students, teaching associates, and book reviewers (Jon Hufnagle, Illinois State University; Marylou Pausewang Gelfer, University of Wisconsin, Milwaukee; E. Charles Healey, University of Nebraska, Lincoln; and Celia R. Hooper, University of North Carolina) for their critical insights of previous editions of this book with specific recommendations for improving the effectiveness of this sixth edition. Reviewers recommended that the basic format of the book stay the same. Accordingly, we have kept the format the same but have done extensive revision and expansion of the previous text to incorporate more recent literature and research findings. Chapter 1 has changed the least, taking a look at how the voice is influenced by the larynx in its ever-changing biologic, emotional, and linguistic roles. Anatomy and physiology of the larynx and airways responsible for the respiration–phonation–resonance required for normal voice are developed in Chapter 2, which includes a number of new illustrations. Descriptions of voice disorders are found in Chapter 3, with some emphasis given to identifying causal factors and describing particular voice symptoms of specific disorders. In the CD that accompanies this text, the student may hear the voices and case presentations of ten voice patients with various disorders as they are described in Chapter 3. Color photographs of various laryngeal disorders are included at the end of this disorders chapter. Neurogenic voice disorders are no longer described in Chapter 3 but are now included in a new chapter on neurogenic voice disorders, Chapter 4. A brief working scheme is presented about the normal nervous system and its role in voice production, which is then followed by descriptions of neurogenic voice disorders with emphasis given to their management by the speech-language pathologist and other professionals.

A new look at instrumental evaluation contrasted with perceptual evaluation is presented in the new Chapter 5, The Voice Evaluation. In this chapter, instrumentation and procedural application is given for aerodynamic assessment, acoustic evaluation, structural and physiological assessment of respiratory–phonatory–resonance components of voice, along with observational and perceptual scaling of the patient and his or her voice. Chapter 6, Voice Therapy, begins with a table listing twenty-five facilitating therapy approaches. One reviewer wrote that this table is "probably the most famous and most photocopied table in the history of this discipline!"; it lists the facilitating approach with the probable parameter of voice affected by application of that particular approach. Validation of particular techniques in the voice disorders literature has been slow in coming, primarily because the voice clinician rarely uses one approach for a particular disorder. Rather, the voice clinician blends various approaches together to meet the needs and the voice-ability level of the particular patient. Various therapy approaches are cited on the CD, along with listening to the patient's voice before and after voice therapy. The facilitating approach list remains at twenty-five by adding to, or by combining, or dropping approaches listed in the fifth edition.

Management and voice therapy for particular problems of voice are presented in Chapter 7. The voice problems of particular populations, such as in aging or in professional users of voice, are considered from the point of view of optimizing vocal function. Faulty voice usage and respiratory-based voice problems are given particular attention, with medical management/voice therapy suggestions for particular laryngeal problems, such as cysts and granuloma. In response to our reviewers and our colleagues who use this book as a text, we have restored and developed a new chapter on management and therapy for various voice problems related to laryngeal cancer. Chapter 8 looks at various management approaches for laryngeal cancer, including methods of insufflation testing, TEP, traditional esophageal speech, and the use of various voice prostheses. In the new Chapter 9, consideration is given to deviations in both oral and nasal resonance. We discuss advances in instrumentation for measuring aspects of nasalance, as well as using this same equipment in therapy for direct feedback to the patient.

The sixth edition of *The Voice and Voice Therapy* represents a major revision by the authors. This would not have been possible without the tireless literature search of two doctoral students at the University of Nevada at Reno, Shelley Von Berg and Marie Sterkel. Manuscript scrutiny and organization of references and the reference bibliography were made possible by the efforts of Paul S. McFarlane and Casey Oliver in Reno. Diagnostic and trial therapy regimens in Tucson were made possible by Kay Wiley, Anthony Defeo, Ph.D., Julie Barkmeier, Ph.D., and Stan Coulthard, M.D., all at the University of Arizona. Case illustrations throughout this text were made possible by our Arizona and Nevada patients with voice disorders. A critical review of the total manuscript by Tom Watterson, Ph.D., University of Nevada was much appreciated.

We were urged by several reviewers and our executive editor at Allyn & Bacon, Stephen D. Dragin, to add a clinical CD to this new edition of the text. We agree that a clinical CD will greatly enhance the teaching value of what we have written here. On the inside cover of this book, the reader will find a clinical CD, presenting 12 voice patients of various ages, each with a different voice problem. The causal factors of the problem are first presented, followed by a recording of the patient's pre- and posttreatment voice. The therapy techniques that were used with that particular patient are then presented. It should be noted that each patient received a combination of several facilitating approaches as part of his or her treatment. Rarely will one therapy technique alone optimize the patient's vocal performance. The listener will then hear the patient's voice at the end of therapy.

The sixth edition of this book has been shaped by the feedback we have received from our colleagues and reviewers, by an expanding clinical and research literature, and from our continuing involvement with both voice patients and students. Looking closely at voice therapy outcomes tells us that the typical voice problem is resolved faster than most other communication problems that we face as speech–language pathologists. Identifying and modifying causal factors of the voice problem followed by behavioral voice therapy, as detailed in this sixth edition, seems to work. Please continue to give us your feedback.

Daniel R. Boone
Stephen C. McFarlane

CHAPTER

1

The Voice and Voice Therapy

We use our voices in many different ways. Vegetatively, our voices may signal biologic states, such as signaling our physical discomfort from hunger or pain. Emotionally, from infancy throughout life we unmask, with and without our conscious permission, our emotions by the sound of our voices. Linguistically, our voice (phonation) carries the message of segments and the vocal rhythm (prosody) that supports those segments. Paralinguistically, our voicing quality colors the meaning of the words that we say, so much so that it is not always *what* we say but *how* we say it.

The primary function of the airway (lungs, larynx, pharynx, oral and nasal cavities) is the biologic role of maintaining and ensuring survival through breathing in oxygenated air and exhaling out carbon dioxide-loaded air. The larynx sits as a guardian below the oral and pharyngeal cavities, guarding the vital airway structures below it from intrusion of liquids, foods, phlegm, and other foreign bodies. As we shall see in this book, the emotional state of many mammals is often revealed by the sound of their voices (from dogs barking at an intruder to the intruder yelling his or her fear at the dog). However, the human being appears to be the only mammal species that has added complicated linguistic voicing to the biologic–emotional roles of the airway. We shall see how human voicing in infancy and early childhood plays a primary role in the acquisition and development of spoken language. Voicing continues to play a vital role in spoken communication throughout the life span. At the other end of the phonation scale is artistic voicing, in which we see the mechanisms of respiration, phonation, and resonance used in incredibly artistic ways, such as the voice of the Shakespearean actor or the high notes sung by an operatic tenor. The best speakers and singers are often those people who, by natural gift or training or by a studied blend of both, have mastered the art of optimally using these vocal mechanisms.

Although the vast majority of people experience normal function of the airway, some people have trouble within their nasal–pharyngeal cavities, or in the larynx, the trachea below it, the lungs, or with the muscles of respiration that make breathing possible. Any compromise of these airway structures or their function can cause voice disorders. And we shall see in this book, this airway compromise can be the result of anatomic deviation, disease, emotions overriding normal vocal function, or a change of vocal function because of abuse–misuse of vocal mechanisms. In much of this text we will look at voice disorders and the various management and therapy approaches available to children and adults with voice disorders.

In Chapter 2 of this book we will look at the normal airway structures and their functions that are required for normal voice. Before we go there, however, we will take a closer look at the larynx (the actual producer of voice), looking closer at its biologic role, its emotional function, and the role it plays in generating voice as part of one's overall linguistic function. We will then take a look at the people with voice disorders who experience problems in everyday communication, as well as those professional voice users whose problem voices may disrupt their job performance. We will then take an overview look at various voice disorders and some of the management and voice therapy approaches used to minimize or overcome such voice disorders.

The Biological Function of the Larynx

A description of the biological aspects of laryngeal function provides us an early hint of how the biological demands of the airway and the larynx will always take precedence over artistic or communicative vocal production. When the brain signals the body's need for renewal of oxygen in the breath cycle, we automatically take in a breath. Oxygen-laden air flows through the passages of the upper airway into the lungs, followed by the outgoing carbon dioxide-loaded air flowing out of the body through the airway. This transportation of air into and out of the lungs is the primary function of the airway. Protecting the airway for an unobstructed passage of the air supply is the larynx. The primary biological function of the larynx is to keep fluids and foods from going into the airway (aspiration).

The larynx sits in a vital site at the front, bottom of the throat (pharynx), and at the top of the windpipe (trachea). As fluids and chewed food (bolus) come down the posterior throat, they are diverted from the lower throat (hypopharynx) into the open esophagus, where they continue their journey through the esophagus down into the stomach. As part of the swallowing act, the laryngeal mechanism rises high (elevating the esophagus and trachea with it) in the neck. As the swallow progresses, the tongue comes back, the epiglottis cartilage of the larynx, which acts as a cover, closes over the open larynx.

Whenever the larynx plays this sphincteral role of closing off the airway to permit the posterior passage of liquids or food, the entire laryngeal body rises. Also, in fear situations, the larynx may reflexively elevate as part of its primary role in protecting the airway. Some voice patients, sometimes those with excessive fears, will attempt voice with the larynx in its elevated "protector" posture. Such excessive laryngeal elevation is not a good posture for producing a normal voice.

Besides the elevating capability of the larynx, which helps prevent aspiration, airway closure is aided by three laryngeal muscle valves, described in Chapter 2 as the aryepiglottic folds, the ventricular folds (false folds), and the thyroarytenoid muscles (the true vocal cords, or vocal folds). The most vertical of these valve pairs in the larynx are the aryepiglottic folds, which are considered part of the supralarynx. Under vigorous valving conditions, such as severe coughing, they begin to approximate (adduct) each other. Below them are the ventricular folds; only during vigorous adductory activities, like the cough, do they approach each other. The lowest and more medial of the three laryngeal valves are the thyroarytenoid muscles, the true vocal folds. During swallow, they always adduct to prevent possible aspiration. Also, the individual has fine control of the true folds with some capability of altering their shape, length, and tension, producing various voicing changes.

When an individual breathes naturally, all three valve sites are open. The vocal folds are in an open position on inspiration, the vocal folds separate a bit more (abduct) and, on expiration, they move slightly toward (adduct) each other. If the individual were to cough, all three valve sites would adduct medially, closing off the airway. In Chapter 2, we discover that normal voice is achieved by the true vocal folds adducting with the outgoing airstream passing between them, setting them into vibration. The vertical changes of laryngeal height and the degree of adductory or abductory positioning can have a profound influence on the sound of the voice. We will see in Chapter 3 that inadequate adduction can lead to no voice (aphonia); excessive vocal fold adduction produces an extremely tight-sounding voice (spasmodic dysphonia).

The Emotional Function of the Larynx

As early as three months old, the infant seems to express emotions by making laryngeal sounds. Certainly, the caregiver can soon detect differences in the emotional state of the baby by changes in the sound of the baby's vocalizations: A cry from hunger may sound different from a cry of discomfort or the vocalization of anger. Contentment (after a full stomach or being held) can be heard in the cooing responses of the baby. From early infancy throughout the life span, the sound of one's vocalization often mirrors one's internal emotional state.

Our voice can sound happy or sad, contented or angry, secure or unsafe, placid or passionate. How one feels affectively may be heard in the sound of the voice as well as in changes of the prosodic rhythm patterns of vocalization. Our emotional status plays a primary role in the control of respiration; for example, nervousness can be heard in one's shortness of breath. Our emotional state seems to dictate the vertical positioning of the larynx, the relative relaxation of the vocal folds, the posturing and relaxation of the muscles of the pharynx and tongue.

One's emotionality can be heard in the voice, a fact that can be threatening to the professional singer, or harmful to sales for the nervous salesperson, or embarrassing to someone who sounds like he or she is crying when actually happy. Our mood state can be harmful to voice. Many voice disorders are the result of various affective excesses; for example, a young professional woman attempts to use normal conversational voice when her larynx is postured in a high, sphincterally closed position, resulting in a tight, tense voice. Her problem may be more related to unchecked and unrealistic fear than it is to faulty use of the vocal mechanisms per se.

Because emotionality and vocal function are so closely entwined, effective voice therapy often requires the treatment of the total person and not just fixating on the remediation of voice symptoms. Therefore, as we will see in ensuing chapters, getting to know the patient is an important prerequisite to taking a case history or making an instrumental–perceptual voice evaluation. Voice clinicians have long recognized that the patient in the office may not resemble the same person in play settings; the patient's voice will change according to his or her mood state. To assess voice realistically, we have to observe and listen to the patient in various life settings.

The Linguistic Function of the Voice

Voice seems to hold spoken language together. From the primitive emotional vocalization that may color what we say to the skilled use of voice stress to emphasize a particular utterance, the voicing component of spoken language plays a primary role. It is not always what we say that carries the message, but how we say it.

New interest in infant vocalization is producing a fascinating literature. By the time typical one-year-old babies utter their first word, they have already used their voice in highly elaborate jargon communication. While human babies all seem to babble about the same way from four to six months of age, babbling becomes more language differentiated beyond that age. That is, babies no longer sound alike after six months; rather, they begin to sound like the primary language they have been hearing. The melody of the parent language, or its prosody, begins to color the vocalizations of the baby. The jargon of Chinese babies begins to sound like the sweeping tonal patterns of the Chinese language; the pharyngeal sounds of an Arab language begin to be heard in the jargon of Arab babies.

These prosodic vocal patterns exist far beyond the individual word or segment. Such voicing is known as *suprasegmental phonation.* In young babies, suprasegmental vocalization far exceeds the voicing of actual word segments. As babies acquire new words, they often place them in the proper place of their ongoing voicing rhythm. If they want to say *milk*, rather than say the word in isolation, they are far more likely to say the word at the end of a jargon phrase, such as "gawa na ta milk." The jargon leading up to the word is suprasegmental voicing. The jargon voice carries an uncoded message with no specific meaning but seems to convey some general meaning by the overall sound of it. The mood and need state of the baby influence the sound of the vocalization. And it appears that the sound of our voice colors the meaning of what we say for a lifetime.

Although jargon speech appears to diminish after the first eighteen months of life, we continue to use suprasegmental vocalization in all aspects of spoken communication. We add vocal stress patterns to augment the meaning of what we say. The actual words we say are only part of the communication. The "how we say it" is conveyed by various vocal stress strategies, such as changing loudness, grouping words together on one breath, changing pitch level, changing vocal quality and resonance to match our mood. These stress changes of the suprasegmentals of what we say can be produced with or without intent. That is, if it serves our purpose, we can sound angry by talking louder, or we may sound angry despite our best efforts to hide our anger from our listener. Once again, the voice carries much of the message. The same words spoken or written may convey different messages (as any lawyer taking depositions will tell you) depending on the stress patterns given the words by the speaker, with or without intent.

Considering the role of the voice in both emotional and linguistic expression, it is no wonder that people with voice disorders may find themselves handicapped in their communication. A young girl with vocal nodules, for example, may have developed them in part from excessive emotional vocalization (such as constantly yelling). Once the nodules were developed, however, she may be unable to use the vocal suprasegmentals and stress patterns she had previously used in communication. As anyone knows who has ever suffered a complete loss of voice from severe laryngitis, the lack of voice prevents you from being you. Somehow whisper and gesture do not carry the communication effectiveness that normal voice allows you to add to the words you say.

While a primary role of the human larynx appears to be biological (guarding the airway), laryngeal voicing plays a vital role in the expression of both emotional and linguistic communication. When we add the voicing dimensions of acting and singing as laryngeal functions, we can truly appreciate the amazing artistic capabilities of the vocal tract (that a few people are fortunate to have and sometimes use). The role of the human larynx is obviously more complex and more subtle than the way the larynx functions as an airway protector in most other mammals.

Physical disorders of the airway, larynx, and resonating cavities can affect all of these functions: biological, emotional, linguistic, and artistic. We will look at various physically caused voice disorders in Chapter 3, such as a disorder of vocal cord paralysis. With unilateral paralysis, typically the patient cannot bring his or her vocal folds together adequately, preventing the production of normal voice.

Voice Disorders in the Normal Population

It is difficult to establish normative incidence data on voice disorders for several reasons. For example, voice can become temporarily disordered from a common cold that changes laryngeal tissue vibration and may fill resonating sinuses with infected mucus; almost everyone at some time of life has experienced some voice change (phonation or resonance) as a result of a cold. Or some people experience continuing voice problems. Therefore, if we were to take a large segment of the population and determine the present and past incidence of a voice disorder, our incidence reporting would be near 100 percent. Such incidence data would be meaningless. Rather, if we took a segment of a population, such as airline pilots, and looked back at the occurrences of hoarseness (dysphonia) in a certain time period, we would determine some prevalence data for that particular group. Even this data would have far more meaning if the pilots' voices were compared with the voices of matched controls (matched, for example, by gender and age). Let us look at a few recent voice prevalence/incidence studies.

Looking at the voices of 259 children in primary school, Lecoq and Drape (1996) found that 10 percent of the children at the time of examination had dysphonic voices related to laryngeal or resonance disorders. If one asked the children's parents whether the child had experienced dysphonia in the past, the incidence data would be close to 100 percent. While incidence data might well include every encounter (brief or long) of voice problem that someone ever experienced over time, the prevalence data would probably be limited to a problem at the time the study was done. If one were to generalize from the papers and books that report incidence of voice disorders in the past twenty years, one might generalize (and not be too far off) that about 7 percent of an existing population of school-aged children experience continuing voice disorders; in the adult population, we might speculate that about 3 percent of people over 18 years experience continuing voice symptoms.

It would appear that studying particular groups, such as teachers or salespersons who make heavy use of their voice, can yield useful prevalence data. One such study by Smith and others (1997) found that, comparing 237 teachers with 178 nonteachers, over 20 percent of the teachers, had missed work in the past because of a voice disorder, while no control subject missed any work because of a voice problem. The total group of teachers averaged two or more voice symptoms, while the nonteachers reported no voice symptoms. Teaching appears to be among the highest voice risk groups that have been studied. Looking at how voice disorders can affect one's quality of life, Smith and others queried 174 patients with voice disorders, compared them with 173 adult control subjects, and found that 75 percent of voice patients and only 11 percent of the controls felt that social interactions were "adversely affected by voice problems." In a different study, negative findings were found among questionnaires from 237 female teachers who often reported that their voice symptoms limited their teaching effectiveness and "that their voice was a chronic source of stress or frustration" (Sapir, Keidar, and Mathers-Schmidt, 1993, p. 177). Cheerleaders as a group appear particularly vulnerable to voice disorders according to Case (1996), who summarized several of his studies looking at school cheerleaders before and after cheerleading camp, at the end of the cheerleading season, before and after one game, and so forth. Case found that the prevalence of immediate vocal fold tissue change from continued vocal yelling (measured before and after one game) was as high as 75 percent in twelve cheerleaders (six males, six females). While most of our prevalence data is based on special populations who experience unusually heavy use of voice resulting in some voice problem, there are many other kinds of voice disorders that are not primarily related to abuse or misuse of voice.

Kinds of Voice Disorders

There are many causes of voice disorders. In this book, we will classify voice disorders according to one of three primary causal factors: organic, neurogenic, or functional. That is, the presenting voice symptom may have one or several causes. In an organic voice disorder, hoarseness may be caused by a physical problem, such as a web growing between the vocal folds that prevents normal fold vibration. Or hoarseness heard in a neurogenic voice disorder may be caused by the vocal folds not moving properly, perhaps the result of paralysis of one of the folds. Or hoarseness heard in a functionally-caused voice disorder may be the result of poor vocal fold vibration after continuous heavy use, misuse, or abuse of the voice. The evaluation and diagnosis of the voice disorder, such as presenting hoarseness, should identify the causal factors of the disorder. The cause of the disorder will dictate the specific management and/or voice therapy steps required for that particular problem.

In Chapter 2 we will look at the physical components of the normal voice (respiration, phonation, and resonance). The reader should keep these normal processes in mind as we now consider the different kinds of voice disorders. A particular voice problem may affect primarily one of the processes, such as respiration, which in turn could cause problems of phonation and resonance. We shall look now at the impact on respiration–phonation–resonance caused by organic, neurogenic, and functional voice problems.

Organic Voice Problems

Many voice problems are the result of organic structural problems of the vocal tract. This is why it is important that any voice problem that lasts more than a week be investigated medically for possible physical causation and treatment. Sometimes the required treatment may be medical–surgical with voice therapy only helping to find and maintain the best possible voice. Some organic voice problems are static, relatively fixed, and not responsive to medical treatment; for these problems, voice therapy may be the only remediation possible.

Impairment in Respiration.   The respiratory system functions as the activator of the voice. The expiratory airflow pressures and volumes passing between the approximated vocal folds sets the folds into vibration, which produces voice. Therefore, any compromise of respiratory function can have a negative effect on speech (decrease in number of words said per breath) and voice (poorer voice quality). Lung volume may be reduced through space-occupying lesions, such as various forms of cancer or fluids in the lung; a reduction in air volume will reduce the amount of air the speaker can use for voice. Diseases of the airway, such as bronchitis or emphysema, can decrease lung elasticity and make it more difficult for the patient to sustain airflow and voicing. Although organic disease of the respiratory system may require medical treatment, voice therapy can often help patients develop the best respiratory control possible for speech and voice.

For example, the case of Charles illustrates a speech–voice problem, caused by two organic diseases, pulmonary emphysema and laryngeal leukoplakia:

> Charles, a fifty-eight-year-old chef, began to experience a shortness of breath that allowed him to say only about five words per breath. Physical examination indicated that he had severe pulmonary emphysema, probably directly related to his smoking about three packs of cigarettes daily. In fact, he reported to his doctor that in his twenties and thirties, he had smoked four packs a day, but he had cut back because the continuous smoking interfered with his preparing meals in his restaurant. Extensive pulmonary and respiratory testing revealed that Charles had lost most of his lung elasticity, which was confirmed by his inability to empty his lungs quickly on various tests. When asked to count as far as he could on one breath, he could count only to five; he could prolong a vowel for only eight seconds. Endoscopic examination showed that Charles had additive growth along the glottal margin of the vocal folds, a condition diagnosed as leukoplakia. Although no medical treatment was recommended for Charles's pulmonary emphysema, much of the leukoplakia was removed surgically. In voice therapy, Charles practiced extending his expirations. With practice, he could count to fifteen on one breath, extend vowels for over fifteen seconds, and say eight to ten words on one expiration. Functionally, despite the irreversible lung disease, Charles was able to increase his ability to say more words with less shortness of breath. Following the surgery on his vocal folds, he received some voice therapy to help establish a voice pitch level he found acceptable.

The speech–language pathologist must deal with other respiratory problems that affect voice, and these are described in Chapters 3 and 7.

Impairment in Phonation.   We will now consider causal organic factors of problems in phonation. How well the vocal folds come together plays a primary role in the sound of the voice. That is, the vocal folds in their total length are brought together (adducted) by active muscular forces. (Any muscle movement problem we will consider in the next section, Neurogenic Voice Problems). As the two vocal folds approximate one another, the outgoing airstream passes between them, setting them into vibration, producing voice. How fast and how well the folds vibrate is related to their relative tension and their mass. Any interference between the two folds, such as a laryngeal web growing between the two folds or a tumor sticking between them, may produce serious changes in voice. It is more often the membranous cover of the vocal folds that is affected by organic diseases of the vocal folds such as cysts, papilloma, granuloma, webbing, or laryngeal infection. Perhaps the most common involvement of the laryngeal cover is in the severe head cold: The infected vocal fold tissue swells, resulting in hoarseness or what may be perceived as laryngitis. Some laryngeal diseases, such as advanced granuloma or carcinoma, involve not only the membranous cover of the vocal folds but include the vocal fold ligament and muscle structures underneath the cover, resulting in severe involvement of phonation. These organic laryngeal problems and their management will be considered in greater detail in Chapters 3 and 7.

The management of organic voice problems is primarily medical–surgical. The speech–language pathologist (SLP) plays an important but secondary role, such as measuring voice performance and any change in it, teaching the patient to use a compensatory voice, or helping the patient develop a vocal hygiene program, i.e., temporary but complete voice rest.

Impairment in Resonance.   The majority of resonance problems are related to excessive nasality (hypernasality) or insufficient nasality (hyponasality or denasality). Although some people are hypernasal for wholly functional reasons (they have learned to sound this way), the majority of people with hypernasal voices speak that way for physical reasons. Obvious effects, like an unrepaired cleft palate or a short palate, will allow excessive coupling between the oral and nasal cavities, which results in an escape of air and sound waves through the nose. Some patients with hypernasality have difficulty moving the muscles of the pharynx and soft palate because of weakness, loss of coordination, or paralysis of these muscles, a neurogenic voice problem discussed in Chapters 4 and 9.

The opposite problem, insufficient nasal resonance or denasality, is usually caused by an obstruction in the nasopharyngeal and nasal cavities. Allergies, enlarged adenoidal tissue, and severe head colds are typical physical problems that may cause denasality. The primary treatment and management of patients with denasality is medical–surgical; voice therapy for denasality is rarely helpful.

The SLP plays a primary evaluative–diagnostic role in the management of resonance disorders. Measuring airflow, assessing competence of velopharyngeal closure, determining the amount of nasality in the acoustic evaluation of voice, and assessing speech articulation are among the evaluative tasks administered by the SLP. The SLP works closely with his or her dental and medical associates to determine the effectiveness of various dental–medical procedures used for correcting resonance problems. Once structural adequacy is achieved and normal resonance is possible, voice therapy can be most effective in establishing improved resonance.

Neurogenic Voice Problems

The muscle control and innervation of the muscles of respiration, phonation, and resonance may be impaired from birth or secondary to injury or disease of the peripheral or central nervous systems. Such communication disorders are classified etiologically as neurogenic disorders. Although Chapter 4 in this text is wholly devoted to neurogenic voice disorders, let us look now at how such disorders may affect the processes of respiration, phonation, and resonance.

Impairment in Respiration.   Any compromise by disease or trauma to the neck, spinal column, or brainstem, including the medulla, may cause some neurogenic impairment of respiration. For example, damage to the high spinal cord and medulla may have devastating effects on breathing. At this high level of involvement, the patient may require ventilator assistance to maintain minimal respiration competency; without the assistance of the ventilator, the patient could not breathe sufficiently to sustain life. In sudden trauma situations like injury to the high breathing centers in the medulla in an automobile accident, the patient would require immediate assistance for breathing, perhaps requiring a tracheostomy (a surgical opening of the neck directly into the trachea). In spinal cord injury, the higher the injury (such as within the cervical vertebrae) the greater the possible involvement of the diaphragm and the respiratory muscles of the neck, shoulders, and ribcage with a resulting lowering of respiratory competence. The lower the spinal injury (such as damage to the lower thoracic and lumbar vertebrae) the less likely that there would be involvement of the muscles of the ribcage, resulting in lower breathing volumes affecting voice.

   Also, central motor problems, such as observed in most forms of cerebral palsy, may prevent the patient from developing the needed inspiratory–expiratory control required for normal voice. For example, the child with athetoid cerebral palsy may experience such torso twisting and flailing of arms that sustaining expiration for speech and voice may be seriously impaired. Some form of postural stabilization and possible bracing of extremities may be required before some control of voice and speech can be taught. Diseases of the central nervous system (CNS), such as observed in myasthenia gravis or Parkinson's disease, may have a generalized effect of lowering inspiratory and expiratory muscle control, affecting the patient's voice. The medical treatment of such CNS disorders through use of various medications, combined with voice therapy efforts of the SLP can often improve the functionality of the patient's breathing, enabling the patient to have a better-sounding voice. As we shall see in Chapter 4, whether the neurogenic voice disorder is the result of lower motor neuron (we will define these terms in Chapter 4), upper motor neuron, or mixed involvement will determine the severity of the respiratory disorder and influence the limitations and successes of its treatment and therapy.

Impairment in Phonation.   The most common neurogenic voice problem seen by the SLP is unilateral vocal fold paralysis. Usually the result of surgical trauma, the innervating nerve to five of the intrinsic muscles of the larynx, the recurrent laryngeal nerve, is inadvertently cut. This leaves the patient with a paralyzed vocal fold, usually in the open paramedian position. Because the paralyzed vocal fold cannot meet the normal fold in the midline, the patient will experience a complete absence of voice (aphonia) or a weak, hoarse voice (dysphonia). Such a case may be seen in this 42-year-old woman who experienced a unilateral vocal fold paralysis during the surgical removal of her thyroid gland (thyroidectomy):

> Mary was referred three days after a thyroidectomy by her surgeon to a speech–language pathologist for "a left vocal fold paralysis following thyroid surgery that has left the patient with a complete aphonia." A subsequent voice evaluation found Mary to have "normal breathing patterns, visual confirmation of the left vocal fold paralyzed in the paramedian position, aphonia, with all oral communication limited to whispered speech." It was subsequently discussed with the patient by the SLP that any decision for long-term management and treatment of the vocal fold paralysis should be deferred for, at least, six months as "there was a good chance that the paralyzed vocal fold would in time have a complete return of function" (the severed nerve would regenerate). Until voice function returned, however, the SLP could help the patient with voice therapy to develop a temporary voice. Mary experienced a functional temporary voice by "increasing breath support, elevating her voice pitch one note, and speaking with harder glottal attack." About eight months after onset of the paralysis, she experienced a total recovery of nerve function (the severed nerve had regenerated) with a complete return of normal voice.

In Chapter 4 we will consider some other medical–surgical and voice therapy options that might have been offered to Mary had she not experienced a spontaneous recovery of recurrent laryngeal nerve function.

One of the most disturbing neurogenic voice problems is **spasmodic dysphonia** in which the patient experiences a voice that sounds strangled, using great effort to "push" the voice out of an overadducted pair of vocal folds. Sometimes called "the laryngeal stutter," the patient may experience normal voicing while laughing or singing, but when attempting to speak the vocal folds become tightly compressed, with only the strangled voice emerging. Voice therapy has never been particularly successful in reducing the voice symptoms of spasmodic dysphonia; however, there are some medical–surgical management procedures offering some help (as shown in Chapter 4), often combined with voice therapy.

Other neurological diseases may cause voice problems. The patient may experience not only problems in breathing and phonation, but difficulty in speech articulation, controlling rate of speech, and maintaining the normal prosodic patterns of a language. Such neurogenic speech–voice changes are classified as dysarthria (an alteration of speech–voice caused by disease or injury of the nervous system) or anarthria (a complete absence of speech due to a neurogenic lesion). In head injury, there is sometimes a dysarthria; generally, the lower the lesion in the brain and the greater the presence of bilateral damage, the more severe the dysarthria. Diseases that may contribute to dysarthria may include stroke, myasthenia gravis, Parkinson's disease, multiple sclerosis, amyotrophic lateral sclerosis, and others (see Chapter 4).

Impairment in Resonance.   Various neurogenic disorders may cause problems in both oral and nasal resonance. Oral resonance is primarily shaped by the opening of the mouth, the position of the tongue, and the posture of the pharynx. A bilateral stroke low in the brain may alter the function and shape of all of these oral structures, affecting the resonance of the voice. Diseases like multiple sclerosis and amyotrophic lateral sclerosis will often result in a back-focus of the voice, caused by faulty nerve innervation of the tongue and pharynx. A child with cerebral palsy may sound as if "its voice is stuck way down in the throat." The voice evaluation for a neurogenic disorder will assess the appropriateness of oral resonance. If oral resonance problems are found, voice therapy is often helpful in helping the patient produce better oral resonance (see Chapters 6, 7, and 9).

The most obvious neurogenic resonance problems are connected with excessive hypernasality, often connected with velopharyngeal incompetence (VPI). The velum (soft palate) and pharynx do not make sufficient contact to shut off the oral and nasal cavities from one another. Consequently, this VPI opening allows excessive amounts of airflow and voice to enter the nasal cavities, contributing to excessive hypernasality. The muscular movements of the velum and pharynx are insufficient to allow the rapid closure patterns required for normal oral–nasal resonance. The most severe VPI disorder may be heard in patients with bulbar palsy (the result of disease or trauma to the medulla and the lower four or five cranial nerves), which will not only produce severe symptoms of hypernasality, but problems in articulation, breathing, chewing, and swallowing.

Strokes (such as pontine artery hemorrhage), diseases (such as amyotrophic lateral sclerosis), or head trauma that involve lower brain tracts are often the causes of severe forms of hypernasality. The voice evaluation should include some assessment of nasal resonance. Problems of nasal resonance can often be helped by dentists (who can design corrective prostheses), surgeons (who can surgically correct some defects), and the SLP (who can provide needed voice and resonance therapies).

Functional Voice Disorders

Most voice disorders are not related to organic or neurogenic problems but are related to misusing the vocal mechanisms, producing a functional dysphonia. People with functional dysphonias produce their faulty voices in different ways. Some do not coordinate their breathing patterns with what they want to say. Toward the end of an utterance, instead of renewing their breath, they may continue talking on the same breath, squeezing out the last few words and sometimes experiencing some laryngeal strain. Some instruction in learning how to coordinate breathing with voicing is often successful, enabling the voice patient to develop good breath support for voice. At the vocal fold level, many patients misuse their voices by speaking excessively loud, speaking with hard glottal attack (speaking with abrupt onset of voice), using inappropriate pitch levels, or never resting their voices. Or the vocal folds are abused by excessive yelling, coughing, smoking, throat clearing, or excessive crying.

When excessive patterns of vocal misuse and abuse are found, they are usually part of a problem of vocal hyperfunction. Vocal hyperfunction is defined in this text as the involvement of too much muscle force and physical effort in the systems of respiration, phonation, and resonance. Continued vocal hyperfunction can often lead to tissue changes of the vocal folds, such as an overall thickening of the inner margins of the folds, or vocal nodules (bilateral nodes resembling callus on the inner margin of each vocal fold) or a vocal polyp (unilateral soft growth on inner margin of one fold). Voice therapy is usually the preferred treatment for reducing or eliminating both vocal nodules or polyps. Although functional problems of resonance are less common, they can be observed in excessive carriage of the tongue (too forward or too far back), which can negatively influence overall voice resonance. Another functional resonance problem can be heard in the voice that sounds like it is coming from "deep in the throat" (at the level of the larynx), often remediated by helping the patient "place" the voice higher in the "facial mask" (discussed in Chapter 6).

Impairment in Respiration.   The regulation of breathing for phonation is basically involuntary and highly automatic in everyday speech; however, public speakers or actors or singers learn to take in quick breaths and then extend them over a prolonged period of continuous voicing. Singers, for example, require an additional supply of air in excess of that obtained in normal inhalation and are able to replenish their air supply quickly and efficiently. Singers must be able to sustain prolonged expiration.

Unusual force or muscle tension (hyperfunction) can be observed in various phases of respiration among both normal persons and clinical voice patients. Although normal speakers without vocal pathology can tolerate vocal stresses related to inadequate and inefficient respiration, patients with vocal pathology usually cannot tolerate such respiratory inefficiency Perhaps the most common problem of respiration observed among voice patients is the attempt to speak on an inadequate expiration. The inspiratory phase may be inadequate for the phonatory task. Untrained singers may elevate their shoulders, using their neck accessory muscles for inhalation.

Some voice patients literally use chest and abdominal muscles in competition with each other. Rather than contracting or expanding the chest (thorax) in direct coordination with contraction or expansion of the abdomen, these two anatomical sites may be "pulling and pushing" against each other. Lecturers or singers, in their need to get in a "big" breath, to take a maximum inhalation, may display obviously distended abdomens, fixed thoraxes, elevated shoulders with the associated neck accessory muscles in a hypertonic state, and possibly heads thrust forward. Although such "deep breathers" may have increased their air volume, they are in no position to parcel out their exhalations for a controlled sustained phonation. More commonly, perhaps, we see patients who suffer not from too little or too much inhalation, but from improper utilization of their expirations. A speaker may let out so much expiration early in a verbal passage that, by the end of the sentence, he or she is short of breath.

Normal speakers demonstrate adequate inspiration–expiration for the daily needs of voice, generally speaking. Professional users of voice demonstrate much more vigorous respiration and show much muscular participation in large, quick inspiration followed by steady expiration that can produce vocal beauty and intensities not possible from untrained speakers or singers. Many voice patients have problems with inspiration–expiration movements as well as poor timing and control of sustained expiration—symptoms of voice that are related to lack of respiratory control.

We discuss normal respiration and its role in supplying expiratory air pressures and volumes needed for normal phonation in Chapter 2, and consider some of the respiration problems of patients with voice disorders. In Chapter demonstrate several therapy approaches that have been found helpful for imp ing respiratory function and control.

Impairment in Phonation.   In functional voice disorders, the natural vibratory characteristics of the vocal folds are interrupted or altered in various ways. For example, in the voice perceived as excessively breathy, the vocal folds are usually too laxly approximated, permitting excessive airflow between them. The excessive airflow is perceived as breathiness. Or the folds may be so firmly together that their normal vibration is inhibited, contributing to the perception of harshness.

Voice authorities disagree about the influence of inappropriate pitch level or fundamental frequency on the development of various vocal pathologies. For some patients an inapproriately low or high pitch level might appear as a primary etiologic factor in a vocal disorder, but for other patients faulty pitch levels have developed secondarily from the increase of vocal fold mass due to early polypoid or nodule growth. That is, sometimes the inappropriate pitch level produces the dysphonia, and sometimes the prolonged dysphonia produces vocal fold tissue changes and thus alters pitch. It is important for any speaker or singer to use the vocal mechanism optimally with regard to fundamental frequency. Speaking or singing at an inappropriate pitch level requires excessive force and contraction of the intrinsic muscles of the larynx, which leads to vocal fatigue or the hoarseness related to a tired vocal mechanism.

A common pitch deviation may be the inappropriately low pitch of young professional males, such as teachers or clergy members, who speak at the bottom of their pitch ranges in an attempt to convey some extra authority through their voices. Young professional women may also speak at fundamental frequency values well below the normative values of the average adult female. An inappropriate pitch level, whether too low or too high, requires unnecessary muscle energy to maintain the necessary vocal fold adjustments of length and mass to produce the "artificial" voice. Of the many variables we identify as hyperfunctional voice behaviors, inappropriate pitch level is one of the easiest of the disorders to remedy. Sometimes, just by raising or lowering the fundamental frequency slightly, patients will experience a lessening of the energy they employ to speak, which will result in a noticeable decrease in their dysphonia.

Initiation of phonation at the beginning of words is known as *glottal attack.* We often hear *easy* or *soft glottal attack* in voicing patterns that are considered typical of a southern accent, or in what is called a *legato* in music—the soft, uninterrupted voicing pattern that seems to flow without break. Words begin softly, and a blend of unvoiced air gradually becomes voiced. In southern dialect the words not only begin softly, but most of the vowels in the utterance are prolonged as well. Soft glottal attack as a vocal style appears to be easy on the vocal mechanism; however, a politician or performer with such an easy attack may sound a "bit boring and too passive" in overall presentation.

The opposite type of voicing mode is known as the *hard glottal attack.* Phonation is abruptly initiated, so that often each word sounds like an individual entity with its own initial stress and stresses put on the beginning of words. We often hear hard glottal attack in the voicing patterns of people in such large eastern cities as New York or Philadelphia. Their overall speaking patterns appear much faster, for example, than what we hear in southern speech. Speaking with hard glottal attack is often characterized as vocal hyperfunction. Voice therapy may entail a patient's deliberately attempting an easier vocal attack to take the "work" out of voicing.

Vocal abuse and vocal misuse can contribute to voice problems. By *vocal abuse* we mean that the laryngeal mechanisms are used excessively in various nonverbal abusive ways, such as continuous coughing, throat-clearing, laughing, crying, or smoking. Such abusive behaviors can have negative effects on laryngeal function and sometimes on vocal production as well. Vocal misuse may consist of excessive or inappropriate voicing, such as speaking with excessive vocal hard attack, speaking at the wrong voice pitch, speaking too loudly, or speaking too much. The additive nature of the vocal fold edema (swelling) or tissue engorgement that may result from excessive voicing, such as screaming or yelling, enlarges the vocal folds. This vocal fold enlargement changes the sound of the voice. The patient, in turn, reacts to the vocal change and begins to employ other vocal behaviors to compensate for the changed vocal mechanism. These compensatory behaviors further contribute to what is perceived as some kind of voice problem.

Functional abuse (such as excessive throat-clearing) and vocal misuse (speaking with hard glottal attack) can lead to actual tissue changes (nodules or polyps) of the vocal folds. The following description of a young boy with vocal nodules illustrates a hyperfunctional voice disorder that is frequently observed in a young primary school population.

Eli, age seven, was described by his parents as a boy "who was always talking, yelling, and letting the family know that he was around." For the past year Eli often demonstrated a low-pitched, hoarse voice, particularly toward the end of the day, after many hours of noisy play. His hoarseness was noticed by his pediatrician, who subsequently referred him to an ear–nose–throat specialist, an otolaryngologist. Initial attempts by the otolaryngologist at indirect laryngoscopy were unsuccessful because of the boy's intolerance for the laryngeal mirror. After a second visit, however, the physician was able to see Eli's vocal folds, and he found small bilateral vocal nodules. Eli was then referred to the speech–language pathologist in the same hospital, who took a thorough case history from both the parents and the boy. A number of abusive noises the boy produced were heard, and a gross determination was made of how often these abuses occurred. The speech–language pathologist saw Eli for several sessions, during which he provided graphic materials that showed Eli in language he could understand how abusing his voice had produced the "little bumps he now had on his vocal folds." The counseling was coupled with requests that Eli make serious attempts to curb his yelling and funny noises. Each time he found himself making a noise, he was asked to chart it on a time graph the clinician gave him to take home. After several weeks of monitoring his yelling behavior with the help of his parents, Eli returned for another visit with the otolaryngologist. This time laryngoscopy showed that Eli's nodules were much smaller. It appeared that curbing his vocal abuses lessened the laryngeal strain he was experiencing, which reduced the size of his vocal nodules.

The management of Eli's voice problem required a few sessions of counseling specific to his vocal abuses. If he had needed voice therapy over a longer period of time, the focus of his therapy would have been to discover what kind of abuse or misuse was present and then to design a program to reduce that abuse. We would also have searched with him for the best voice he could produce.

The voice clinician must continually search for the patient's best and most appropriate voice production. This searching is necessary because so much vocal behavior is highly automatic, particularly the dimensions of pitch and quality. The patient cannot deliberately break down vocalization into various components and then hope to combine them into some ideal phonation. Voice therapy techniques are primarily vehicles of facilitation; that is, we try a particular therapy approach to see if it facilitates the production of a better voice. If it does, then we utilize it as therapy practice material. If it does not, we quickly abandon it. As part of every clinical session, we must probe and search for the patient's best voice. When an acceptable production is produced, we use this "best" voice as the patient's voice target. The easiest achieved and/or best-sounding voice is often used as the patient's target in voice therapy.

Impairment in Resonance. Much of the beauty or quality of the voice is produced by the resonating chambers of the airway, beginning within the larynx itself, and extending into the pharynx, the oral cavity, and the nasal cavity above. Functional influences on resonance are generally related to change of cavity size and configuration, achieved by the action of various muscle contractions and relaxations. For example, the quality of oral resonance is often directly related to the opening of the mouth, achieved by mandible posturing and the relative height and placement of the tongue within the oral cavity. A tongue too far forward in the mouth is often the primary cause of a baby-sounding voice (Boone, 1997). Practicing more posterior tongue carriage by various self-practice methods can replace the thin baby quality with fuller oral resonance. Conversely, excessively posterior carriage of the tongue can give the voice a posterior oral focus (Boone, 1997), like the voice of the "country bumpkin" or, more recently, the voice of TV's Alf; bringing tongue carriage more forward through practice exercises can give the voice a more normal oral resonance.

Although most excesses of nasal resonance described earlier in this chapter are organic or physical in origin, occasionally people with hypernasal voices speak this way for totally functional reasons. If there is no organic basis for the hypernasality, the patient can elect to develop greater oral resonance with voice therapy (as outlined in Chapter 9 in this text). Denasality, the lack of nasal resonance, is usually the result of nasopharyngeal blockage, preventing normal nasal resonance within the nasal cavities. Generally, correction of denasality requires medical–surgical intervention and is not responsive to voice therapy per se. Another nasal resonance problem not previously mentioned in this chapter is *assimilative nasality* (vowel production "next" to nasal consonants is excessively nasal). If the patient elects to eliminate assimilative nasality, voice therapy focused on improving oral resonance (see Chapter 9) is often effective.

Management and Therapy for Voice Disorders

Successful management of a voice disorder first requires identification of the cause of the disorder. We have grouped causal factors of voice disorders into three major categories: organic, neurogenic, and functional. The typical sequence of events begins with the patient experiencing some kind of voice problem in breathing, voice, or resonance. Breathing and resonance problems are often long-standing, perhaps experienced by the patient over time. Phonation problems, like hoarseness, are more likely to have occurred more recently. We often counsel that, unless the patient is experiencing hoarseness (dysphonia) as part of an allergy or severe upper respiratory infection (URI), he or she should wait no more than seven days to have a medical evaluation of the problem. The physician best trained to evaluate the phonation problem is the otolaryngologist (a physician trained in the identification and treatment of ear–nose–throat disease).

The physician in turn refers the patient to the speech–language pathologist who by training is able to evaluate and diagnose the voice problem and its respiration–phonation–resonance components. The SLP takes a detailed history, observes the patient closely, uses instrumental–noninstrumental assessment approaches (as discussed in Chapter 5), and usually tries a few remediation approaches (therapy techniques used in the initial evaluation are often called diagnostic probes). Once causal factors and various aspects of the problem are measured, the SLP outlines a treatment plan. For organic voice problems, the SLP may work closely with other specialists, such as medicine or respiratory therapy, depending on the particular problem. For example, a preschool youngster with a growth in the airway called papilloma (caused by a virus) may require the clinical services of the surgeon, a respiratory therapist, extra nursing care, and the close watching of the SLP, who may need to work with the child in breathing, language, and voice therapy. The voice therapy goal with such a child may be solely to develop the best voice possible with a vocal mechanism heavily laden with multiple papilloma growths. When such papillomas become large enough to impinge on the airway, the surgeon excises or reduces them, as needed, to restore breathing function.

Neurogenic voice problems come in many varied forms as we will see in Chapter 4. The SLP may be the first professional person to see a patient who is just beginning to experience voice symptoms. For example, a recent patient was seen in our clinics because he felt he was experiencing a new problem pronouncing occasional words. A subsequent evaluation by the SLP found evidence of tongue tremor and a problem in tongue *diadochokinesis* (he could not move his tongue rapidly when making alternating movements, such as saying "ta-ka" in a rapid series). A subsequent referral by the SLP to a neurologist confirmed that the patient was showing beginning signs of amyotrophic lateral sclerosis. Or the neurologist may be the first professional to see the patient with a neurogenic disorder, referring the patient to the SLP for detailed assessment of breathing, phonation, and speech. The SLP sends his or her evaluation back to the neurologist, and together they may develop a management plan for the patient. Such a plan will frequently include medications for improving the patient's motor functions with specific goals for the patient to achieve with the SLP in voice therapy.

Most patients with functional voice problems work directly with the SLP. A growing number of people, particularly professional voice users, such as salespeople and teachers (Titze, Lemke, and Montequin, 1997), seek the services of the SLP for general voice improvement in such dimensions as loudness, quality, strength, or overall effectiveness. For such people, the voice is evaluated and a specific program is designed for voice improvement. Other people may experience loss or symptoms of voice for which the SLP can find no organic or physical cause; accordingly, the presenting symptom of aphonia or dysphonia is classified as a functional voice disorder, which is usually very responsive to voice therapy.

Excessive misuse, overuse, and abuse of the voice, vocal hyperfunction, once identified can be reduced and often eliminated by voice therapy alone. Continued vocal hyperfunction is considered the primary cause of vocal nodules and polyps; such lesions, once discovered, are responsive to voice therapy. Benninger and Jacobson (1995) found in their study of 115 patients with vocal nodules that 94 percent of them experienced resolution of their problem, concluding that "with appropriate voice modification and care delivered by voice and speech–language pathologists, nodules will generally resolve with return of normal vocal function" (p. 326). Much of Chapter 6 in this text is devoted to procedures of voice therapy that are used by the SLP in the treatment of such functional voice disorders.

Summary

In this introductory chapter we have looked at the role of the voice in the biologic survival of the person, in the expression of emotion, and the complicated voicing required in linguistic oral communication. We have seen that voice problems of respiration, phonation, and resonance may be related to one or more of three causal factors: organic, neurogenic, and functional. The speech–language pathologist evaluates the patient and the voice problem by various instrumental–noninstrumental approaches, attempting to identify the causal factors of the voice problem. Using the evaluation findings, the SLP then develops an individualized management and voice therapy plan for the patient and the particular voice disorder.

CHAPTER

2

The Normal Voice

This chapter describes the normal voice and its characteristics. It is important to understand the range of the normal voice in order to be able to diagnose and plan treatment for a disordered voice. Few things are so difficult to define or understand as, "What is normal and what constitutes normal limits?" Voice therapy is often "antagonistic" therapy. We are trying to undo what patients have done to their voice through "overworking" the normal mechanism. In order to help someone to return to the range of normal and to abandon the abnormal functions, one must know the characteristics of the normal voice. To be effective in voice evaluation and therapy clinicians must have a good working knowledge of the structures involved in phonation. Also, they must have a knowledge of the normal function of these structures.

Normal Aspects of Voice

Normal voice may be characterized by five aspects. These constitute a functional description of normal voice. First, the normal voice must be loud enough to be heard. In a word, loudness. We may refer to this as adequate carrying power. Adequate loudness is a key component of speech intelligibility. This means that the normal voice can be heard over the noise of most everyday environmental sounds such as the TV, air conditioning, computer typing, and so on. Secondly, the normal voice must be produced in a manner that does not produce vocal trauma and thus laryngeal lesions. Again, in a word, hygienic voice production. The production of normal voice should not hurt or cause damage to the speaker's vocal mechanism. Third, the normal voice should be pleasant to listen to or in keeping with one-word descriptors, pleasing in vocal quality. Fourth, the normal voice should be flexible enough to express emotion. We often say a great deal with the emotional tone of our voice. The sentence, "I am so happy for you," can be said in such a manner as to be sincere or sarcastic just by the tone of voice while the words remain the same. The expression, "Oh wonderful," can be said with excitement or with scorn. The normal voice should represent the speaker well in terms of age and gender. We should not be surprised to meet someone for the first time after speaking to him or her on the phone. Our voice should not portray us as either older, younger, or as less mature than we are. Nor will we likely be pleased if we are mistaken for the opposite gender. The normal voice could be said to represent the speaker faithfully.

Using these five aspects of loudness, hygiene, pleasantness, flexibility, representation, we can begin to address the area of normal voice. A normal v[c] for a seven-year-old boy will be quite different from that of a seventy-year-o[female but both can be normal and can be adequately loud, hygienic, pleasan[t] enough to not be distracting, have the flexibility to express the speaker's emotion and allow the listener to judge the speaker's age and gender.

This chapter presents the anatomical structures and physiological functions necessary for normal respiration, phonation, and resonance with a current view of the clinical physiology of these events. It is these structures and functions that underlie normal voice.

Normal Processes of Voice Production

Separating the normal speaking voice into three individual processes (respiration, phonation, and resonance) for purposes of study is helpful but we must remember that the three components of voice production are highly interdependent. For example, without the expiratory phase of respiration there would be no phonation or resonance. Also, these three processes are constantly changing simultaneously. Let us first consider the structures and function of respiration, particularly as they relate to production of voice.

Respiration

For speech to be possible, humans have learned to use respiration by sustaining their exhalations for phonation purposes. Both speaking and singing require an outgoing air stream capable of activating vocal fold vibration. When "training" their voice, speakers or singers frequently focus on developing conscious control of the breathing mechanism. This conscious control, however, must not conflict with the physiological air requirements of the individual. When a problem occurs with respiration, it is often the conflict between the physiological needs and the speaking–singing demands for air that causes faulty usage of the vocal mechanism. Our dependence on the constant renewal of oxygen supply imposes certain limitations on how many words we can say, how many phrases we can sing, or how much loud emphasis we can use on one expiration.

Respiration Structures. Inspired air enters through the nostrils and passes into the nasal cavities into the nasopharynx through the open velopharyngeal port into the oropharynx. For mouth breathers, the air would enter through the open mouth, pass through the oral cavity over the surface of the tongue and into the oropharynx. The air would then flow through the hypopharynx. From the hypopharynx, the inspiration would flow into the larynx (Figure 2.1), pass between the ventricular or false vocal folds, and pass between the true vocal folds down into the trachea or windpipe. At the bottom end of the trachea, the airway divides into the two bronchial tubes shown in the accompanying photograph of the lungs and tracheal bifurcation (Figure 2.2). The bronchial tubes further branch into divisions known as the bronchioles, and they eventually terminate in the lungs in little air sacs

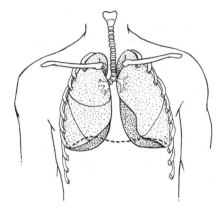

CHAPTER 2

FIGURE 2.1 The Respiratory Tract
Note the resting level of the diaphragm as outlined in the diaphragm contour.

known as the alveolar sacs. Some of the bronchioli are visible in the upper picture of Figure 2.2, but most of the bronchioli and all the alveoli are covered by the pleural membrane that covers the lungs.

The ribs connected to the twelve thoracic vertebrae and their connecting muscles play an important role in respiration, as we shall see when we discuss respiratory function. The thorax can move in several ways. For example, the rib cage wall expands for inspiration of air and collapses for expiration. Sometimes the accessory muscles in the neck assist in deep inspiration when they contract because they elevate the shoulders and increase the vertical dimension of the thorax. At the base of the thorax is the important diaphragm muscle, a composite of muscle, tendon, and membrane that separates the thoracic cavity from the abdominal cavity. As the diaphragm contracts, it descends and increases the vertical dimension of the thorax; as the diaphragm relaxes, it ascends back to its higher position. The diaphragm has direct contact with the lungs, and only the pleural space comes between the lungs and the diaphragm. The shape of the diaphragm, its superior contour, can be seen on the lower surface of the cadaver lung in Figure 2.2. The relaxed diaphragm is high in the chest within the rib cage, and the stomach and liver lie directly below it. As the diaphragm contracts and descends, it pushes from above on the contents of the abdomen below, often displacing the abdominal wall by pushing it outward on inspiration. The abdominal wall is composed primarily of the abdominal muscles that sometimes play an active role in expiration. This is especially true in singing, in loud speech, when laughing (thus the term *belly laugh*) or when producing a very long phrase. We identify those muscles of the thorax in the abdomen that relate to respiration as we discuss respiration.

Respiration Function. The respiratory tract functions much like a bellows. When we move the handles on the bellows apart, the bellows becomes larger and the air within it becomes less dense than the air outside it. The outside air rushes in due to the lower pressure of the less dense air in the bellows and the greater pressure in the more dense outside air. The inspiration of air into the bellows is achieved by active enlargement of the bellows's body. Similarly, in human respiration, the inspiration of air is achieved by active movement of muscles that enlarge the thoracic cavity. When the thorax enlarges, the lungs within the thorax enlarge. The air within

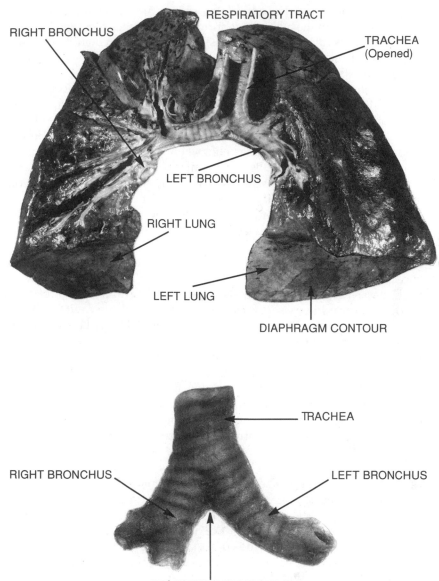

RESPIRATORY TRACT

RIGHT BRONCHUS

TRACHEA
(Opened)

LEFT BRONCHUS

RIGHT LUNG

LEFT LUNG

DIAPHRAGM CONTOUR

TRACHEA

RIGHT BRONCHUS

LEFT BRONCHUS

TRACHEAL BIRFURCATION

FIGURE 2.2   Lungs and Tracheal Bifurcation *An illustration of the tracheal bifur-cation that introduces air into the lungs by way of the left and right bronchi. At the bottom end of the trachea, the airway divides into the two bronchial tubes. The bronchial tubes further branch into divisions known as the bronchioles, and they eventually termi-nate in the lungs in little air sacs known as the alveolar sacs. Some of the bronchioli are visible in the upper picture, but most of the bronchioli and all the alveoli are covered by the pleural membrane that covers the lungs.*

the lungs becomes less dense than atmospheric air, and inspiration of air begins. The air is expired from the bellows by bringing the handles together, decreasing the size of the bellows's cavity, thus compressing the air and forcing it to rush out. In human respiration, however, much of expiration is achieved by passive collapse of thoracic size and not by active muscle contraction. This is an extremely important fact and can be valuable information for voice clinicians. Much of expiration is passive. Hixon, Mead, and Goldman (1973) have described human respiration as having two types of forces that are always present: passive forces (such as the elastic lungs) and active, volitional force (such as contraction of muscles of inspiration). The pleural membrane that covers the lungs clings almost adhesively to the inner wall of the thorax. As the thorax expands by muscular contraction, the lungs within it expand. The inherent elastic force of the lungs is always there. Their elastic recoil will be as fast as thoracic collapse allows. In fact, in at-rest expiration (the expiration during the quiet breathing of sleep, for example), the expiratory phase of respiration is wholly accomplished by the elasticity of the inherent or passive forces.

Passive Components.   Much of the air pressure or "power" required for normal speech can be supplied by the passive factors of respiration (passive exhalation). Such passive factors as lung tissue elasticity, gravity, visceral recoil, and rib untorquing provide passive factors that reduce the lung cavity size during expiration and thus contribute to outward air flow, which may be used in speech. While there may always be some level of active muscle function during "passive" respiration for voice production, no muscle action is required to supply this breath power, thus, there is no tendency to "overdo" (hyperactivity) the effort. When a long phrase or other speaking task (such as increased loudness when singing) requires more effort or "breath power," we make up the difference between the power provided by passive factors and the needed amount of breath power by using the abdominal musculature. The mechanism of passive components can be understood by examining the concept of the relaxation pressure curve.

Relaxation Pressure.   The best (most efficient and most pleasing vocal quality) voice is produced at mid air-pressure levels and mid lung-volume levels of air, as shown in the relaxation pressure curve in Figure 2.3. To demonstrate this, simply take about a half-breath and produce an /i/ vowel for five seconds at a medium loudness level. Then listen to the vocal quality. Now take a very deep breath and produce the same /i/ vowel for five seconds at medium loudness. The vocal quality will generally be poorer with the effort required to control the greater air volume and higher air pressure, thus contributing to the perception of poorer voice quality. Finally, produce the same /i/ vowel for five seconds at medium loudness immediately after releasing three-fourths of your air supply. Again, the vocal quality will suffer as you try to compensate for the low air pressure and low lung volume. The excessive muscular contraction required to phonate at this low lung volume will also be seen in the "overvalving," in the larynx, giving rise to the rougher voice quality.

This exercise demonstrates how vocal quality is affected by extremely high or low air pressure at high or low lung volume. It translates into an excellent clinical stimulation technique. We can often change the vocal quality of our dysphonic patients by instructing them to use the midrange of air pressure and lung volume. Teaching a shortened phrasing pattern may be important to teaching breath-stream

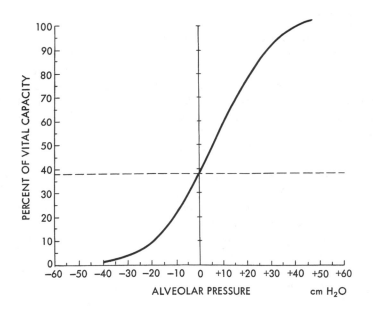

FIGURE 2.3 **The Relaxation Pressure Curve** *The passive forces of exhalation tend to generate force during inhalation that works to restore the lung and rib cage system to the normal resting state or equilibrium. After active inhalation, these passive forces of exhalation rebound to provide some of the expiratory force needed for speech. There is a nearly linear relationship between relaxation pressure and lung volume in the range between 20% and 70% of the vital capacity. This curve represents the pressure generated by the passive factors of the respiratory system.*

management. Except in singers or actors this generally is all the "respiration training" that needs to be given by the speech–language pathologist. All of the emphasis placed on breathing exercises and respiration training in the past seems unproductive and unnecessary for nearly all of our patients with dysphonias. The clinical facilitation technique of glottal fry (discussed in Chapter 6) makes use of this information because glottal fry is produced with little air pressure and little airflow.

Active Components.   A key problem for many voice disordered patients is the tendency to "squeeze" the glottis closed in order to produce the needed power, rather than to increase air pressure and airflow by contracting the abdominal muscles. We can better understand this "mistake" by a simple analogy. If we are watering flowers in a garden and we want to reach the far row of plants, we can either place a thumb over the end of the hose and squirt the water further (increase the power), or we can increase the water power by turning the faucet on further. When we squeeze the glottis closed, we are "putting a thumb over the end of the hose." When we contract the abdominal muscles, we are "turning the faucet further on" and increasing the airflow. Even though squeezing the glottis tends to increase the vocal power, vocal quality is diminished because the voice sounds strained. If this method is habitual, the excessive effort becomes the basis of a hyperfunctional voice disorder. Such effort may lead to vocal nodules, contact ulcers, vocal polyps, recurring laryngitis, or loss of voice. We often see this type of voice production in politicians who are campaigning and frequently speak loudly to make a point. If they use too much effort in over adducting the larynx to achieve the loudness, vocal strain and laryngeal swelling edema will likely result. This was seen in the voice of President Clinton during his campaign speaking. Indeed he demonstrates a hoarse voice during long speeches, such as the State of the Union speech. He frequently resorted to voice rest between speeches to allow the swelling in his larynx to reduce and the resultant laryngitis to subside. When we need increased power to speak louder, to stress words, or to extend a phrase when singing or speaking, we should use the larger muscles of the abdomen and "turn on the faucet" controlling the source of air. Thus, the pressure at the valve (the larynx) is not excessive, and vocal quality is improved with delicate laryngeal tissue not subjected to stress and strain, which produces laryngeal edema and laryngitis. Vocal quality is not diminished, and adverse tissue change is avoided. Voice clinicians can use this water analogy to teach patients how to monitor breath control by properly using expiratory reserve volume (see definition of terms below) via the abdominal muscles, rather than using excessive glottal valving in the larynx.

Muscles of Respiration.   We now need to consider the muscles of respiration that contribute active, volitional force in inspiration, as shown in Figure 2.4. The primary muscle of inspiration is the diaphragm, as already noted. Perhaps the external intercostals play the next most important role in inspiration. Because of their oblique angulation, when they contract, they lift the rib below, enlarging the rib cage on a somewhat horizontal plane. Slight elevation of the upper thorax is achieved with contraction of the pectoralis major and minor, the costal elevators, the serratus posterior, and the neck accessory muscles (primarily the sternocleidomastoid). The primary inherent elasticity and recoil of thoracic structures come into play when the active muscles of inspiration cease contracting and relax, but some muscles of expiration can and do assist in expiration. These muscles of expiration may contract in some conditions of talking, singing, and forced expiration, such as we use in playing wind instruments. The primary muscles of expiration are the four abdominal muscles, the internal oblique abdominal, external oblique abdominal, transverse abdominal, and the rectus abdominal. Some thoracic decrease can also be achieved by active contraction of the internal intercostals (they slant upward in the opposite direction of the external intercostals) and the posterior inferior serratus.

   In passive respiration, the kind of breathing we do when sleeping, the active contraction of inspiratory muscles produces the inspiration, and the expiration phase of the respiratory cycle is wholly related to the passive (nonmuscular) collapse properties of the thorax. These passive factors may include lung elasticity, rib untorquing, visceral recoil, and gravity's pulling the ribs down to a resting position. When we add the function of expiratory muscles to the passive expiration, we alter

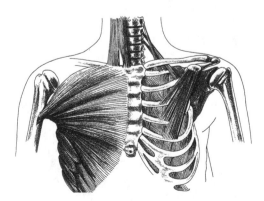

FIGURE 2.4   The Thoracic Surface Muscles of Respiration *Muscles shown include the pectoralis major, the external and internal intercostals, the scalene, pectoralis minor, and the sternocleidomastoid muscles. Bones readily identified include the clavical, sternum, scapula, and ribs 1 to 8.* (J. M. Palmer, *Anatomy for Speech and Hearing.* [New York: Harper & Row, 1972], p. 149.

the duration and force of the expiration. For example, while speaking long passages, we may well begin with passive expirations; active contraction of expiratory muscles comes after passive expiration has begun. Any time we prolong the expiration beyond a simple tidal volume (see definitions below), we have added some active muscle contraction of the expiratory muscles. When patients tell us that they "Have to work hard to talk" or that "It is such an effort to speak," we should be alerted to hyperfunction in the respiratory and phonatory (laryngeal level) processes.

Figure 2.5, the simple tracings of a pneumotachometer, shows the relative time for inspiration–expiration for a passive, tidal breath, for saying the numbers "1, 2, 3, 4, 5," and for singing the musical passage, "I don't want to walk without you, baby," from the old song by that title. Note that the inspiratory time during normal tidal breathing is much longer than the quick inspiration for speech and singing. This is indicated by the rapid rise of the tracing from a resting baseline in

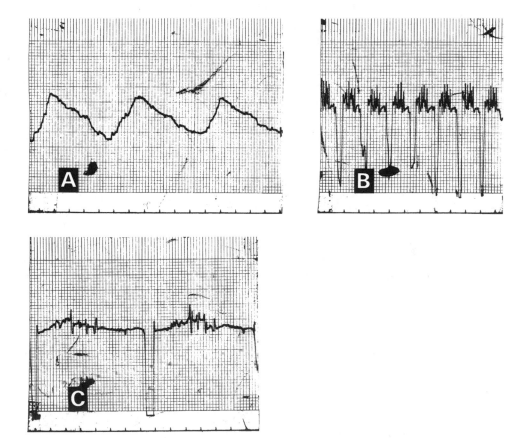

FIGURE 2.5   Pneumotachometer Tracings Measure Airflow over Time *Note the relative time for inspiration as opposed to expiration for three conditions: tracing A (three tidal breaths) produces an inspiration–expiration time ratio of about 1:2; tracing B (counting from one to five on eight trials) produces a ratio of about 1:3; tracing C (singing twice, "I don't want to walk without you, baby") yielded an inspiration–expiration ratio of approximately 1:10.*

an almost vertical move. In the tidal breath the rise from the baseline is gradual and sloped rather than vertical. We will now define the terms we will use in following discussions to describe aspects of respiration. (Methods for evaluating respiratory volumes and capacities will be discussed in Chapter 5.)

Lung Volumes and Capacities.   **Tidal volume** (TV) is the amount of air inspired and expired during a typical respiratory cycle. It is determined by the oxygen needs (not the speaking or singing needs) of the individual. For a young, healthy adult male the volume is about **750 cc.** at rest.

Inspiratory reserve volume (IRV), known also as complemental air, is the maximum volume of air that can be inspired beyond the end of a tidal inspiration. This volume is about **1500–2500 cc.** in a healthy adult male.

Expiratory reserve volume (ERV), known also as supplemental air, is the maximum volume of air that can be expired beyond the end of a tidal expiration and averages between **1500–2000 cc.** or more in a young, healthy adult male.

Residual volume (RV) is the volume of air that remains in the lungs after a maximum expiration. No matter how forceful the expiration, the residual volume cannot be forced from the lungs and averages between **1000–1500 cc.** in the young adult male. A common error made by many is to state that a speaker is using residual air, which is impossible because residual air cannot be expelled. What one is referring to when excessive effort is used to "get the last bit of speech out on the exhaled air stream" is excessive respiratory muscle effort at the end of the expiratory reserve volume.

Vital capacity (VC) is the total amount of air that can be expired from the lungs and air passages following a maximum inhalation. It represents the total volumes previously listed, with the exception of residual volume (which cannot be expired). Vital capacity in the young adult male averages between **3500–5000 cc.**

Total lung capacity (TLC) represents the total volume of air that can be held in the lungs and airways after a maximum inspiration. It can only be measured by special volume displacement tests (not by measuring the total expiratory volume).

In the normal inspiratory–expiratory cycle of tidal volume, the relative timing of inspiration–expiration, is only slightly longer for expiration. Human beings appear to have a slight bias toward longer expirations, which is apparently quite compatible with the need to extend expiration for purposes of vocal communication. The respiratory system supplies the power for phonation, as described in the myoelastic theory of phonation later in this chapter.

Influencing types of respiration are the interactions and pragmatics between the speaker and the listener, the type of utterance being produced, the background noise in the setting, the relative arousal level of the autonomic nervous system, the comfort of the speaker, and so forth. Therefore, some of the ensuing descriptions of the physiology of respiration, when lifted out of speaking or singing context, often appear to be deceptively simple. For example, when an individual begins to speak or sing, the inspiration time unit is often shortened (by employing more vigor to the muscles of inspiration) and the expiration time is obviously extended. Hixon, Mead, and Goldman (1973) have studied the dynamics and function of the thorax, rib cage, diaphragm, and abdomen during speech and have concluded that there are marked differences in respiratory function according to body position and type of speech task. For example, utterances that required nearly total use of a patient's vital capacity activated different activity zones, depending on whether the patient was in an upright or supine body position. The inspiratory activity "was governed predominantly by the rib cage and the abdomen in the upright body position and the diaphragm in the supine position" (p. 297). It appears that, during the inspiratory phase preceding speech, we shorten our inspiration and then use the chest wall and the abdomen in different ways for the expiratory phase (when we are actually speaking). We renew inspiration and "catch up" on inspiration during conversational passages, tucking in the abdomen with a slight elevation of the rib cage. Hixon and Abbs have written that the "importance of this shape is that it forces the diaphragm—our major inspiratory muscle—into a highly domed position where its action results in the development of great amounts of inspiratory force very rapidly" (1980, p. 63).

Normal speakers adjust inspiration–expiration to match the linguistic utterances they wish to make. Inspiration during conversation, public speaking, and even singing happens quickly, and it is usually masked from the view of all but the searching eye. After a quick inspiration, normal speakers then begin the passive expiration, quickly using the tidal volume and adding the sustained expiration of the expiratory reserve. Fluctuations of expiratory airflow, to meet a speaker's demand for vocal stress and changes in vocal intensity, are apparently made by slight chest wall adjustments. Increases in airflow and subglottal pressure are made quickly and with little visible effort to match the linguistic or artistic needs of speakers or singers. Gifted talkers or singers also learn to take little quick "catch-up" inhalations sandwiched within what appears to listeners to be a continuous expiratory flow. When breath support or perhaps breath control is a problem in a voice disordered patient, it is often related to failure to take these "catch-up" breaths at appropriate places. At other times, the tendency to push too hard in extending the expiratory reserve volume produces the strained vocal quality discussed previously in this chapter.

Phonation

The airway requires various protective structures to prevent the infiltration of liquids, the aspiration of food particles and fluids during deglutition (swallowing), and the inhalation of foreign bodies during respiration. In most higher mammals, particularly humans, the larynx serves as the basic valvelike entryway to the respiratory tract. All incoming and outgoing pulmonary (lung) air must pass through the valving glottal opening of the larynx. The primary biological roles of the larynx are, **first,** to prevent foreign bodies from moving into the airway and, **second,** to fixate the thorax by stopping the airflow at the glottal level, which permits the arms to perform heavy lifting and extensive weight-supporting feats. This primitive valvelike action appears to be the primary function of the human larynx. Using the laryngeal valving mechanism for phonation has required the development of intricate neural controls that permit humans to use the approximating valvelike vocal folds for the precise phonations required in speaking and singing. The valving action of the larynx functions because, first, we have a fixed framework (the laryngeal cartilages); second, we are able to open (abduct) and close (adduct) the valve, primarily by using the intrinsic muscles of the larynx;

and third, the valving mechanism receives external support from the extrinsic muscles of the larynx.

Laryngeal Structures.   Prominent above the trachea (windpipe) is the larynx, with its large, protective thyroid cartilage housing the individual cartilages, muscles, and ligaments that compose the total laryngeal structure. In some people, particularly in adult males, the thyroid cartilage (called the "Adam's Apple") is so prominent that it can easily be seen rising high in the neck during swallowing, dropping low during conversational speech, and rising slightly on high notes during singing.

Photographs of the five primary laryngeal cartilages (cricoid, thyroid, paired arytenoids, and epiglottis) are shown in Figures 2.6 through 2.9. Two other small paired cartilages, the corniculates (small cone-shaped bodies that sit on the apex

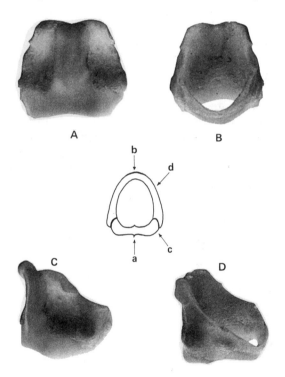

FIGURE 2.6   Four Views of the Cricoid Cartilage *In all photographs, ligaments and muscle attachments and the membranous covering have been removed, showing the bare cartilage. This line drawing shows the overall superior contour of the cricoid, and the anatomical site of the four cricoid photographs indicates that photograph A was taken from that view. (A) Posterior surface of the cricoid; the difference in texture (smooth and rough) is related to ossification; the smooth portions represent the ossification; (B) anterior view; (C) right lateral view of the cricoid ring with the cartilage tipped upward, exposing the superior rim of the signet portion of the cartilage; the two arytenoid cartilages rotate on this clearly defined rim; (D) right lateral view of the cricoid; note the contrast in thickness between the thin anterior portion of the ring and the high signet posterior portion. This difference in size is also shown in (B).*

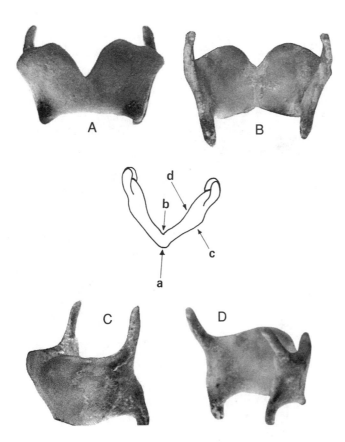

FIGURE 2.7   Four Views of the Laryngeal Thyroid Cartilage *The letters in the line drawing of the superior view of the thyroid cartilage indicate the side of the cartilage photographed. (A) Direct frontal view of the thyroid; (B) posterior view of the cartilage (note the clear extension of the inferior and superior horns on each side); (C) primarily the thyroid cartilage wall; (D) the thyroid posteriorly from a three-fourths view. The size and shape of the thyroid cartilage can be extremely variable in normal individuals. Asymmetry is often seen in normal individuals.*

of the arytenoids extending into the aryepiglottic folds) and the cuneiforms (tiny cone- or rod-shaped cartilage pieces under the mucous membrane covering the aryepiglottic folds), apparently play only a minimal role in the phonatory functions of the larynx. Read the legends under each of the cartilage photographs thoroughly, observing some of the other structures that are also identified.

The three major cartilages seem to play separate roles, and each one is dependent on the others, primarily by muscle action and ligament attachment. The **cricoid** appears almost as an enlarged and complete tracheal ring, forming the solid base of the larynx (other tracheal rings are incomplete or three-quarter rings). It is circular in shape, and the two "pyramid-shaped" arytenoids sit on top of its high posterior (signet-shaped) wall. We shall see later that the arytenoids rock, slide, and rotate on their articular facets on the cricoid by action of the intrinsic laryngeal muscles. Partially surrounding the cricoid and arytenoids, on three sides, is the U-shaped thyroid cartilage, which has two points of articulation with the cricoid cartilage below. All the laryngeal cartilages (similar to cartilage throughout the skeletal system) are coated with a tough leathery covering (the perichondrium), which gives the lateral view of the larynx in Figure 2.10 such a waxy look. This perichondrium covering had been removed in the series of photographs of the separate cartilages.

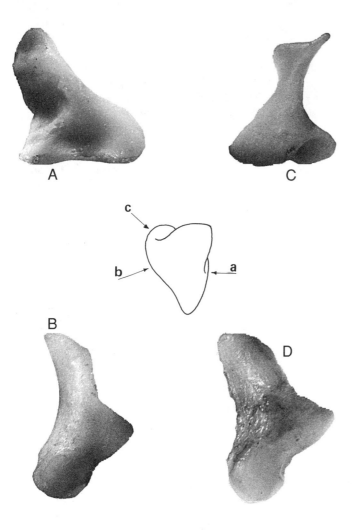

FIGURE 2.8   Four Views of an Arytenoid Cartilage after Removal of Ligament, Muscle, and Membrane Attachments *(A) Lateral view of the indentation (fovea) toward the base, which receives the attachment of the thyroarytenoid muscles (vocal folds); the higher indentation on the left margin receives the ventricular fold; the muscular process to which the posterior and lateral cricoarytenoids are attached is visible at the right base; (B) medial view of an arytenoid that has been tilted up slightly to the left; the right angular corner is the vocal process; (C) posterior-lateral view of the muscular process at the base; note toward the right base the cricoarytenoid articular facet (point of joint articulation); (D) camera lens picks up the base of the cartilage as well as its medial wall; the curving base of the arytenoid allows it to rotate, slide, and rock on the cricoid rim below during adduction and abduction and tensing of the vocal folds. (D is not shown in the line drawing.)*

There are two main groups of muscles of the larynx: the extrinsic and the intrinsic. The extrinsic laryngeal muscles have one attachment to the larynx and another attachment to some structure external to the larynx. The extrinsic muscles give the larynx fixed support and elevate or lower its position in the neck. Functionally, the extrinsic muscles (all but the cricopharyngeus) may be divided into two groups, elevators and depressors:

elevators	**depressors**
digastrics	omohyoids
geniohyoids	sternohyoids
mylohyoids	sternothyroids
stylohyoids	
thyrohyoids	

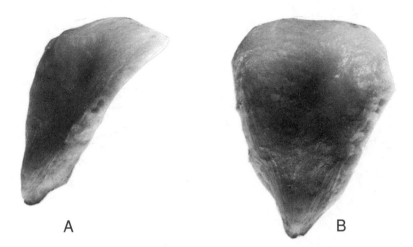

A   B

FIGURE 2.9 **Two Views of the Epiglottis** *The epiglottis has been removed from its attachment on the lower, internal surface of the anterior portion of the thyroid cartilage. For purposes of photography, the cartilage has been denuded, excising away its ligament and muscle attachments and its membranous cover-ing. (A) Epiglottis from a frontal-lateral view; the rotation of the cartilage per-mits us to see the concave epiglottal contour; (B) epiglottis in its whole anterior dimension, which represents the lingual surface.*

These elevators and depressors are well pictured and described in anatomi-cal texts such as Zemlin (1998) and Palmer (1993).

The extrinsic elevators lift the larynx high during swallowing and slightly during production of high singing notes (especially in untrained singers). The depressors lower the larynx after deglutition and after high-note singing; they also lower the larynx a bit for production of low singing notes. Actually, normal speakers should experience only minimal vertical excursion of the larynx. Trained singers keep the height of the larynx nearly constant while singing a range of high and low notes (Sataloff, 1981).

The other extrinsic laryngeal muscle (other than the elevators and depressors) is the cricopharyngeus, which is a part of the lower portion of the interior pharyn-geal constrictor. This cricopharyngeus muscle serves as the new source (neoglottis) of vibration in esophageal speech production. The sphincterlike fibers of the cri-copharyngeus, originating from the posterior wall of the cricoid cartilage, help anchor the larynx in the fixed position in which it usually lies. In her fourth edition of *The Voice and Its Disorders*, Greene (1980) writes that "the steadying influence of the cricopharyngeus on the larynx during phonation is of importance" and that the cricopharyngeus "is in fact an antagonist to the cricothyroid muscle" (pp. 36, 38). The distance between the larynx and the hyoid bone, as determined by the function of the extrinsic muscles, is often the focus of instruction by singing teachers in the production of a good singing voice. However, it does not appear that the good speaking voice requires much active muscle movement from either elevators or depressors. Indeed, the larynx should "float" rather freely, suspended between the

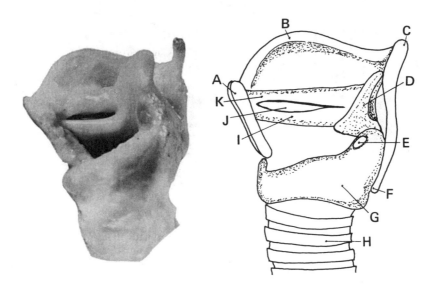

FIGURE 2.10   A Lateral Left View of the Larynx, with the Left Half of the Thyroid Cartilage Removed *The unretouched photograph shows a remarkable view of the ventricle opening between the true folds and the false folds. (A) Cut edge at lamina of thyroid cartilage; (B) arch of the thyroid cartilage; (C) superior horn of the thyroid cartilage; (D) arytenoid cartilage, right; (E) articular facet of the cricoid and arytenoid cartilage; (F) inferior horn of the thyroid cartilage; (G) cricoid cartilage; (H) tracheal ring; (I) vocal fold, right; (J) ventricle; (K) ventricular fold or false fold.*

elevators above and the depressors below. The sphincteric action of the larynx and its phonatory capabilities appear to be the function of the intrinsic muscles of the larynx, which we consider in more detail than we did the extrinsic laryngeal muscles.

The larynx has six intrinsic muscles. Four of them are clearly identifiable in the photographs and drawings in Figure 2.11. One pair of muscles, the posterior cricoarytenoids (PCA), is known as the lone vocal fold abductor (these muscles open the glottis by separating the folds at the posterior larynx). The other five intrinsic muscles can be classified as adductors (they close the glottis by bringing the posterior portion of the vocal folds together), although they have other functions. The following brief descriptions identify each muscle in Figures 2.11 and 2.12.

Posterior Cricoarytenoids.   This lone abductor muscle (E in Figure 2.11) is the largest laryngeal intrinsic muscle. The fibers originate from a middle depression on the posterior surface of the cricoid and angle up, inserting in the muscular process of the arytenoid on that side (right-sided fibers go to the right muscular process, and so on). This paired muscle is innervated by the recurrent laryngeal nerve. Its primary function is to abduct the folds by rotating laterally the vocal process of the arytenoids.

Lateral Cricoarytenoids.   This paired muscle (F in Figure 2.11) functions as a direct antagonist to the posterior cricoarytenoid as it plays its adductor role. The lateral

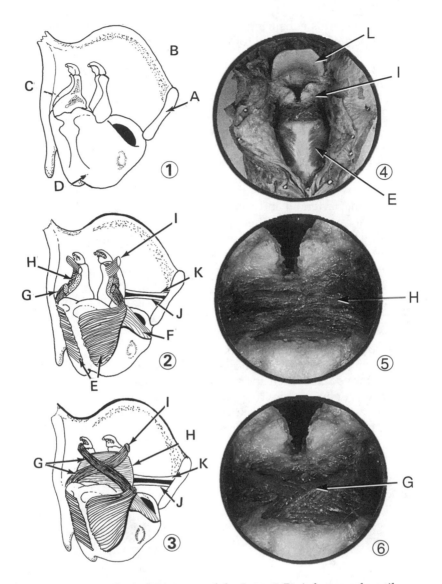

FIGURE 2.11   Intrinsic Structures of the Larynx Basic laryngeal cartilage structures: *(A) cutaway of right thyroid wing; (B) left thyroid cartilage wall; (C) left arytenoid cartilage; (D) posterior of cricoid cartilage. Intrinsic muscles; (E) posterior cricoarytenoid; (F) lateral cricoarytenoid; (G) oblique arytenoid; (H) transverse arytenoid; (I) aryepiglottic; (J) thyroarytenoid (vocal fold); (K) ventricular fold; (L) the epiglottis.*

cricoarytenoid originates from the upper border of the arch of the cricoid cartilage and inserts into the muscular process of the arytenoid on the same side. [Innervation is also by the recurrent laryngeal nerve.] When this muscle contracts, it rotates the muscular process forward and at the same time causes the vocal process of the arytenoid (and the attached posterior part of the vocal fold) to "toe in" at the midline, thus enhancing adduction of the vocal processes and their corresponding portion of the vocal folds.

Transverse Arytenoids.   These muscle fibers (H in Figure 2.11) originate from the lateral margin and posterior surface of one arytenoid and insert on the same sites on the opposite arytenoid. The transverse arytenoids are not paired muscles, per se. They transverse the distance between the two arytenoids. Innervated bilaterally by the recurrent laryngeal nerves, when these muscles contract, they approximate the bodies of the arytenoid cartilages together, functioning as adductor intrinsics as well as fold compressors.

Oblique Arytenoids.   This muscle (G in Figure 2.11) originates from the muscular process of one arytenoid and courses obliquely upward and across to the apex of the opposite cartilage. The fibers actually continue obliquely to the lateral border of the epiglottis and are known as the aryepiglottic muscles after they leave the arytenoid apex. The aryepiglottics become part of the aryepiglottic folds, which also include some cuneiform cartilage and membrane. These folds are active in the swallowing mechanism. The oblique arytenoid muscles are innervated bilaterally by the recurrent nerves and are active in bringing the vocal folds closer together by approximation of the apex of each arytenoid cartilage.

Thyroarytenoids.   The paired thyroarytenoids, shown in Figure 2.12, form the bulk of the muscular portion of the vocal folds. The inner section of the thyroarytenoid is known as the vocalis section and the larger, more lateral fibers are known as the thyromuscularis, or external thyroarytenoids (Zemlin, 1998). As Figure 2.12 shows, the fibers originate on the inner surface of the thyroid cartilage and extend posteriorly to where they insert in the vocal process (vocalis fibers) and the lateral surface

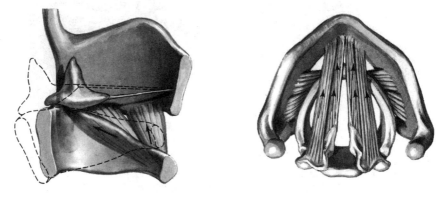

FIGURE 2.12   The Cricothyroid Muscles *The cricothyroid muscles can be seen in the drawing on the left, angling from the inner superior surface of the cricoid cartilage up to the thyroid cartilage. The medial fibers of the vocalis section and the lateral section of the thyroarytenoids are seen in the drawing on the right. (Reprinted with permission from* The CIBA Collection of Medical Illustrations, *illustrated by Frank H. Netter, M.D. All rights reserved. Copyright © 1986, CIBA Pharmaceutical Company, Division of CIBA-Geigy Corporation.)*

(external thyroarytenoid) of the arytenoid cartilages. The inner border of the vocal fold contains the vocal ligament that originates at the anterior commissure and extends to the vocal process end of the arytenoids.

In summary, the vocal folds include both sections of the thyroarytenoids, the inner surface of the arytenoid cartilage, and the vocal ligament. The whole apparatus is covered with a tough white membrane known as the **conus elasticus.** Figure 2.13 shows the white membranous covering of the vocal folds (as they appear to the eye during endoscopy), with the folds in an open abducted position. The muscular aspect of the folds, the thyroarytenoids, are also innervated by the recurrent laryngeal nerve, and they seem to have a dual function. They shorten themselves as required for producing lower phonation frequencies, and, by their own muscular tension and elasticity, they work as glottal adducting structures.

Cricothyroids.   Figure 2.12 shows the anteriorly placed paired cricothyroid muscles that lie external to the laryngeal cartilages. This muscle pair is made up of two parts or portions: the obliqua and the recta. The fibers originate from the anterior-lateral arch of the cricoid cartilage and end in two distinctly different insertions. The lower fibers (obliqua portion) insert near the lower horn of the thyroid cartilage, and the more superior fibers (recta portion) course to the lower margin of the lateral thyroid cartilage wall. This pair of muscles is innervated by the superior laryngeal nerve (SLN). When these muscles contract, they increase the distance between the thyroid and arytenoid cartilages, thus contributing to pitch elevation by stretching the vocal folds; the tensing of the vocal folds (by elongating them) is also a minor adducting action. When the superior laryngeal nerve is impaired the larynx is canted or slanted, thus making the glottis run obliquely across the larynx rather than in a straight anterior-posterior direction.

Figure 2.14 contains four photographs, A, B, C, D. Photograph A is of an adult male with normal larynx in the adducted position. Photograph B is of an adult male with unilateral superior laryngeal nerve paralysis. Note the canting of the larynx that causes the glottis to rest in an oblique position rather than in a straight anterior–posterior direction. Also, the patient has difficulty making pitch shifts when there is superior laryngeal nerve paralysis. This is not true for pure

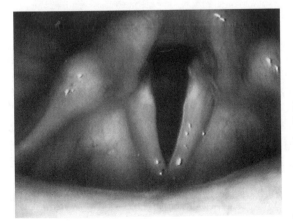

FIGURE 2.13   Normal Vocal Folds in Abducted Expiratory Position
Normal vocal folds in abducted expiratory position, as viewed with oral video endoscopy: The anterior commissure (V) is at the bottom of the picture, the glottis is the dark V portion, and the right vocal fold is on the left side of the picture.

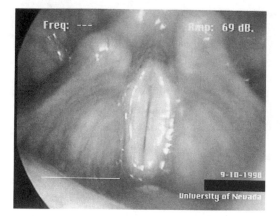

FIGURE 2.14A An adult male larynx with the vocal folds in the adducted position.

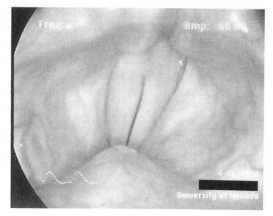

FIGURE 2.14B An adult male larynx with a unilateral left superior laryngeal nerve lesion.

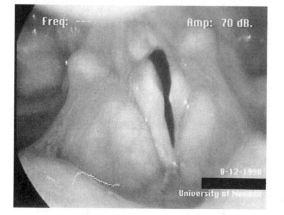

FIGURE 2.14C An aging female larynx showing bowing and some partial fold wastage.

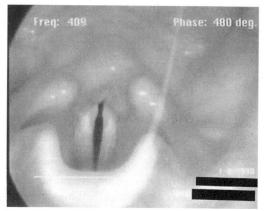

FIGURE 2.14D The normal larynx of a seven-year-old child.

recurrent laryngeal nerve paralysis. Photograph C is of an elderly female larynx. Note that the vocal folds demonstrate some bowing and the partial wastage of the folds due to aging make the vocal processes appear more prominent. In the final photograph, D, is the larynx of a child.

Phonation Function and Mucosal Wave

It is difficult to discuss the cartilages and the muscles of the larynx without some description of laryngeal function. Before we further describe function and laryngeal physiology, we should describe the important functional organization of the laryngeal structures that give rise to the mucosal wave. In Figure 2.15 is a stroboscopic photograph demonstrating the mucosal wave. The surface cover of the

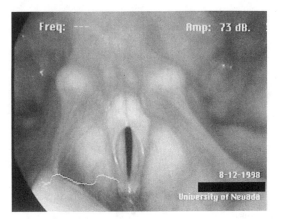

FIGURE 2.15   A stroboscopic photograph demonstrating a mucosal wave.

vocal fold is raised in a wave that travels across the vocal fold from the medial edge to the lateral margin of the vocal fold near where the vocal fold is overlapped by the false vocal cord.

Hirano (1981) has described the functional structure of the vocal folds themselves in such a way as to explain the mucosal wave that occurs with vocal fold vibration. The cover (epithelium and superficial lamina propria, Reinke's space) over the vocal fold body (intermediate and deep layers of lamina propria and vocalis muscle) slides and produces a wave that moves or travels across the superior surface of the vocal fold about two thirds of the way to the lateral edge of the fold. The wave will generally dissipate before reaching the inner surface of the thyroid cartilage. When the vocal folds fail to vibrate properly, there is an abnormal or absent mucosal wave. This can be seen in the post surgical (stripped) vocal folds of patients who present with aphonia following removal of large portions of vocal fold mucosa. While the cords may look white and the medial edge may be straight, they do not vibrate. The mucosa that has recovered on the folds after surgery is adherent to the underlying tissue and is also stiff. Without the differences in density between the cover and body relationship described by Hirano (1981), vibration does not occur. When vocal folds that have been overinjected with teflon as a treatment for unilateral paralysis are viewed stroboscopically, they frequently may also fail to vibrate (Watterson, McFarlane, and Menicucci 1990). The first description of this failure of overinjected vocal folds to vibrate, demonstrating an absent mucosal wave was reported by Watterson, McFarlane, and Menicucci. Scarring can also create a disruption in the cover of the vocal fold and produce an interrupted mucosal wave. McFarlane and colleagues (1991) demonstrated that teflon injected vocal folds can produce poorly perceived vocal quality compared to the results from voice therapy and from muscle nerve reinnervation surgery in cases of unilateral vocal fold paralysis. Watterson, McFarlane, and Menicucci (1990) demonstrated that teflon injected vocal folds may be adynamic and not vibrate during phonation. A mass such as teflon, a nodule, cyst, or underlying carcinoma or swelling (edema) can all produce a visible alteration of the normal mucosal wave. This is why videostroboscopic evaluation is such an important tool for the study and diagnosis of the vocal folds and of voice disorders.

TABLE 2.1   Functional Structure of the Vocal Fold

Vocal Fold Physiology

Cover

Epithelium
Superficial lamina propria (Reinke's space)

Transition

Intermediate and deep layers of lamina propria (Vocal ligament)

Body

Vocalis muscle

Figure 2.16 shows the actual structure of the vocal fold and clearly demonstrates the difference in density from the least dense outer cover through the more dense transition to the most dense body of the vocal fold vocalis portion of the thyroarytenoid muscle.

The myoelastic aerodynamic theory of phonation (Van den Berg, 1968) is generally regarded as the most accurate model to explain the mechanics of phonation. Phonation begins basically with an expiration (air volume and air pressure changes), setting the approximated (closed or adducted) vocal folds in vibration as the airflow passes between the folds (transglottal pressure drop). In the prephonation period, the vocal folds may be abducted in the expiration position (Figure 2.17A). The folds approximate one another for phonation as phonation begins (Figure 2.17B). The five laryngeal adductor muscles contract to bring the vocal folds together.

Two of the adductors—for example, the lateral cricoarytenoid and the thyroarytenoids—have very rapid contraction times, sometimes as fast as fifteen msec, which Martensson (1968) has written is "exceedingly fast and surpassed only by the extrinsic eye muscles" for speed. It would appear that vocal fold adduction is achieved in milliseconds, prior to the onset of voicing. As the folds approximate, they begin to obstruct the airflow passing through the glottal level of the airway. This obstruction or glottal resistance is accomplished by the vocal folds as a function of the medial compression action of the adductor muscles of the larynx. Vocal fold adduction need not be complete for phonation to occur. Zemlin (1998) states: "If the glottal chink is narrowed to about 3 mm, a minimal amount of airflow will set the vocal folds into vibration." (p. 144).

The subglottal pressure builds up when the folds are approximated. The volume of expired air leaving the lungs is impeded at the level of the glottis, resulting in an increased velocity of airflow through the glottis. Subglottal pressure increases (with respect to the supraglottal air pressure), and the vocal folds are blown apart, equalizing supraglottal and subglottal pressure (the opening phase of one cycle of vibration). Because of the mass of the folds (their muscle and ligament covered with a membrane) and the Bernoulli effect, they come back together again

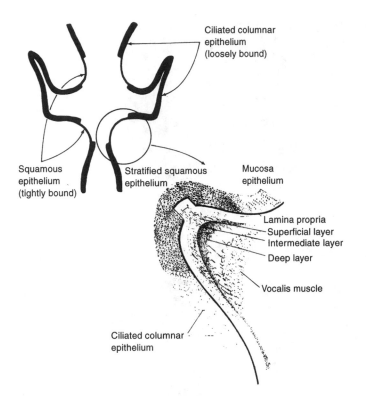

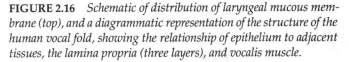

FIGURE 2.16 *Schematic of distribution of laryngeal mucous membrane (top), and a diagrammatic representation of the structure of the human vocal fold, showing the relationship of epithelium to adjacent tissues, the lamina propria (three layers), and vocalis muscle.*

From Zemlin, W. R. (1998). Speech and Hearing Science: Anatomy and Physiology *(4th ed).*

to their previous approximation line (the closed phase of the phonatory cycle, transglottal pressure drop). The Bernoulli effect occurs when the velocity of subglottal air is increased while approaching and passing through the constricted glottis. This increased velocity of airflow will create a negative pressure between, and just below, the medial edges of the vocal lips. The vocal folds will then be "sucked" back together producing the repetitive vibratory cycle of folds "blown" apart and "sucked" back together hundreds of times per second. The Bernoulli effect results in a "suction action" (negative pressure under the vocal lips relative to a positive pressure above the vocal lip) that draws the folds together.

The vibratory cycle of the vocal folds can be summarized as follows: The intrinsic adductors approximate the folds as expiration begins. Subglottal pressure increases. The airflow velocity increases as it passes through the glottal opening and blows the folds apart. The static mass of the folds and the Bernoulli suction effect bring them back together again. The vibratory cycle then repeats itself. This is repeated approximately 125 times per second in the phonation of an adult male and 225 times per second in an adult female.

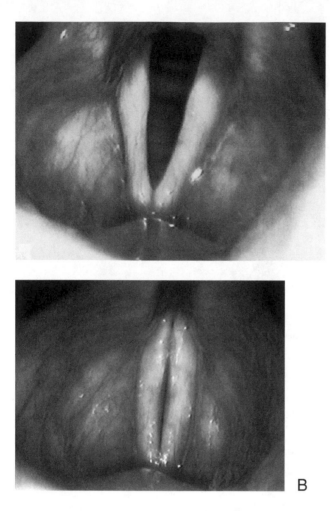

A

B

FIGURE 2.17   Two Photographs of the Vocal Folds *In (A) the vocal folds are open (abducted) in the expiratory position. In (B) the folds have approximated (adducted) and are in the phonation position.*

During normal phonation, the vocal folds approximate one another in their total anterior–posterior dimension. Some normal females sometimes demonstrate a slight posterior glottal chink or gap during phonation. The vocal folds appear slightly shorter during phonation and whispering; that is, the vocal folds are always longer in the open abducted position than in the closed adducted one. The configuration of the glottis for whispering is characterized by an open, posterior chink, with the arytenoid cartilages and their vocal processes angled in an open, inverted Y position. Although the vocal folds are parallel to one another during whispering, they do not firmly approximate. This lack of adduction, particularly in the posterior chink, produces frictional sounds when the outgoing airstream passes through, producing what we perceive as turbulence or whispering.

During at-rest breathing, the vocal folds appear to be maximally long. They are shortened somewhat during phonation. In fact, at the lower end of an individual's pitch range, at the level where conversational phonation is generally found, the vocal folds are considerably shortened compared to their length during expiration.

Pitch Mechanism

In speaking about the length and thickness of the folds, we refer to the mechanism that controls fundamental frequency, or the pitch of the voice that we hear. Fundamental frequency is directly related to how many vibratory closings and openings (cycles) the vocal folds make in one second. The rate of vibration is related to their thickness, length, and elasticity. A short, thick, somewhat lax fold vibrates at a much slower rate (producing a low pitch) than a long, thin, tense fold, which will produce a higher pitch. As the length of the vocal folds increases, there is a corresponding increase in frequency that proceeds in an almost "stair step" fashion. By using X-ray laminagraphy, which permits cross-sectional, coronal viewing of the vocal folds, Hollien (1962) found that the mean thickness, or mass, of the folds systematically decreased as voice pitch increased. It appears, then, from the multiple studies conducted on vocal fold length and thickness by the Hollien group, that fundamental frequency, or voice pitch level, is directly related to the length and thickness of the individual's vocal folds.

The relative differences between men and women in vocal fold length (approximately 17–20 mm for men and 12–17 mm for women) and vocal fold thickness appear to be the primary determinants of differences in voice pitch. The typical fundamental frequency for men is around 125 Hz; for women, around 225 Hz. Table 2.2 shows examples of normal pitch values, including pitch range and fundamental frequency. The speaker's age also has an effect on fundamental frequency. For example, at age 6 or 7 years boys and girls have similar fundamental frequencies near 285–295 Hz. By young adulthood, males descend to a fundamental frequency of about 125 Hz while females at this age demonstrate a fundamental of about 220 Hz. In advanced age, women will drop in fundamental frequency to 190–200 Hz while men will rise to about 145–150 Hz. When individuals phonate at increasingly higher pitch levels, they must lengthen the vocal folds to decrease their relative mass and increase their tension. Increases of pitch, therefore, appear to be related to lengthening of the vocal folds, with a corresponding decrease of tissue mass and an increase of fold tissue elasticity. Lowering the pitch is directly related to shortening (and thus relaxing) the vocal folds.

It would appear that both the cricothyroids and possibly the cricopharyngeus play active roles in elongating the vocal folds, which in turn increases their elasticity. The vocal folds are stretched by the action of the cricothyroids, which increase the distance between the arytenoids and the thyroid cartilage by drawing the cricoid cartilage up toward the thyroid, which in effect lowers the posterior cricoid rim on which the arytenoids sit. A review of Figure 2.12 will be helpful at this point. The drawing at the left in Figure 2.12 demonstrates the vocal fold stretching due to action of the cricothyroid muscle (the only intrinsic laryngeal muscle with superior laryngeal nerve supply). The cricopharyngeus, when contracted, can pull the cricoid slightly posterior, adding to vocal fold stretching and thus increased elasticity. For a detailed description with accompanying drawings of the elongation functions of the cricothyroid muscles, see the phonation chapter in *Speech and Hearing Science* (Zemlin, 1998). Relaxation of the cricothyroids with the simultaneous contraction of the thyroarytenoids appears to be essential for shortening and thickening the folds, which lowers the pitch of the voice. Greene

TABLE 2.2   Normal Fundamental Frequency (F_0) and Pitch Range for Four Voices (Bass, Tenor, Alto, and Soprano)

Note on Piano	Physical Hz	Typical F_0 and Pitch Range			
		(Bass)	(Tenor)	(Alto)	(Soprano)
C_6	1,024				1,040
B	960				
A	853				
G_5	768				
F	682			700	
E	640				
D	576				
C_5	512		550		
B	480				
A	426				
G_4	384				
F	341	340			
E	320				
D	288				
C_4	256				$F_0$256
B	240				
A	213			$F_0$200	
G_3	192				
F	170				170
E	160				
D	144		$F_0$135	140	
C_3	128				
B	120				
A	106	$F_0$100			
G_2	96		95		
F	85	80			

(1980) has suggested that the cricopharyngeus may play an antagonist (shortening) role to the cricothyroids.

Near the upper end of the natural pitch range, increased elasticity of the vocal folds results in increased glottal resistance, requiring increased subglottal air pressure to produce higher frequency phonations. Increased tension of the vocal folds requires greater air pressure to set the folds into vibration. Van den Berg (1968) has written that the average person must slightly increase subglottal air pressure in order to increase voice pitch; however, because increasing subglottal pressure has an abducting effect on the vocal folds, the folds must continue to increase in tension (longitudinal tension) to maintain their approximated position. Although the primary determinants of pitch seems to be the length, mass, and tension adjustments of the vocal folds, increases in pitch level are usually characterized by increasing subglottal pressures, increased medial compression, and increased glottal airflow rates.

Table 2.2 demonstrates the piano note and corresponding physical frequency in Hz for four voices (bass, tenor, alto, and soprano).

Falsetto. The vocal folds can elongate and stretch only so far. If singers want to extend their pitch range beyond what normal vocal fold stretching can do, they are forced to produce a falsetto voice. Zemlin (1998), in describing the vocal folds during falsetto production, says "the folds appear long, stiff, very thin along the edges, and often somewhat bow-shaped" (p. 167). We might describe the production of the falsetto voice in this manner: The folds approximate with tight, posterior vocal process adduction. The posterior cartilaginous portion is so tightly adducted that little or no posterior vibration occurs while the anterior portion vibrates rapidly. The lateral portions of the thyroarytenoid do not actively vibrate to produce the falsetto voice. The mucosal wave is confined to the medial edge of the vocal folds. Thus there is a high frequency, low amplitude, and limited lateral excursion of the mucosal wave. The amplitude and height of the mucosal wave is greatly reduced generally in high pitch and even more reduced in the production of falsetto. The inner vocalis segment of the muscle is extremely contracted (and thus thinned out) along the vocal ligament. As the membrane wraps the ligament, the membrane itself may become the primary vibrating structure during falsetto. In falsetto the vocal folds may remain somewhat open, although parallel, which gives falsetto its characteristic "breathy" quality. At times there may also be a posterior chink during the production of falsetto that contributes to the breathy quality of falsetto voice. Falsetto has been described (called the "loft" register by Hollien, 1962) as a production of the vibrating membrane of the anterior two-thirds surface of the glottal margin. This limitation of the mucosal wave to the anterior two thirds of the vocal folds has the effect of making the cords functionally shorter and thus the higher pitch of falsetto.

Glottal Fry. The kind of pitch opposite from the falsetto in both quality and airflow rate is the low glottal fry. Greene (1980) described the fry as the pulse register, the "lowest range of notes and synonymous with vocal fry, glottal fry, creak and strohbass" (p. 81). The glottal fry sounds something like the sputter of a low-powered outboard motor or, as we tell our patients, the sound of a stick being dragged along a picket fence. Zemlin (1998) wrote that fry is produced when the folds are approximated tightly with a flaccid appearance along the glottal margin. Moore and von Leden (1958) found that during fry a double vibration of the folds is followed by a prolonged period of approximation (almost two thirds the duration of the vibratory cycle). Vocal fry may well be the normal vibratory cycle we use near the bottom of our normal pitch range. It is normally produced near the end of a long phrase when subglottal air pressure and airflow rate are both low and lung volume is less. The normal nontense larynx makes use of this last end of the air supply by relaxing the vocal fold medial margins to phonate on the last available air of the expiratory reserve volume. Some speakers may add fry to their phonation, to give, in their minds, an authoritative quality to what they are saying or to give a perception of being extremely relaxed or calm. Although glottal fry does not appear to be a vocal abnormality, some voice patients successfully work to eliminate it by elevating their pitch levels slightly and increasing subglottic air pressure slightly. We describe the use of glottal fry as a clinical facilitation technique (Chapter 6) that we often employ in therapy with hyperfunctional voice disorders such as vocal nodules.

Related to the production of voice pitch and the pitch range of any individual is voice register. It appears that a particular register characterizes a certain pattern of vocal fold vibration, and the vocal folds are approximated in a similar way (vibratory mode) throughout a particular pitch range. Once this pitch range reaches its maximum limit, the folds adjust to a new approximation contour (or mode of vibration) that produces an abrupt change in vocal quality. Van den Berg (1968) describes three primary forms of voice register: chest, midvoice, and falsetto. We would add to these three the vocal fry register at the lower end of the normal pitch range.

The frontal, coronal view of the folds sketched in Figure 2.18 shows the thickened folds of the chest or normal register contrasted with the thin folds of the falsetto register. From the perceptual viewpoint, voice register is confined to the similar sound (quality) of an individual's voice at various pitches. Although this similar quality is undoubtedly related to the similarity in vocal fold approximation and vibration characteristics (mode of vibration), teachers of voice strive to blend the various registers, so that the difference in quality of voice becomes almost imperceptible as the singer goes from one register to the next. Some singers seem to have only one register; no matter how they change their pitch, their voice always seems to have the same quality, with no discernible break toward the upper part of the pitch range. This is no small accomplishment and requires considerable voice training. It is a highly regarded attribute in the professional singing voice. Such persons' frontal X-rays would probably show a relatively stable contour in the approximations of the vocal folds. An excellent review of the literature and detailed

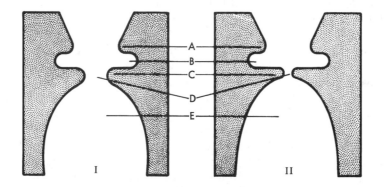

FIGURE 2.18   Line Tracing of a Tomogram *A line tracing on a tomogram that presents an X-ray frontal view of the vocal folds showing vocal fold approximation contours for (I) chest register, and (II) falsetto register: (A) ventricular fold; (B) open ventricle; (C) vocal fold; (D) glottis, opening between folds; (E) trachea. Note the thicker fold approximation for the chest register, as opposed to the thinner, superior approximation of the two folds during the production of the falsetto register.*

description of voice register may be found in the old but valuable reference by Luchsinger and Arnold (1965).

Loudness Mechanism. The intensity of the voice, perceived as loudness of the voice, is directly related to changes in subglottal and transglottal air pressure drops. Hixon and Abbs (1980) have written: "Sound pressure level, the primary factor contributing to our perception of the loudness of the voice, is governed mainly by the pressure supplied to the larynx by the respiratory pump" (p. 68). It appears that the trained voices of actors or singers increase intensity by increasing both subglottal pressure and airflow rate (similar to the water hose analogy), with only minimal increase of glottal tension (Bouhuys, Proctor, and Mead, 1966). At very loud levels untrained voices often increase in pitch as part of the loudness. It is difficult for untrained voices to produce loud sounds at very low pitch levels, which is the reason for the extent of vocal abuse in low- as opposed to high-pitched voice production. This may account for the reported excessively low-pitched voice associated with contact ulcer development. The trained voice of the bass singer has no trouble being very loud indeed while retaining a healthy larynx.

As voice intensity increases, the vocal folds tend to remain closed for longer periods of time during each vibratory cycle (see Figure 2.19), and the greater intensity of voice is characterized by greater excursion of the vibrating folds. It would appear that, as intensity increases, increased glottal tension impedes the rate of airflow, increasing subglottal pressure. At lower pitch levels this tension during intense phonations is minimal. It causes singers, for example, to run out of air sooner when producing varying intensities at low pitches than at high ones.

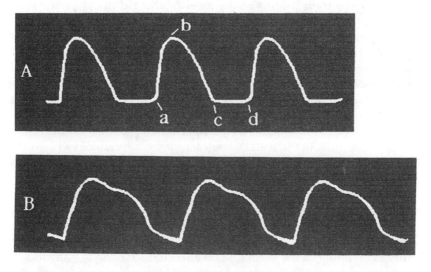

FIGURE 2.19 Laryngograms *The two laryngograms represent (A) a prolonged vowel /i/ at 125 Hz normal intensity and (B) at a louder intensity. The letter a represents the beginning of the closing phase as the cords come together; at b the cords are completely together and beginning to open; at c the cords are open; at d the open phase is completed and another cycle begins. The closed phase (b to c) is much longer in the louder production (B). The open phase (c to d) is shorter in the louder production (B).*

Evidently, speakers or singers who continually require a loud voice could use their vocal mechanisms more optimally by developing their expiratory skills and relying more on increased subglottal air pressure and increased airflow rates, and less on increased glottal elasticity, to achieve louder intensities.

Quality Mechanisms.   Besides pitch, loudness, quality, and register as measurable dimensions of voice, Perkins (1983) has added constriction and vertical as well as horizontal focus to the concept of voice quality production. He describes the feeling of constriction on a continuum of open (the yawn) to closed (the swallow). The clinical facilitation technique of yawn–sigh discussed in Chapter 6 demonstrates the clinical value of these physiological configurations of the supraglottal vocal tract. Imagery or feeling is used to determine the vertical focus of the voice, "the perception associated with the placement of the focal point of the tone in the head" (Perkins, 1983, p. 113). At the low end of the vertical focus, speakers or singers feel their voice is being squeezed out of the throat, whereas at the high end the focus seems to be high in the head. The sensation is described as if the tone were "floating in the head." Vocal efficiency seems to occur best at the higher end of the vertical placement. The clinical facilitation technique of focus discussed in Chapter 6 makes use of these observations. It has been our experience that subjects given these instructions relative to the imagery of constriction and verticality produce voices with greater aperiodicity (hoarseness) at the low end of the vertical scale and greater vocal clarity at the high end. In time Perkins's construct of constriction and horizontal as well as vertical focus may well have greater measurement potential and utilization. Vocal quality may well be related primarily to supraglottal resonance, but important components of the spectrum of the laryngeal tone have their origins at the level of the glottis. How the vocal folds are approximated together, laxly or tightly, in part determines the quality of the voice as well as the filtering done by the supraglottal vocal tract. Many individuals can produce several different voices, all at the same pitch level, by varying the approximation characteristics of the vocal folds. A breathy voice is often produced by adding phonation to the ongoing expiration, with the folds only laxly approximating one another. Spectrographic analysis of the breathy voice shows us that noise and aperiodicity produced by the turbulent airflow typify the first part of the utterance, and that phonation (greater periodicity) comes in after some delay. The four spectrograms in Figure 2.20 contrast the breathy voice (with much aperiodicity and noise) with the harsh voice (with hard glottal attack) with the hoarse voice (combined hard glottal attack with breathiness) and the normal voice.

Each of the spectrograms was produced by the same normal speaker prolonging an /i/. In hard glottal attack, the opposite kind of vocal onset is observed. Here the first voicing patterns begin abruptly with the onset of expiration. The glottis seems to be held tightly until a sudden release of air sets the folds into vibration. Faulty positioning of the vocal folds is also characteristic of patients with adductor spastic dysphonia. (While we use the term *adductor spastic dysphonia,* Watterson and McFarlane (1992) make a case that the *abductor* and *adductor* types are actually different disorders, not two types of the same disorder.) These patients bring the folds so tightly together that they act like a valve, almost totally preventing the flow of air from traveling through the glottis. The patient's voice is strained and has a strangled

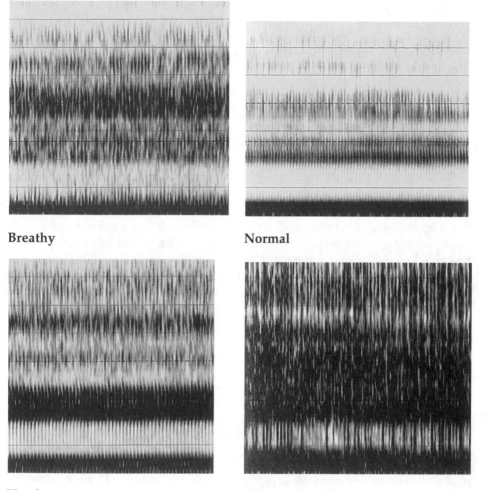

Breathy   **Normal**

Harsh   **Hoarse**

FIGURE 2.20   Spectrograms *Four spectrograms of the same speaker producing the /i/ vowel under four conditions: breathy, normal, harsh, and hoarse. The relative spacing of the formants stays the same as the signal source changes.*

quality. How the folds are approximated has much to do with how voices sound. Study of the vocal fold "set" aspect of phonation has been limited to such methods as high-speed film, viewing the larynx through indirect laryngoscopy, or employing spectrograms displaying visually the voices that we hear. Even though we know something about the extreme of breathiness and hard glottal attack, our knowledge of vocal fold physiology for most of the voices we hear is relatively lacking in regard to vocal fold approximation and its effect on quality. The development of flexible videoendoscopy with stroboscopic light sources and glottographic instruments has allowed us to study the production of these aspects further. McFarlane and

Lavorato (1984) have discussed the use of videoendoscopy in the study of voice disorders. We discuss this topic in detail in Chapter 5, where we present evaluation procedures. Likewise, Watterson, McFarlane, and Menicucci (1990), McFarlane (1988), Watterson and McFarlane (1991), and Tyler and Watterson (1991) have all addressed aspects of glottal closure and its effect on voice quality.

Resonance

The fundamental frequency produced by the vocal folds would be a weak-sounding "reedy" voice without the additional component of resonance. Years ago one of the authors observed a patient who had been cut from ear to ear with a massive wound that opened immediately superior to his thyroid cartilage. Before the wound was sutured, we heard the patient's feeble attempts at phonation. Much of his airflow and sound waves escaped through the wound. The result was a voice that was truly unique. Someone even likened it to the thin bleat of a baby lamb. Apparently, what is perceived as the quality, timbre, richness, fullness, and loudness of the voice is largely produced by the supraglottal resonators. Even though the structures of the chest and trachea may play some role in resonance, this role is not as clearly defined as that of the supraglottal resonators of the pharynx, oral cavity, and nasal cavity.

Figure 2.21 shows a line drawing and cadaver head that demonstrate the F-shaped vocal tract.

Structures of Resonance

The vocal tract begins, for all practical purposes, at the level of the glottis. The airflow and sound waves probably have some beginning passage in the ventricular space (B in Figure 2.21) between the true folds (A) and the ventricular folds (C). In Figure 2.21 the cavities of the vocal tract have been shaded darker. The epiglottis (D), by its concavity, probably serves as a deflector or sounding-board resonator as sound waves travel between the aryepiglottic folds (E) into the hypopharynx (F). The hypopharynx is the cavity directly above the esophagus (G). Its anterior border comprises the structures and opening of the larynx (G); its sides and back wall are composed of the inferior pharyngeal constrictors (G). The oropharynx (U) begins at the tip of the epiglottis and extends to the level of the velum and hard palate. The small angular spaces between the front of the epiglottis and the back of the tongue (L) are called the valleculae (I). Cutting away the mandible (K) in a lateral view is the great body of the tongue, which occupies most of the oral cavity and forms the constantly changing floor of that cavity. The hard palate is designated (O), with the soft palate or velum (N) forming the roof of the oral cavity. The lips, teeth, and cheeks play obvious front and lateral roles in shaping the oral cavity. The middle and superior pharyngeal constrictors form the lateral and posterior muscular wall of the oropharynx (H). The site of the velopharyngeal closure, necessary for the separation of the oral and nasal cavities required for oral resonance, is the Passavant's pad (M) area of the superior pharyngeal constrictor; most subjects do not have much Passavant area enlargement. As shown in Figure 2.21, superior to the velopharyngeal contact point, the posterior pharyngeal wall makes a sharp angulation forward, forming the superior wall of the nasopharynx (P) and continuing on as the superior wall of the nasal cavity. We make no further structural breakdown of the nasal cavities (Q) as a prelude to our discussion of resonance. Note that Figure 2.21 also shows the lateral walls, pillars of fauces, and muscles of the palate, pharynx, and tongue. If we look again at the overall lateral view of the vocal tract, we see that the total darkened areas look something like a large letter F. The vocal tract in the photograph resembles an F because the velopharyngeal port is open, connecting the oral and nasal cavities together. If the port were closed at the velopharyngeal contact point (M), the vocal tract opening available for voice resonance would resemble the letter r, formed only by the pharynx and the oral cavity opening above the surface of the tongue.

Mechanism of Resonance

A vibrator, such as the string of a violin or the vocal folds, originates a fundamental vibration (or sound waves), which by itself produces weak, barely audible sounds. This vibrating energy is usually amplified by a resonating body of some type. For example, a violin string, when plucked, will set up a fundamental vibration; this vibration becomes resonated by the bridge to which the strings are attached, which then sets into vibration the sounding board below and in turn the main resonating body of the violin (the chest), which provides open cavity resonance. When all the violin parts are working together in harmony, the fundamental tone of the involved string becomes louder, richer, and fuller in quality. The same string stripped out of its mount on the violin and then plucked (even with the same amount of tension to the string) will sound less intense, less rich, and thinner in quality.

The violin provides a ready example of the two main types of resonance, the sounding-board effect and the open-cavity effect. When a particular string of the violin is bowed, the airwaves that develop are low in amplitude and barely audible; however, because the vibrating string is stretched tightly over the bridge of the violin, it sets the bridge itself into vibration. The bridge functions as a sounding board. The sounding board then vibrates, setting into vibration the air over a much larger area, increasing the loudness of the tone. The sounding-board vibration also introduces the sound waves into the violin cavity itself. The main body, or chest, of the violin provides cavity resonance to the source sound of the vibrating string. The string vibrating alone, which is similar to laryngeal vibration without supraglottal resonance, produces a barely audible tone. The cavity resonance provided by the body of the violin increases the volume or intensity of the vibrating string. The size and overall shape of the resonating cavity has an obvious relationship to the resonance of a vibration.

Every frequency of vibration has an ideal resonating cavity size and shape. The ideal is represented by the cavity that seems to give the loudest tone and the tone with the fullest amount of amplification to its overtones. This may be thought of as acoustic efficiency. This observation can be easily tested by placing a tuning fork over a large glass and varying the amounts of water in the glass. At a particular level of water, the glass will provide optimum resonance, heard as increased loudness and richness of the sound. The lower the frequency of the vibrating wave, the larger the size of the resonating cavity. The thinner string of the violin

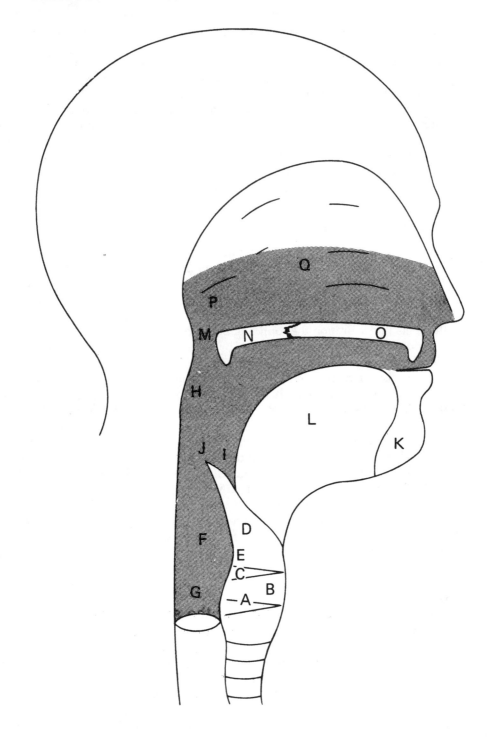

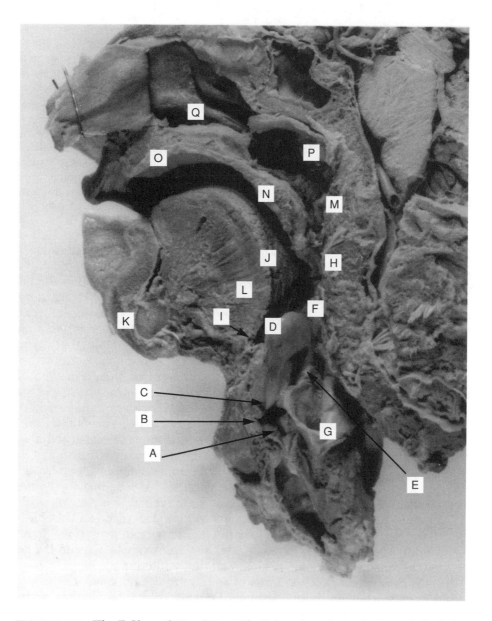

FIGURE 2.21   The F-Shaped Vocal Tract *The F-shaped vocal tract is shown in both the line drawing on the left and the photograph of a cadaver head on the right. Letters A through O identify various structures of the vocal tract: (A) True folds; (B) ventricular space; (C) ventricular folds; (D) epiglottis; (E) aryepiglottic folds; (F) hypopharynx; (G) inferior pharyngeal constrictors; (H) middle pharyngeal constrictors; (I) valleculae; (J) oropharynx; (K) mandible; (L) tongue; (M) Passavant's pad; (N) soft palate (velum); (O) hard palate; (P) nasopharynx; (Q) nasal cavity.*

requires a much smaller resonating body than the larger string of the bass viola, which requires a resonating body as tall as the person who plays the instrument.

The human vocal tract is continually changing. As Minifie (1973) has written:

> During the production of vowels the vocal tract may be viewed as a tortuously shaped tube open at one end (the opening between the lips) and bounded at the other end by a vibrating valve (the vocal folds) which has the effect of closing off the tube at the larynx. The three-dimensional geometry of this tube may be altered through the contraction of muscles which regulate the movements of the tongue, velum, pharynx, mandible, lips, epiglottis, and larynx. These structures may be moved individually or in various combinations. The combination of structures which move during the production of a particular speech sound will determine the unique vocal tract configuration, and hence, the unique acoustical filter for that sound (p. 243).

Some areas of the vocal tract, depending on their configuration, are compatible with the periodic vibration coming from the vocal folds and amplify the fundamental frequency and its harmonics. For example, a fundamental frequency of 125 Hz will resonate harmonic frequencies at 250, 375, 500 (each subsequent harmonic frequency is a whole number multiple of the fundamental), and so on. For a more detailed description of vocal tract acoustics the reader is referred to sources such as Daniloff (1985), Baken (1987), Baken and Daniloff (1991), Borden, Harris, and Raphael (1994), and Minifie (1994). The continuous vocal tract tube is constantly interrupted at various sites from the intrusion and movement of various structures. Some of the interruptions or constrictions may be severe, such as carrying the tongue high and forward in the oral cavity. Any movement of mandible, tongue, or velum, for example, will greatly alter the opening of the oral cavity. Some of the movements have no effect on the fundamental or sound source; some of them filter or inhibit the fundamental. What finally comes out of the mouth or the nasal cavity perceived as voice has become a complex periodic signal with the same fundamental frequency as the vocal fold source, but highly modified in its overall sound characteristics. We can hear several familiar voices all saying the same few words at the same fundamental frequency, and still be able to differentiate each voice and assign it to each familiar person. Even if we do not know the speaker, we can fairly accurately tell the approximate age and the gender of the speaker. Perhaps even more importantly, by filtering the glottal tone we can tell if the person has a cold, is upset or angery, tired, frightened, or the meaning could even be changed by the change in quality or emphasis while saying the same words. The vocal characteristics related to the individualization of each person's vocal tract will have given each voice its own unique characteristics (vocal quality) as the result of the amplification and filtering unique to each vocal tract.

The F configuration of the supraglottal vocal tract is constantly changing. What happens in any one portion of the tract influences both the total flow of air and sound wave through the total tract and the sound that eventually issues out from the mouth (or nose). By action of the pharyngeal constrictors and other supraglottal muscles, the overall dimensions of the pharynx are always changing. The membranes of the pharynx and the degree of relaxation or tautness of the pharyngeal constrictors have noticeable acoustic filtering effects. Higher frequency vocalizations seem to receive their best resonating effects under a fairly high degree of pharyngeal wall tension. Lower frequencies appear to be better amplified by a pharynx that is somewhat larger and more relaxed. This appears to be related to the short wave length of high frequency sounds and the long wave length of the low frequency components.

The oral cavity, or mouth, is as essential for resonance as the pharynx. Of all our resonators, the mouth is capable of the most variation in size and shape. It is the constant size–shape adjustment of the mouth that permits us to speak or, more accurately, allows us to be understood. Our vowels and diphthongs, for example, are originated by a laryngeal vibration, but shaped and restricted by the size and shape adjustment of the oral cavity. The mouth has fixed structures (teeth, alveolar processes, dental arch, and hard palate) and moving structures (tongue, velum, and lips). We are most concerned with the moving structures, primarily the tongue, velum, and mandible, in our study of voice resonance. It is the mouth and other supraglottal resonators that give us the perception of a regional dialect to help identify the speaker and, more importantly, that allows for the formation of distinguishable vowels.

The tongue is the most mobile articulator, and it possesses both extrinsic and intrinsic muscles to move it. Each of the extrinsic muscles can, on contraction, elevate or lower the tongue at its anterior, middle, or posterior points and extend it forward or backward. The intrinsic muscles control the shape of the tongue by narrowing, flattening, lengthening, or shortening the overall tongue body and elevating or lowering the tongue tip. The various combinations of intrinsic and extrinsic muscle contractions can produce an unlimited number of tongue positions with resulting size–shape variations of the oral cavity. In addition to the tongue movements, the lowering and closing of the mandible contributes to the formation of specific vowels. The relationships of these cavities to vowel formants have been well described in several references, such as the Peterson and Barney study (1952), and in chapters by Netsell and Daniloff (1973), and Minifie (1994).

The structural adequacy and normal functioning of the velum are also important for the development of normal voice resonance. The elevation and tensing of the velum, as well as some pharyngeal wall movement, are vital for achieving velopharyngeal closure. A lack of adequate palatal movement, despite adequacy of velar length, can cause serious problems of excessive nasality. Although the velum probably serves as a sounding-board structure in resonance, it plays an obviously important role in separating the oral cavity from the nasal cavity. The movement and positioning of the velum changes the size and shape of three important resonating cavities: the pharynx, the oral cavity, and the nasal cavity. Therefore, any alteration of the velum (such as a soft-palate cleft or velar weakness) may have a profound influence on resonance. Velar movement is only one component contributing to velopharyngeal closure (Zwitman, Gyepes, and Ward, 1976). Closure patterns that separate the oral and nasal cavities from one another may include velar action coupled by posterior pharyngeal wall movement, or velar action with active lateral and posterior pharyngeal wall movement. Watterson and McFarlane (1990) describe five classes of velopharyngeal closure and their various effect on speech and voice. Regardless of the type of closure pattern (velar–posterior–lateral pharyngeal wall), the site of closure is generally in the Passavant's area (designated as M in Figure 2.21). More will be said of nasal resonance and treatment of hyper-nasality and hyponasality in Chapter 7.

The fundamental frequency that comes from the vocal folds is modified throughout the vocal tract. Movements and constrictions within the tract contribute to the overall amplifying or filtering or modification of the voice signal produced by the vibrating vocal folds. Faulty use of the structures of the vocal tract often leads to disorders in vocal quality and resonance.

Summary

This chapter reviewed the respiratory, phonatory, and resonance aspects of voice and also discussed the five aspects of voice, loudness, hygiene, pleasantness, flexibility, and representation. We found that the outgoing airstream is the primary driving force of voice. The efficient user of voice develops good expiratory control. The value and magnitude of respiratory volumes were discussed. A description of the physiology of phonation reviewed the structures and mechanisms of normal phonation, including frequency, intensity, and quality shaping mechanisms. Supraglottal structures and functions specific to quality and resonance were also reviewed. The entire vocal tract contributes to the amplification and filtering of the fundamental frequency into the final unique voice of any speaker. The understanding of these processes provides the underpinning for effective voice therapy for patients with a variety of dysphonias.

3   Voice Disorders

Voice is the sound produced by the vibrating vocal folds. This sound is shaped by the vocal tract into a unique acoustic form that allows the listener to recognize the speaker. Voice disorders result from faulty structure or function somewhere in the vocal tract, in the processes of respiration, phonation, or resonance. When one or more aspects of voice such as loudness, pitch, quality, or resonance are outside of the normal range for the age, gender, or geographic background of the speaker, we say a voice disorder exists. In Chapter 2 we discussed five aspects of voice that characterize or identify normal voice: Loudness, Hygiene, Pleasantness, Flexibility, and Speaker Representation. When any one or more of these aspects is outside the normal range, the voice is disordered. For example, if the voice is too loud or too soft or is produced with trauma to the mechanism, sounds strange, is unpleasant, is unable to express emotion or meaning by pitch variations, or leads the listener to misjudge our age or gender, we are said to have a voice defect. Long ago Van Riper said that speech is defective if it interferes with communication, draws undue attention to itself or causes the speaker to be somehow maladjusted. The same may be said for voice.

When the voice changes in any negative way, it is said to be disordered or dysphonic. Such changes have many different common names: hoarseness, harshness, huskiness, stridency, thinness, to name only a few. Unfortunately, there is little common agreement about what these terms mean among different listeners. In this text, we use a more generic term, dysphonia, which means any alteration in normal phonation. The lack of a common vocabulary for the various parameters of voice production and voice pathology is perhaps related to the number of different kinds of specialists who are concerned with voice, the laryngologist, the singing teacher, the speech–voice scientist, the speech–voice pathologist, and the voice-and-diction teacher. The laryngologist is primarily interested in identifying the etiological and pathological aspects for purposes of treatment; the singing teacher uses imagery in an attempt to get the desired acoustical effect from the voice student; the speech–voice scientist has the laboratory interest of the physiologist or physicist; the speech–voice pathologist often attempts to use the knowledge and vocabulary of all three of these disciplines to bring about voice improvement through treatment of the voice; and the voice-and-diction teacher assesses the dynamics of voice production and uses whatever is necessary to "get" the best voice. It is no wonder that interdisciplinary communication among voice specialists breaks down, considering the number of individuals involved.

Tolerance by the public or an indifference to voice problems makes the early identification of voice pathologies difficult. Hoarseness that persists longer than several days is often identified by the laryngologist as a possible symptom of serious laryngeal disease, and it may be. Hoarseness is certainly the acoustic correlate of improper vocal fold functioning, with or without true laryngeal disease. The distinction between organic disease of the larynx and functional misuse has been a prominent dichotomy in the consideration of phonatory disorders. It is important for the laryngologists, in their need to rule out or identify true organic disease, to view the laryngeal mechanism by laryngoscopy in order to make a judgment about organic-structural or neurological involvement. In the absence of observable structural deviation or neurological involvement, the laryngologist generally describes the voice disorder as functional. It has become important for the speech–voice pathologist to view the larynx as part of the voice evaluation and in designing the voice therapy (McFarlane and Lavorato, 1984; McFarlane, Watterson, and Brophy, 1990; Watterson and McFarlane, 1991). Indeed, the joint action of the AAO (American Academy of Otolaryngology) and ASHA (American Speech and Hearing Association) has resulted in a statement that affirms the practice of visualization of the larynx by both otolaryngologists and speech–language pathologists (1998). It is an important milestone for speech–language pathologists to be able to count laryngeal visualization and imaging as within their scope of practice. More will be said about the joint statement and the role and scope of the speech–language pathologist's practice of visualization of the larynx and VP mechanism in Chapters 5 and 9.

A traditional, although artificial, way of looking at voice disorders has been to divide them into two etiologic (causal) categories: functional or organic. Functional voice disorders are usually caused by faulty use of a normal vocal mechanism. Organic voice problems are related to some physical abnormality in structure at various sites of the vocal tract. A few problems with this historical manner of classification will be discussed prior to presenting our organizational system in this chapter.

Functional versus Organic Dilemma

The terms *functional* and *organic* may be too broad to account for and describe the etiological factors in a group of voice disorders, or even in a single voice disorder. Functional aphonia, for example, may be a wholly functional voice problem. The patient may exhibit normal breath flow and an adequately open pharynx and oral cavity for normal resonance, but totally lack voice. When functionally aphonic patients attempt to use voice, they may whisper through very incompletely approximated vocal folds or make a very weak shrill, high-pitched breathy whistle of a voice. The result is basically a form or variation of a whisper. As a result, some have called functional aphonia *whisper aphonia*. This voice disorder may indeed be referred to as a functional voice disorder and can be fit into a functional category quite well.

On the other hand, a patient can also functionally misuse the vocal tract (such as by inadequate breath support or excessively hard glottal attack or by closing down the supraglottal mechanisms), which, in time, may lead to organic changes of structure, such as bilateral vocal nodules or contact ulcers. Such nodules might well have been caused by excessive vocal abuse and misuse and thus be seen as having a functional etiology. Once the nodules develop, however, they contribute to the poor voice, characterized by low pitch, excessive breathiness, and severe hoarseness. This may be a functional disorder in terms of etiology but now the faulty functional behavior is also complicated by the presence of organic tissue change. The presence of organic tissue (the nodules) may now be more responsible for the resultant voice that we hear than the functional etiological component.

Many structural organic alterations of the larynx (such as cancer, granuloma, or web) can have profound effects on the larynx and the vocal folds in particular, which can result in serious alterations of voice. It is no doubt that these are examples of organic voice disorders, although we have seen some patients who have these organic disorders and yet produce only mild voice disorders. Importantly, we have been able to use clinical stimulation, even in the presence of organic tissue change, to get the patient to produce normal sounding voice. The function of the larynx was altered by clinical stimulation to such a degree as to override the organic nature of the voice disorder. The point is that function and structure overlap and interact. Organic and functional do not always separate into two neat categories.

A normal voice requires relatively normal usage of respiratory, phonatory, and resonance mechanisms. Conversely, poor use of these mechanisms can produce faulty voice. Some poor voices result from faulty respiratory timing and control; for example, the patient may "run out of air" in the middle of a verbal passage. Instead of renewing the breath with some kind of catch-up inspiration, the patient continues to attempt to vocalize. The resulting insufficient airflow, low lung volume, and inadequate subglottal air pressure can be heard in the dysphonic voice toward the end of the utterance. The excess effort required at these low lung volumes and low air pressure levels result in the poor voice quality noted at the end of a very long phrase. This manner of phonation can be habituated in a type of hyperfunctional voice disorder. Similarly, changes in the mass, size, and tension of the vocal folds can result in changes of frequency, also characterized by fluctuations in voice pitch.

As described in Chapter 2, normal phonation requires that, in addition to proper mass–size adjustments, the two vocal folds approximate one another optimally along nearly their entire length (from the anterior commissure up to, and including, the vocal process). An exception can be observed in cases of posterior glottal chink and, as noted in Chapter 2, where an incomplete glottal closure of about 3 mm may be closed enough to produce vocal fold vibration. The easy imitation of several different voices by some actors suggests that individuals are able to vary the strength of fold approximation and other vocal adjustments. Consistent with this observation is the further one that most functionally caused dysphonias are related directly to under- or overadduction of the vocal folds and to alterations in airflow. In underadduction, the folds are too lax in their approximation, resulting in a breathy type of phonation. Sometimes, after prolonged hyperfunctional use of the voice, the folds will show an open chink posteriorly; actually, this posterior chink is the incomplete adduction of the vocal processes. Overadduction of the folds results in the tight valving of the glottal mechanism, so much so that the individual may be unable to phonate for speech.

Often, conditions that increase the mass–size of the vocal folds—that is, cord thickening, nodules, or polyps—will, by their size, and the irregular shape of the vocal fold edge, make the optimum adduction of the vocal folds impossible. Glottal growths, such as nodules (McFarlane and Watterson, 1990) and polyps, interfere with the approximating edges of the vocal folds, and they often produce open chinks between the approximating folds on each side of the growth. Any structural interference between the approximating edges of the vocal folds usually results in some degree of dysphonia and air wastage. However, some patients may actually attempt to cope with this air wastage by overadducting the folds and producing too little airflow. This gives rise to a strained, tight, squeezed-off voice rather than a breathy voice quality.

Neurological Factors

Spastic dysphonia (adductor type) is a severe overadduction problem likely due to neurological causes that are not completely understood at this time. While the etiological factor or factors are not well understood at present, there is considerable agreement among voice specialists about the sounds and vocal qualities that are a part of the diagnosis of this disorder (Watterson, Gibbons, and McFarlane, 1998). The voice sounds strained, like the kind of phonation we hear from someone attempting to talk while lifting a heavy object; the valving action of the larynx (fixed, tight adduction) overrules the individual's desire to phonate, and phonation becomes nearly impossible.

A person with another type of neurological dysphonia such as unilateral vocal fold paralysis has a completely different sounding voice. This voice disorder usually demonstrates excessive airflow rate, low loudness, short phonation time, and often hoarseness (McFarlane, Watterson, Lewis, and Boone, 1998). On the basis of the neurological etiology alone, the voice quality of unilateral vocal fold paralysis should sound like the exact opposite of adductor spasmodic dysphonia. This is not always the case and many patients present with voices that are a combination of the results of neurological etiologic factors and functional factors. These patients often compensate for inadequate glottal closure produced by the vocal fold paralysis and produce excessive false fold activity (squeezing of the pharynx), and may even produce diplophonia. These are functional components that may overlay a neurological voice disorder. This involvement of functional components can be seen in organic (tissue change) voice disorders, as mentioned earlier, and can just as well be present in neurological voice disorders.

On nasoendoscopy (McFarlane, Watterson, and Brophy, 1990), we often observe resonance being altered by surprisingly large movements of supraglottal structures (false folds, aryepiglottic folds, pharyngeal walls, tongue). For example, the tight voice of spastic dysphonia is not only produced by tight sphincteric closure of the vocal folds, but by pronounced supraglottal shutoff or valving as well. By watching the movements of the oro- and hypopharynx during nasoendoscopy (McFarlane and Lavorato, 1984; Pershall and Boone, 1986), we have come to appreciate the dynamic role that these structures have in both vocal quality and resonance. Supraglottal structures play an important role in the production of both normal and abnormal voice.

For these reasons and more we have elected to revise our classification system in this edition of the text. In this chapter we will consider a three-way classification of voice disorders: functional, neurological, and organic. We will also look at the various sites of the vocal tract to see how they may be contributing to the various voice disorders.

Table 3.1 lists voice disorders in three columns, some primarily the result of misuse of vocal mechanisms, some due to neurological etiology, and some the direct result of organic changes and disease of the vocal mechanism. The left column lists voice disorders whose etiology appears to be primarily functional; the names of many of these functional voice disorders describe, in effect, the vocal changes they cause. The center column lists neurological voice disorders, and the right column lists organic conditions of the vocal tract that may contribute to various vocal pathologies. The organic disorders are more often labeled by etiology or the tissue change they may cause than by the acoustic alterations they may produce. One could make a case for including a fourth column for "psychogenic" disorders but we have resisted this and will instead comment on the possible psychogenic aspects of individual disorders as they are discussed in this and other chapters. One quick example would be functional aphonia, which could be considered as a conversion aphonia (psychogenic) or it could be considered as functional with some psychological aspects.

Voice Disorders Related to Faulty Usage: Functional Etiology

In this section, we consider the voice problems listed in the left-hand column of Table 3.1. These voice disorders result from using a normal vocal mechanism in a faulty manner. For reader convenience, we consider separately each of these functional voice disorders, including their possible etiology and management, in the order in which they appear in Table 3.1.

TABLE 3.1 Etiology of Disorders

Functional	Neurological	Organic
Falsetto	Paradoxical movement	Sulcus vocalis
Functional aphonia	Essential tremor	Contact ulcer
Functional dysphonia	Spastic dysphonia	Cancer
Muscle tension	Vocal fold paralysis	Leukoplakia
Fold thickening	Dysarthria: ALS, MG,	Endocrine change
Diplophonia	MS, MD, PD	Hypothyroidism
Reinke's edema		Granuloma
Polyp		Hemangioma
Nodules		Hyperkeratosis
Traumatic laryngitis		Infectious laryngitis
Ventricular dysphonia		Laryngectomy
Phonation breaks		Papilloma
Pitch breaks		Pubertal changes
		Webbing

Falsetto

Other names for falsetto are puberphonia, mutational falsetto, and incomplete mutation of voice (discussed later in this chapter). The sound of falsetto is high-pitched and is also breathy in quality. There are frequent downward pitch breaks in the person using falsetto voice. The too-high pitch is produced as discussed in Chapter 2 with only the anterior portions of the vocal folds vibrating and the posterior part of the folds open or gapped. The folds approximate with thin vocal lips and do not completely touch in the midline. The result vocally is a voice that is too high for the speaker and draws attention to itself. The voice pitch and quality are inappropriate except in some singing roles. The perception is of a small, young, immature speaker. Males with falsetto voice are often mistaken for females on the phone or in situations where the listener is unable to see the speaker. They are frequently referred to as "madam" by the caller on the other end of the telephone. Falsetto is the upper end of the normal range and represents the highest register of voice. It is a voice disorder when used as the major mode of vibration or voice by either male or female adults. Use of this voice projects a female quality for male speakers and a juvenile or immature impression when used by female speakers. However, the social penalty for this type of voice is greater for the male speaker. Falsetto is nearly always due to functional causes and is generally very responsive to treatment by voice therapy. An ENT (ear, nose, and throat) examination is always in order to rule out the unlikely possibility of an endocrine or structural etiology. We have very rarely felt the need to refer these patients for counseling or psychotherapy. McFarlane (1988) reports an exception of a patient who was undergoing psychotherapy simultaneously with voice therapy whose response to voice therapy was less successful. We have never had a patient relapse into a falsetto voice after completion of voice therapy. Case (1996) notes that this is a disorder that is "easily corrected" and in which he has also not experienced "relapse."

Therapy for falsetto voice takes the general approach of lowering the pitch and improving the vocal quality. This is accomplished by digital pressure to produce a lower pitch, using "glottal fry to a tone," and extending the cough or throat clearing, which are almost always at a dramatically lower or more appropriate, pitch level. Other techniques that are helpful are inhalation phonation and masking. Aronson (1990) advocates massage of the larynx and manual lowering of the high tense laryngeal position during falsetto production. These techniques are discussed in the chapter on voice therapy facilitation techniques (Chapter 6).

Track
6 & 13

Functional Aphonia

The unique aspect of this disorder is that patients with functional aphonia speak with a whisper. In order to rule out some form of organic laryngeal involvement, such as vocal fold paralysis, these patients must be examined by either indirect laryngoscopy or videoendoscopy of the larynx (McFarlane, 1990). When functional aphonic patients are requested to say "ah," their vocal folds simply are not set adequately in vibration.

Functional aphonia has no organic cause. In fact, it is frequently described as a hysterical or conversion symptom, according to Aronson, Peterson, and Litin

(1966), who found these two terms used by various laryngologists for twenty functional dysphonic and aphonic patients they had observed. Although functional aphonia may well be a form of conversion hysteria, Brodnitz (1971, p. 65) recommends that we avoid using the term in the "presence of the patient because of the social stigma attached to it." Usually patients have had several temporary losses of voice before the disorder becomes permanent. In our experience, they may also have had a recent bout of the flu or an upper respiratory infection (URI) prior to onset of functional aphonia. Temporarily aphonic patients may derive some reinforcing gains from their loss of voice, such as not having to give speeches or not being able to preside over meetings. Aphonia may even become permanent after moments of acute stress by maintaining itself for various reasons. Aronson, Peterson, and Litin (1961) report that in ten out of twenty-seven patients they studied, the onset of functional dysphonia or aphonia was associated with an event of acute stress; in thirteen of the twenty-seven patients it was associated with stress over a longer period of time. The onset of functional aphonia is sometimes related to the patient's having experienced some laryngeal pathology or other disease. For example, Boone (1966b) described the physical origin of functional aphonia in two patients, one who became aphonic after a meningitis attack, and the other after a laryngeal operation, when she could not end the voice rest imposed on her by the laryngologist. Both of these aphonic patients were highly responsive to voice therapy. We once successfully treated a patient who developed functional aphonia suddenly during his testimony as a witness in a courtroom trial.

A more unusual case history involved a female Navy member who could not or would not return to voice use during and after a dozen voice therapy sessions with three skilled voice clinicians. She continued to whisper in all situations at work on the U.S. Navy base, at home, and with her husband, her baby, her sister, and her parents. She whispered under conditions of auditory masking and following counseling. Coughing and throat-clearing produced voice, but she would not extend these. Even when gargling, she produced whisper rather than voice while bubbling the water. Even though she was under considerable stress, she refused psychological counseling referrals. After one year and one month, she returned to voice therapy but did not produce voice after twelve sessions. Four months after termination of the second course of voice therapy, she resumed voice use. There appeared to be some **secondary gain,** in the form of attention, for the functional aphonia. Attention was largely negative in tone but was nonetheless better to her than being ignored. Again, this case is the exception rather than the rule in that she was not responsive to voice therapy rather quickly.

Track 6

Patients with functional aphonia communicate well by gesture and whisper or by a high-pitched, shrill-sounding weak voice. Typical aphonic patients whisper with clarity and sharpness. Aphonic patients rarely avoid communication situations; conversely, they communicate effectively by using facial expressions, hands, and highly intelligible whispered speech. What they lack in communication is voice. Embarrassed and frustrated by lack of voice, aphonic patients generally self-refer to a physician or speech–language pathologist. Despite Greene's (1980) warning that many patients with functional aphonia may require psychological counseling, most aphonic patients, in our experience, completely recover their normal voice, with voice therapy alone (usually in the first session of therapy). Aphonic patients as a group, in fact, have an excellent prognosis. It is almost as if, for whatever reason, the patient has lost the "set" for phonation. The voice clinician's task is to help the patient "find" his or her voice primarily by helping the patient use vegetative phonations, such as coughing or inhalation phonation or sometimes using masking noise (Chapter 6). The patient then extends the vegetative phonation into the production of a vowel, into nonsense syllables, next into single words, then phrases, and so on. Aronson (1990) suggests digital manipulation of the larynx of these patients.

By using behavioral modification approaches, such as those suggested by Eysenck (1961), Sloane and MacAulay (1968), and Wolpe (1987), we have had excellent success in directly working on voice. Typical aphonic patients experience restoration of normal voice in the first, or, at least, in very few voice therapy sessions (McFarlane & Lavorato, 1984). Wilson (1987) described the "sudden and complete recovery" of several teenage girls who responded well to symptomatic voice therapy. Suggested methods of symptomatic voice therapy for functional aphonia will be presented in Chapter 6.

Functional Dysphonia

Some of the most disturbed voices we hear may have no organic or physical cause. Patients may approximate the vocal folds in a lax manner, producing breathiness, or in a tight manner, producing symptoms of harshness or tightness. In addition, patients may close off their voice by bringing the ventricular folds together or by pursing off the larynx by firm, sphinctericlike closure of the aryepiglottic folds. Voice problems that do not result from an organic pathology may be called **functional dysphonia,** a term that conveys very little to the voice clinician other than the important implication that there is no structural pathology present. In fact, the common usage of the term *functional dysphonia* is confined to those dysphonias in which the problem persists independent of any kind of pathology observed on laryngoscopy. After a history of continuing dysphonia, the typical patient is finally examined by laryngoscopy and found not to have any neurological or additive lesion, such as nodules, papilloma, or granuloma (or whatever). In many cases of functional dysphonia, we can hardly visualize the vocal folds by nasoendoscopy because they are often covered by an almost complete supraglottal shutoff (ventricular and aryepiglottic fold adduction). Sometimes this supraglottal shutoff is due to the severe retraction of the tongue. The resultant voice is like that of a muted horn. Functional dysphonia appears to be the product of both laryngeal and supralaryngeal shutdown. In addition, patients complain of many vague disorders—throat "fullness," pain in the laryngeal area or chest, dryness of mouth while talking, neck tightness, and so on—that are usually related to vocal fatigue. The voice frequently just gives out.

Track 9

A functionally caused dysphonia does not necessarily sound different from one that is organically caused. Some of the hoarsest voices are produced by people whose larynges demonstrate no pathology whatsoever. On the other hand, serious organic problems, such as beginning cancer, may produce no alteration of the voice. Anyone with persistent dysphonia (longer than ten days) in the absence of a throat infection or cold (URI) ought to undergo a laryngeal examination to determine the possible cause of the problem and to rule out serious laryngeal disease. While developing critical listening skills is important for the voice clinician, because the same voice sound can be produced by several different laryngeal adjustments or conditions, it is essential that the larynx be visually inspected by a competent ENT physician (otolaryngologist). We suggest that the speech–voice pathologist also visualize the larynx as part of the voice evaluation (ASHA, 1992; McFarlane, 1990; Watterson, 1991). In 1997 the ASHA and the AAO (American Academy of Otolaryngology) produced a joint statement, which asserts that visualization and observation of the larynx is the province of both the otolaryngologist and the speech–language pathologist. The practice of laryngeal visualization is within the scope of practice for both professions although the purpose of the visualization is different for each. The purpose for the laryngologist is for diagnosis of laryngeal disease, while the voice diagnosis and study of faulty voice production is the purpose of visualization for the speech–language pathologist.

Aronson (1990) objects to the term *functional dysphonia* on several grounds, because he thinks that such problems are generally psychogenic in nature:

> A psychogenic voice disorder is broadly synonymous with a functional one but has the advantage of stating positively, based on an exploration of its causes, that the voice disorder is a manifestation of one or more types of psychologic disequilibrium—such as anxiety, depression, conversion reaction, or personality disorder—which interferes with normal volitional control over phonation (p. 131).

As discussed in Chapter 1, we believe that most functional voice problems may be successfully treated symptomatically, by working on dimensions of voice directly to improve the sounds of the voice. In most cases, however, clinicians should offer patients much psychological support in an attempt to minimize their anxieties and concern and should *search*, with the patients, for the best voices they can produce.

The first dimension of voice to be evaluated and worked on if necessary is fundamental frequency. If a patient has no organic problem contributing to dysphonia but has a faulty pitch, the clinician should use various facilitating approaches (see Chapter 6) to develop an appropriate pitch. The vocal intensity of the voice is also measured; if the patient has a loudness problem, direct attempts to change the volume can be initiated. For the occasional patient whose voice loudness is directly related to shyness and insecurity, working on respiratory support and loudness per se may be combined with attempting to improve self-concept and interpersonal relationships as well. The majority of voice patients with vocal intensity problems, however, are quite responsive to symptomatic voice therapy designed to increase their voice loudness. Clinicians help these patients change their pitch and loudness and evaluate how the patients view the changes. The clinicians should observe how the patients respond to direct modification of pitch and loudness. For patients who resist such direct approaches, counseling or concurrent psychotherapy might be appropriate. We have rarely found that professional psychological counseling with the psychologist or psychiatrist is necessary because the vast majority of these patients' voice disorders yield to a symptomatic voice therapy approach. McFarlane and Lavorato (1983) discussed the successful treatment of cases that had a history of failure in previous voice therapy. These resistant cases were successfully treated by a systematic use of symptomatic voice therapy.

Quality of voice is often the primary problem in functional dysphonia. The vocal folds may approximate one another in a faulty manner and produce alterations in quality; words such as *hoarse, harsh, strident,* and *breathy* are applied to these voice quality dimensions of functional dysphonia. Harshness is often the product of overapproximation (excessive medial compression) of the folds when they come sharply together, producing what is also perceived as hard glottal attack. Sometimes harshness is accompanied by inappropriately high levels of loudness, too-high pitch, possible tongue retraction, and contraction of the pharyngeal constrictors. Harshness often indicates a voice that requires a lot of effort and force to produce. The harsh voice is not an **efficient voice.** The opposite problem may be breathiness, produced by folds that may approximate too loosely. Laxity of approximation generally produces an excessive escape of air, perceived as breathiness. Sometimes, as Brodnitz (1971) suggested, the breathy, tired voice appears only after prolonged hyperfunctional voice use. It may emerge late in the day, after a patient has done a lot of phonating, particularly if such phonation has required a good deal of effort and force and the environment is stressful or presents a high level of background noise.

Functional dysphonia often becomes "the" voice of the person:—the way that person talks. For such people, voice therapy should not be initiated until they are made aware of their ability to change and elect to change their voice. For patients who are motivated to change the quality of their voice, and who are accurately diagnosed as having functional dysphonia, voice therapy is remarkably successful.

Track
3 & 9

Muscle Tension Dysphonia

In a type of functional dysphonia called muscle tension dysphonia (MTD) the voice is adversely effected by excessive muscle tension. Koufman and Blalock (1991) describe a classification of muscle tension dysphonia based on 123 patients with tension–fatigue syndromes of the larynx. They describe three subtypes: the partial closure of ventricular folds from side to side, as discussed in the section on ventricular dysphonia. In another form the vocal folds are shortened by the drawing together of the anterior commissure and the arytenoids to make a short anterior–posterior dimension. In a third form they describe a sphincterlike closure of the supraglottal area. This may also be accompanied by a posterior tongue carriage or by the contraction of the pharyngeal constrictor muscles. The tongue base and the epiglottis may be retropositioned in the laryngopharynx. The oropharynx and laryngopharynx may constrict, much as in a swallow. These three forms of hyperfunctional dysphonia, called *muscle tension dysphonia,* are responsive to voice therapy using such techniques as yawn sign, tongue protrusion/i/, aspirate phonation onset, inhalation phonation, and glottal fry as discussed in Chapter 6. Roy, Ford, and Bless (1996) discuss using a manual **palpation** technique to determine the extent of laryngeal elevation, assess focal tenderness, assess the effect on voice of downward pressure on the larynx, and assess the effect of circumlaryngeal massage on the voice.

Track 7

Diplophonia

The term *diplophonia* means **"double voice."** A diplophonic voice is produced with two distinct voice sources, each voicing simultaneously with the other. Occasionally, someone may produce a double voice with one vocal fold in a different mass–size–tension mode than the other fold;—that is, one fold vibrates at a different speed than the other one. For example, a woman with a large unilateral vocal polyp was observed who spoke with a diplophonic voice. Her normal vocal fold vibrated at its normal frequency, while the involved fold (much enlarged with a broad-based polyp) vibrated more slowly and produced the second voice and, thus, the diplophonic voice was a combination of both vibrational patterns. Other possible causes of diplophonia that have been reported are laryngeal web, vocal cord paralysis, ventricular fold vibration simultaneous with true fold vibration, and aryepiglottic vibration added to normal fold vibration and also strictly functional maladjustments of the folds. It is possible to produce diplophonia with normal vocal structures. In other words, one can imitate diplophonia. Theoretically, any bodies (folds or structures) that can approximate in the vocal tract, through which outgoing airflow can pass, have the potential for producing a sound (or voice) when set into vibration.

The treatment of diplophonia is aimed at eliminating the source of the second voice. Sometimes, surgical removal of a unilateral mass or elimination of a laryngeal web will result in a single voice. We have also seen the surgical reduction of a hypertrophied false vocal fold eliminate diplophonia. More often, diplophonia is corrected by voice therapy (which we discuss in Chapters 6 and 7). This is accomplished by reducing the hyperfunction or laryngeal tension that is producing the second sound source. Videoendoscopy is helpful in identifying the source of the undesired vibration and guiding voice therapy in reestablishment of a normal voice production.

Track 7

Thickening (Vocal Fold)

Various inflammatory conditions of the larynx, such as infectious and traumatic laryngitis, may produce irritation and swelling (edema) of the vocal folds. Another form of enlargement along the glottal margin of the vocal folds is known as *vocal fold thickening.* Whereas vocal nodules and polyps are more focal lesions (occupying less space) on the vocal folds, thickening is a broader-based lesion that often covers the anterior two thirds of the glottal margin (the vibrating portion of the vocal folds) or the membrane covering the muscular portion of the vocal fold. There are basically two types of thickening. One represents early tissue reaction (swelling) to vocal fold trauma, often a precursor to vocal nodules or polyps; the second is the result of prolonged (chronic) irritation that often results in extensive polypoid degeneration and more advanced changes of the vocal fold tissue. Another form of chronic vocal fold thickening is called Reinke's Edema. Let us consider each of these thickening changes separately.

Typically, vocal fold thickening results from continuous vocal abuse. Continuous use of loud voice, screaming and yelling, in time may result in some tissue changes along the glottal margin. We have only to observe vocal fold vibration on videoendoscopy and stroboscopy to appreciate the vigorous adduction of the folds and participation of supraglottal structures (ventricular and aryepiglottic folds) that accompany coughing, yelling, or screaming at higher pitches. As a volunteer subject with videoendoscopy, one of the authors witnessed bilateral tissue changes on the glottal margin (beginning of redness) of his own folds after only

five minutes of continuous staccato yelling of the word *peach*. Such yelling is a
benign vocal experience compared to the continuous screaming of some young
children at play or the performance of some rock singers. The cause of early vocal
fold thickening thus seems to be the same as the cause of vocal nodules, primarily
vocal abuse and misuse. However, other reported causes of thickening and vocal
nodules have been summarized by Andrews (1986):

1. Constitutional tendency
2. Chronic upper respiratory problems
3. Psychological living environment—for example, size of family
4. Physical living environment—for example, air pollution
5. Personality and adjustment
6. Endocrine imbalance, especially thyroid
7. Vocal abuse, sudden straining of the voice; continuous use of abusive practices
8. Vocal misuse: incorrect pitch and loudness (p. 107)

To this list we add another:

9. Post surgical thickening of the vocal folds

Certain children and adults are very sensitive to vocally irritating events. For
example, some people can use their vocal folds excessively and never develop any
tissue changes that result in vocal symptoms. Others, with the slightest allergy,
cold, or vocal abuse–misuse, develop aversive glottal margin problems. The emotional and physical environment undoubtedly negatively affects many people. In
the case of children or adults with vocal fold thickening, such environmental
influences cannot be allowed to continue without some attempt at modification.
This makes it absolutely essential to take a careful case history, which will be
developed further in Chapter 5. The overwhelming cause of vocal fold thickening,
however, is vocal abuse and misuse. Until such vocal excesses are identified and
reduced in frequency (they can rarely be totally eliminated), vocal thickening,
nodules, and polyps cannot be successfully treated. In other words, vocal abuse
must be identified and reduced, modified, or eliminated.

Vocal fold thickening can usually be reduced by a voice therapy program
that promotes easy and proper use of the vocal mechanisms (vocal reeducation),
with heavy emphasis on curbing vocal abuse–misuse. This example of a six-year-
old with vocal fold thickening is, unfortunately, typical:

Edith was referred for a voice evaluation because of chronic hoarseness. Indirect
laryngoscopy found that she had bilateral cord thickening with no demonstrable
history of allergy or infections. Her parents were counseled to do what they could to
help Edith eliminate unnecessary crying and yelling, and Edith was sent home. On
a subsequent visit to the laryngologist, no change in cords was observed by laryngoscopy. It was thus decided to "strip" the thickenings surgically. (We must note
here that we never suggest vocal fold stripping except for treatment of malignant
tissue that must be removed, and never in children.) This was done with excellent
results. Three weeks after surgery the child demonstrated clear cords bilaterally,
free of thickening. After a postoperative period of approximately three months, the
family returned to the laryngologist, complaining of the child's recurring hoarse-

ness. Laryngoscopy found that Edith once again had bilateral cord thickening, with the early formation of a vocal nodule on one fold. It was then decided to begin voice therapy. Special efforts were made to identify particular vocal abuses by the child, and a school playground situation was isolated as the cause of continuous vocal strain. Eliminating this and other adverse vocal behavior gradually eliminated the vocal nodule and nearly eliminated the bilateral thickening as well.

The preceding case illustrates that surgical treatment of cord thickening or nodules, without removing the abusive cause of the problem, will not usually be a permanent solution to the vocal problem. Reducing the source of the irritation (such as eliminating an allergy, reducing smoking, or curbing vocal abuse) is probably the best management of the problem. Our strong preference is to have a serious course of voice therapy first. This will generally obviate the need for surgery for this problem and for nodules. Voice therapy likely would have made the surgery in this case unnecessary.

A second form of vocal fold thickening is often more diffuse, because it frequently indicates a more advanced tissue reaction to prolonged laryngeal abuse and misuse. The vocal fold swelling is broader than the anterior–middle third site that is the typical location of nodules or polyps. Rather, the swelling may extend along the glottis from the anterior commissure to the beginning of the vocal process of the arytenoid cartilages. Such swelling, known as *polypoid degeneration,* is characteristic. If, in addition to vocal abuse–misuse, the patient is a heavy smoker or alcohol consumer, the increased mass of the folds can seriously compromise all attempts at vocalization. The primary treatment of extensive polypoid degeneration may be medical–surgical, supplemented by voice therapy. However, trial voice therapy at first is warranted. The primary thrust of voice therapy is to identify possible laryngeal abuses (such as throat-clearing) and voice abuses (such as speaking with excessive glottal attack), to eliminate abuse such as smoking, and then to provide the patient with methods for reducing these aversive behaviors. Many of the voice therapy facilitating approaches presented in Chapter 6 have been effective in reducing overall vocal fold thickening.

Reinke's Edema

Another form of vocal fold thickening with chronic abuse is Reinke's Edema. While some authorities consider polypoid cord degeneration the same as Reinke's Edema, we see the two conditions on a continuum, with polypoid degeneration more severe. In Reinke's Edema the fluid is still watery, while in polypoid cord degeneration the fluid under the vocal fold cover is more jellylike and thicker. This tissue change, Reinke's Edema, gets it name from the accumulation of fluid (edema) under the vocal fold cover in the Reinke's Space. In Chapter 2 we introduced Table 2.1, which showed the functional structure of the vocal folds. The cover is composed of epithelium and the superficial lamina propria and **Reinke's Space.** This space is a potential space and may become filled with fluid in response to repeated vocal trauma. In the case of Reinke's Edema, when vocal folds are examined with stroboscopy, the two vocal folds begin to abduct and the covers of each fold stick together and appear to be pulled slightly away from the body of the folds as the body moves from the midline during abduction. An example of Reinke's Edema is shown in Figure 3.1.

We find that both conditions, Reinke's Edema and polypoid cord degeneration, are often responsive to voice therapy, but the result may not be a normal voice but an improved voice. The voice result is more desirable than the "dry, strained hoarseness" so often seen following vocal fold stripping for these conditions. The scarring following vocal fold stripping is to be avoided at all costs if voice therapy has any chance at all of producing a better and more serviceable voice.

Track 2

Vocal Polyps

Vocal polyps, more often unilateral than bilateral, usually occur at the same anterior–middle third site on the vocal fold(s) as nodules. Polyps and nodules are both related to vocal hyperfunction, and both have some physical similarities. With a polyp the lesion is usually soft, often fluid-filled, and occurs in the inner margin of one vocal fold; because of its softness, it does not irritate the membranous tissue on the opposite fold (as opposed to the bilateral pathology usually observed in vocal nodules). Unlike vocal nodules, which result from continuous or chronic vocal fold irritation, polyps are often precipitated by a single vocal event. For example, a patient may have indulged in excessive vocalization, such as screaming for much of an evening, which produced some hemorrhaging on the membrane at the point of maximum glottal contact. A polyp forms out of such hemorrhagic irritation by eventually adding mass that becomes fluid filled. Once a small polyp begins, any continued vocal abuse, or misuse, will irritate the area, contributing to its continued growth. A typical polyp lies on the glottal margin, interfering with the approximation of the normal fold.

Polyps, which may be either broad-based (**sessile-type** as in Figure 3.2) or narrow-necked on a stem (pedunculated), usually occur in the larynx on the inner margin of the affected fold. An excellent description of polyps, their formation, and their treatment was developed by Kleinsasser (1979), who described the lesions as "gelatinous" and responsive to surgery. The goal of modern vocal fold surgery is to preserve as much mucosa as possible and to disrupt the glottal margin as little as possible. Thus microflap surgery designed to raise a flap of

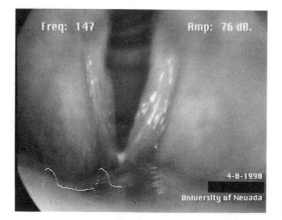

Freq: 147   Amp: 76 dB.

4-8-1998

University of Nevada

FIGURE 3.1   Reinke's Edema

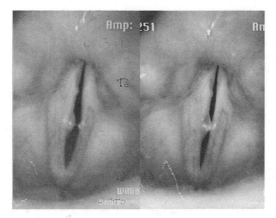

FIGURE 3.2   Sessile or broad-based polyp

mucosa, remove a cyst of gelatinous material via suction, and then lay the flap back down on the vocal fold, is now common and preferred to older stripping techniques. Laser surgery had been thought to be the surgical treatment of choice for vocal fold polyps (Yates and Dedo, 1984). However, it appears that use of the laser for such broad-based tissue lesions does too much damage to the mucosal covering on the vocal fold vibrating edge (Bouchayer and Cornut, 1988). Further, Bouchayer and Cornut (1988) state "We believe that our insistence on voice therapy for all patients with polyps explains why we have yet to see a single recurrence"(p. 462). Unless the causative behaviors are identified and prevented from further occurrence, polyps often recur after surgery. With voice therapy and attempts to use the laryngeal mechanisms more optimally, polyps can be permanently eliminated. We have seen even professional singers return to a singing career with an improved vocal hygiene and improved singing technique after surgery and voice therapy (Lavorato and McFarlane, 1983). We prefer voice therapy as the first approach to treatment of a sessile polyp and surgery followed by voice therapy when initial voice therapy fails to get the desired response.

The voices of patients with unilateral polyps are characterized by severe dysphonia. The normal vocal fold vibrates at one frequency while the additive lesion seriously dampens the vibration of the involved fold, resulting in what is perceived as hoarseness and breathiness, often requiring (or so the patient mistakenly thinks) continuous throat-clearing. Voice therapy requires identifying and reducing vocal abuse–misuse and searching with the patient for the best voice that can be produced using various voice-facilitating approaches (see Chapter 6). Voice therapy was successful in eliminating a unilateral polyp in the following case:

Jane was a 29-year-old teacher who was active in competitive sports. She admitted to doing a lot of yelling during her softball season, when she ended up with a hoarse voice that would not go away. Her teaching schedule required her to give six hours of lectures each day, supervise a study hall, and assist in girls' field hockey events. Finally, by noon each day she had no voice. Subsequent laryngoscopy found her to have a broad-based polyp (about 5 mm in width) on one fold. Voice therapy was initiated that focused on reducing loudness, developing a soft glottal attack, and opening her mouth more as she spoke. An immediate consequence of the therapy was that when she spoke easily, without effort, her voice at first sounded "more hoarse." She kidded her students and colleagues that she would sound worse in the beginning as she learned to use her voice with less effort. In about twelve weeks, the unilateral polyp completely disappeared, and Jane's voice became normal. She then made continuing efforts to avoid any kind of vocal abuse and misuse and has maintained a trouble-free larynx and normal voice.

Vocal Nodules

Track
4 & 10

Vocal nodules are the most common benign lesions of the vocal folds in both children and adults. They are caused by continuous abuse of the larynx and misuse of the voice. These causative abuses are well described by Case (1991), who places "yelling and screaming, making a hard glottal attack, singing in an abusive manner, speaking in a noisy environment, coughing, and excessive throat clearing" (pp. 98–99) at the top of the list of twenty-four vocal abuses–misuses. Nodules, as shown in Figure 3.3, are generally bilateral, whitish protuberances on the glottal margin of each vocal fold, located at the anterior–middle third junction. However, McFarlane and Watterson (1990) demonstrate in their study of 44 cases of vocal nodules that there can be considerable variation in the size, number, and location of vocal nodules in singers and nonsingers. They also demonstrate variation in the nodules of children. Of the variations that can be observed and documented in vocal nodules perhaps the most striking is that nodules can range from singular to two, three, and even four (quad nodules) in number. While these variations are interesting, two important facts remain. First, nodules are responsive to voice therapy, and second, the classic description of number and location (juncture of anterior and middle third) is generally accurate. This nodule site is the midpoint of the muscular vocal fold, involving the membrane that covers the vocal ligament and vocalis muscle inner border of the vocal fold. In the early stages of nodule development, the nodular mass is soft and pliable. With continuous abuse–misuse the lesion becomes more fibrotic and may be slightly larger or may become more focused, smaller, and harder.

The pathogenesis of nodules seems to differ from that of polyps and of cysts. In a review of several studies, McFarlane and Von Berg (1998) point out that "immunohistochemical findings support our understanding of the cause of vocal fold lesions because vocal fold nodules normally develop as a result of chronic vocal

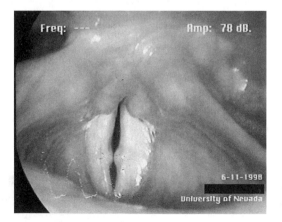

FIGURE 3.3   Bilateral vocal nodules, young adult female

abuse and therefore would present with a thickened BMZ (basement membrane zone) and diffuse healing agents throughout the superficial layer of the lamina propria, probably bilaterally. Vocal fold polyps, on the other hand, are often precipitated by a single vocal event, normally resulting in hemorrhage of the mucous membrane at the point of maximum glottal contact. From this single abusive event, we would not anticipate a thickened BMZ but would expect a fair amount of fibronectin at the point of hemorrhage. Finally, the inconsistent pattern shown by cystic lesions confirms the equally inconsistent basis of these particular lesions."

As the bilateral nodules approximate one another on phonation, there is usually an open glottal chink on each side of the nodule. This open glottal chink (produced by the nodules coming together in exact opposition to one another) results in a lack of complete vocal fold adduction. This faulty approximation leads to breathiness in the voice and air wastage. Also, the increased mass of the nodules added to the vocal folds contributes to a lower voice pitch and increased aperiodicity (usually judged as hoarseness). This leads to a breathy, flat kind of voice that often seems to lack appropriate resonance. Patients complain that they need to clear their throat continually and often that they have excessive mucus or "something" on the vocal folds. Excessive throat-clearing often becomes an identified vocal abuse, which may lead to further enlargement or further organization and consolidation of the nodules. Typical patients with vocal nodules complain that their voices seem to deteriorate with continuous voicing; they may start the day with fairly good voices that become increasingly dysphonic with continuous vocal usage. With prolonged speaking and singing, perhaps coupled with vocal abuse and misuse, phonation rapidly deteriorates.

Small nodules and recently acquired ones can be very successfully treated with voice therapy. Yamaguchi and colleagues (1986), reporting on voice therapy success with twenty adult females with vocal nodules, found that vocal nodules "either disappeared or were reduced in size" after three to four months of voice therapy in 65 percent of the cases. McFarlane and Watterson (1990) reported success in forty-four cases presenting both large and small nodules in children and adults, and in both singers and nonsingers. They also document with pictures the before and after therapy conditions of the larynx of a child and an adult singer. The nodules were completely resolved via voice therapy. Boone (1982) developed a four-point program for adults with vocal nodules that focuses on: identifying abuse/misuse; reducing the occurrence of such abuse–misuse; searching with the patient for various voice therapy facilitating approaches that seem to produce an easy, optimal vocal production; and using the facilitating approach that works best as a practice method. Although we strongly recommend voice therapy as the primary treatment for nodules, we also acknowledge that larger nodules and long-established ones may be treated by surgery, followed by a brief period of complete voice rest and then voice therapy. However, a trial period of voice therapy is an appropriate conservative course of treatment prior to surgery for nodules in nearly all cases. Because voice therapy must follow if surgery is the treatment then why not begin with a period of voice therapy? It is not unusual clinically for new nodules to reappear several weeks after surgical removal of nodules in both children and adults. Unless the underlying hyperfunctional vocal behaviors are identified and reduced, vocal nodules have a stubborn way of reappearing.

Vocal nodules in children before puberty are more common in boys, who are generally aggressive and noisy, busy controlling people with their voices. As boys get older, there is less evidence of nodules, and adolescent females show a higher prevalence of additive lesions related to vocal abuse (Toohill, 1975). The prevalence is also higher in those adult females who, according to Aronson (1990), are "talkative, socially aggressive, and tense, and have acute or chronic interpersonal problems that generate tension, anxiety, anger, or depression" (p. 125). Nodules result from vocal hyperfunction and are therefore often observed in people who in general exhibit "hyperfunctional" personalities. Green (1989) found that children with vocal nodules exhibit more aggressive behaviors than control children as measured with a fifty-item problem behavior checklist. Children with nodules demonstrated more aggressive behaviors, acting out, and disturbed peer relationships (Green, 1989). Although symptomatic voice therapy has been effective in reducing or eliminating vocal nodules, patients with vocal nodules often require strong psychological support by the voice clinician, and sometimes, in a very few patients, psychological counseling and therapy, as well.

Traumatic Laryngitis

In functional laryngitis or traumatic laryngitis, patients experience swelling of the vocal folds as a result of excessive and strained vocalization. The voice sounds hoarse, lacking in volume. Typical functional laryngitis may be heard in the voices of excited spectators after a football or basketball game. In the excitement of the game, with their own voices masked by the noise of the crowd, the fans scream at pitch levels and intensities they normally do not use. The inner glottal edges of the membrane become swollen (edematous) and thickened, an expected consequence of excessive approximation. The increased edema of the folds is accompanied by irritation and increased blood accumulation. The acute stage of functional laryngitis is at its peak during the actual yelling or traumatic vocal behavior, with the vocal folds much increased in size and mass. Brodnitz (1971) wrote that functionally irritated vocal folds appear on laryngoscopic examination to be much like the thickened, reddened folds of acute infectious laryngitis. There is an important difference in treatment, however. For functional or acute, nonspecific laryngitis, which is usually the result of continued irritation by such causes as allergy, excessive smoking and alcohol drinking, and vocal abuse, the obvious treatment is to eliminate the vocal irritant whenever possible. In the case of functional laryngitis secondary to yelling or a similar form of vocal abuse, eliminating the abuse usually permits the vocal mechanism to return to its natural state. The temporary laryngitis experienced toward the end of a basketball game is usually relieved by a return to normal vocal activity and most of the edema and irritation vanish after a good night's sleep.

Chronic laryngitis may typically produce more serious vocal problems if the speaker attempts to "speak above" the laryngitis. The temporary edema of the vocal folds alters the quality and loudness of the phonation; the speaker increases vocal efforts. This increase in effort only increases the irritation of the folds, thereby compounding the problem. Finally, if such hyperfunctional behavior continues over time, what was once a temporary edema may become a more permanent polypoid thickening, which sometimes develops into vocal polyps (more localized) or nodules. For this reason, functional laryngitis should be promptly treated by eliminating the causative abuse and, if possible, by enforcing a short period (two to three

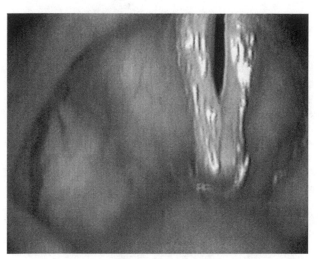

FIGURE 3.4 Ventricular Phonation *As is common in many cases of "ventricular phonation," the vibration of the true folds is dampened by the false folds riding on the true folds.*

days) of complete voice rest. Voice rest in itself is not a "cure" for most voice disorders. This is not true, however, for traumatic laryngitis. Complete or absolute voice rest, which means no phonation or whispering for several days, is usually enough for irritated vocal fold margins to lose their swelling and return to their normal shape. It is important that voice rest designed to promote healing of irritated vocal fold surfaces *not* include whispering; whispering (as most people do it) still causes too much vocal fold movement, and irritation from the rubbing together of the approximating surfaces of each fold is still possible. Studies have shown that during whisper the ventricular folds (see Figure 2.18) often may be brought into function (Pearl and McCall, 1986). The events that cause traumatic laryngitis must be identified and curbed. If such hyperfunctional vocal behavior continues over time, such changes as polypoid thickening, vocal nodules, or vocal polyps may occur.

A dramatic example of sudden (acute) traumatic laryngitis and even aphonia can be seen in the case of the singer or other professional voice user who may overdo on a given vocal activity (e.g., in a song, chairing a committee, etc.). This behavior can lead to **vocal fold hemorrhage** in such a vocal professional. This can be due in part to vocal overuse and the use of aspirin or aspirinlike products during the time of performance. We caution singers not to use such products when they are scheduled to perform. A good view of a vocal fold hemorrhage may be seen in the color plate of vocal fold pathologies at the end of this chapter.

Track 11

Ventricular Dysphonia

Ventricular dysphonia, sometimes known as *dysphonia plicae ventricularis* or false fold phonation, occurs more often than previously indicated (Boone, 1983). While ventricular dysphonia may be produced by the vibration of the approximating ventricular folds, it more often is produced by the true vocal folds vibrating in an abnormal fashion due to the false folds (ventricular folds) riding (or loading) the true folds (see Figure 3.4).

Sometimes the ventricular voice becomes the substitute voice of patients who have severe disease of the true folds (such as severe papilloma or large polyps). The ventricular voice is usually low-pitched because of the large mass of vibrating tissue of the ventricular bands (as compared to the smaller mass of vibrating tissue of the true folds) or from the combined mass of the true and false vocal folds. In addition, the voice has little pitch variability and is therefore monotonous. Finally, because the ventricular folds have difficulty in making a good, firm approximation for their entire length, the voice is usually quite hoarse and may also be breathy. This combination of low pitch, monotony, and hoarseness makes most ventricular voices sound very unpleasant. If no persistent true cord pathology continues to force patients to use their ventricular voices, this disorder usually responds well to voice therapy. Sometimes, however, hypertrophy (enlargement) of the ventricular folds is present, which makes their normal full retraction somewhat difficult. Ventricular phonation is impossible to diagnose by the sound of the voice alone. Laryngoscopic examination during phonation shows the ventricular folds coming together, covering (partially or completely) from view the true folds that lie below.

Some ventricular dysphonias display a special form of **diplophonia** (double voice), in which the true folds vibrate and also drive the ventricular folds to vibrate because the false folds are sitting on the true folds (loading the true cords with ventricular folds). In our experience, more often than not, the ventricular folds do not vibrate as a sole source of sound but load the true vocal folds. The true vocal folds are dampened by the false folds. Identification and confirmation of what vibrating structures the patient is using for phonation can best be made by frontal tomographic X-ray (coronal) of the sites of vibration. Ventricular phonation can also be diagnosed sometimes by nasoendoscopy and endoscopic stroboscopy (McFarlane, 1988; McFarlane and Lavorato, 1984; McFarlane, Watterson, and Brophy, 1990). In ventricular phonation, the true vocal folds will be slightly abducted, with the ventricular bands above in relative approximation and very possibly resting on the true vocal folds. In normal phonation, the opposite relationship between the true folds and the ventricular bands occurs; that is, the true folds are adducted and the ventricular bands are positioned laterally from the midline position. Once ventricular phonation is confirmed by laryngoscopy or X-ray, any physical problem of the true cords that might make normal phonation impossible should be eliminated. We consider both the elimination of ventricular phonation and its occasional need to be taught when we present voice therapy for special problems in Chapter 7.

In many ways ventricular phonation is a symptom of other conditions. For example when one true fold is paralyzed or is too stiff (due to postsurgical scarring) to vibrate the false fold is brought into the phonatory act. We have known ventricular phonation to become habituated after a bout of flu when the true vocal folds were too swollen to vibrate. Ventricular fold phonation in such cases is a compensation used by the patient. It is usually not the best compensation for the problem and is generally responsive to voice therapy such as inhalation phonation or pitch elevation of aspirate voice onset discussed in Chapter 6.

Track
3 & 8

Phonation Breaks (Abductor Spasms)

A phonation break is a temporary loss of voice that may occur for only part of a word, a whole word, a phrase, or a sentence. The individual is phonating with no apparent difficulty when suddenly a complete cessation of voice occurs. Such a fleeting voice loss is usually situational and it usually happens after prolonged hyperfunction. Typical patients with this problem work too hard to talk, often speaking with great effort, and suddenly experience a complete voice break. Such patients usually struggle to "find" their voice by coughing, clearing their throat, or taking a drink of water. In most cases, phonation is restored and remains adequate until the next phonation break, which may occur in only a few moments or not for days. Other than continued vocal hyperfunction, no physical condition seems to cause these phonatory interruptions. They may result from a variety of physiological sources, ranging from reduced subglottal air pressure near the end of a phrase to the "loading" of the true vocal fold by the ventricular fold or mucus on the true fold. Many times these breaks result from excessive laryngeal muscle tension and inappropriate adjustments of the otherwise normal mechanism.

Voice patients who experience phonation breaks or abductor spasms rarely show them during voice evaluation sessions. In their histories, however, such patients report the occurrence of phonation breaks, often with much embarrassment when they occur. Occasionally patients have been told by their employers that they must learn to use their voices correctly (without voice breaks) or they would lose their jobs. Fortunately, the treatment of phonation breaks is relatively simple: taking the "work" out of phonation and elimination of inappropriate vocal behaviors such as excessive coughing and violent throat-clearing. Some of the voice therapy techniques described in Chapter 6, designed to reduce vocal hyperfunction, (tongue protrusion /i/, chant talk, nasal glide stimulation, warble) are most effective in eliminating the phonation break problem. Specific therapy procedures for phonation breaks or more severe abductor spasms are discussed in Chapters 6 and 7.

Pitch Breaks

Track 3

There are two kinds of pitch breaks. One is a developmental phenomenon seen primarily in boys experiencing marked pubertal growth of the larynx, and the other is caused by prolonged vocal hyperfunction, particularly while speaking at an inappropriate (usually too low) pitch level.

The rapid changes in the size of the vocal folds and other laryngeal structures produce varying vocal effects during the pubertal years. Boys experience a lowering of their fundamental frequency of about one octave; girls, a lowering of only about two or three notes. This change does not happen in a day or two. For several years, as this laryngeal growth is taking place, boys will experience temporary hoarseness and occasional pitch breaks. Wise parents or voice clinicians witness these vocal changes with little comment or concern. These mass-size increases of puberty tend to thwart any serious attempts at singing or other vocal arts. Luchsinger and Arnold (1965) point out that much of the European literature on singing makes a valid plea that the formal study of singing be deferred until well after puberty. Until a male child experiences some stability of laryngeal growth, the demands of singing might be inappropriate for his rapidly changing mechanism. Laryngeal strain is a real concern when serious singing is attempted during this period. One of the authors was told by Beverly Sills, the most famous of recent sopranos, that she stopped singing altogether for three years during puberty. Interestingly, Beverly Sills, unlike any other opera singer we know, had only a single voice teacher for her entire child and adult career.

The age and rate of pubertal development varies markedly. From the pediatric literature we find that the main thrust of puberty for any one child seems to take

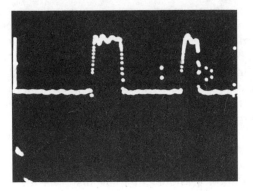

FIGURE 3.5   A Visi-Pitch Tracing of the Voicing Pitch Breaks of a 39-Year-Old Minister *The lower tracing is a prolonged /a/ at about 100 Hz, breaking abruptly to the high tracing at 300 Hz. The pitch breaks occur when he sustains phonation at the lowest voice he can produce.*

place in a total time period of about four years, six months. The most rapid and dramatic changes occur toward the last six months of puberty (this is when pitch breaks, if they occur, may be observed in some boys). Most pubertal changes begin at age twelve in boys, a little earlier in girls, and are completed by age sixteen.

Younger children and adults might experience a different kind of pitch break, related to the voice breaking an octave (sometimes two octaves) up or an octave down when speaking at an inappropriate pitch level. When individuals speak at an inappropriately low frequency, their voice tends to break one octave higher; if they speak too high in the frequency range their voice may break one octave down.

The tracings in Figure 3.5, recorded on a Visi-Pitch, show the inappropriately low fundamental frequency tracings of a 39-year-old minister, suddenly breaking into abrupt upward shifts. His lower F_o value was 100 Hz and his higher (the pitch break F_o) was 300 Hz. We discuss pitch breaks further in the next chapter when we talk about finding a pitch level appropriate for the mass and size of the individual's vocal folds, which can help avoid or eliminate sudden unwanted shifts in vocal frequency.

Pitch breaks can also result from overall vocal fatigue. Heavy users of voice, such as actors after prolonged rehearsals or during long-running performances, may begin to experience pitch breaks after hours of prolonged voicing. Such continued vocal hyperfunction, speaking with too much effort, will sometimes result in either pitch or phonation breaks. Such pitch breaks are usually warnings that the vocal mechanisms are being overworked and being held at an inappropriate pitch level for a prolonged period of time. We refer to such pitch or phonation breaks as "vocal limping," just as one limps when walking with an injured foot. With a little temporary voice rest (two or three days) and initiation of techniques of easy phonation (such as glottal fry or yawn-sigh), fatigue-induced pitch and phonation breaks usually disappear.

Voice Disorders Related to Neurological Factors: Neurologic Etiology

As shown in Table 3.1, the center column represents those voice disorders that are currently thought to have neurogenic causal factors. The neurologic voice disorders are discussed more fully in Chapter 4. As mentioned earlier, there may always be functional or organic components mixed along with causal neurogenic factors.

Paradoxical Vocal Fold Movement (PVFM)

This disorder has been misdiagnosed and confused with other problems, such as asthma and stridor, and can be mistaken for an allergy. Other names for the disorder are *paradoxical vocal fold dysfunction, episodic laryngeal dyskinesia, psychogenic wheezing, Munchausen's stridor,* as well as *vocal cord dysfunction* (VCD). The disorder may have been described first by Christopher, Wood, Eckert, Blager, Raney, and Soutrada (1983). While the causes are not well understood at this time, the disorder can be treated with some success. In our experience, the typical patient is a young (often in her teens) female with a history of multiple hospitalizations in the Emergency Room (ER) for difficulty breathing. While our experience has been with many more females (8:1) than males, the report of Christopher and colleagues (1983) presented with one female and four males. Bless and Swift (1996), in an ASHA paper, indicated a female-to-male ratio of 3.5:1, which is closer to our own experience with gender distribution in this disorder.

The symptoms are wheezing and difficulty maintaining a regular breathing pattern. Patients have been given a mixture of helium and oxygen (heliox), which has improved the symptoms of severe laryngospasm. They have also been treated with epinephrine (epipen).

We have observed that there seem to be at least three subtypes of the disorder. One involves appearing in combination with asthma, one appears to be linked with exercise and perhaps to allergies, and one form seems to be psychogenic or at least strongly exacerbated by psychological stress.

We have had very good success with using a treatment approach that demonstrates that the patient can control the larynx by volitionally shaking the larynx gently with the hand, initiating soft voice, which is breathy, glottal fry, and inhalation phonation. In the presence of these gentle phonation techniques, we reintroduce exercise (jumping jacks, stair climbing), exposure to cold, by going outside or standing in front of an air conditioner, and smells, such as perfume, vanilla, and so on. Ramig and Verdolini (1998), in an article on treatment efficacy for voice disorders, indicate the successful treatment of this disorder by means of behavioral therapy techniques. Our own videolaryngoscopy of these patients showed normal vocal fold function during asymptomatic periods and adduction during inhalation with abduction or continued adduction during phonation. Patients have been able to get off their medications following voice therapy and have not had to have a tracheostomy or a return visit to the ER.

Essential Tremor

This voice disorder, also called *organic tremor* or *familial tremor,* is often confused with spasmodic dysphonia but is quite different in terms of presentation, pathogenesis, and treatment. Essential tremor may be isolated to the voice (and may not appear elsewhere) at a frequency of from 4 to 7 Hz. It may be associated with tremor elsewhere in the body, such as in the head, hand, tongue, or jaw. The tremor is quiet at rest and is present during volitional movement. We find that family members may have also demonstrated similar voice tremor. The disorder seems to be fairly evenly distributed by gender with a slightly larger number being male. It generally appears in the middle to late middle age of life and the onset usually is not sudden. The usually rhythmical tremor may be present in connected speech and is almost always present in sustained vowels. The acoustic result of essential tremor is steady fluctuation in pitch and loudness. The ability to initiate or to terminate a sustained vowel is not usually difficult in essential tremor as it may be in SD cases. We will discuss this disorder more in Chapter 4. While we are not successful at totally eliminating the tremor, voice therapy usually can reduce or mask its acoustic effects. We have used pitch shifts (generally upward shifts) and a somewhat breathy mode of phonation as treatment techniques for the disorder. In more severe cases in which voice arrests may occur and there are other tremors in the body, medications may be tried but we have seen only limited success with medications.

Track 8

Spastic Dysphonia (Spasmodic Dysphonia)

One of the most extreme forms of a neurologic voice disorder is adductor spastic dysphonia (SD). Patients' voices sound strained, choked off with the attempts to voice, as if they are trying to push the outgoing airstream through a tightly adducted laryngeal opening. In a recent study, Watterson, Gibbons, and McFarlane (1998) found that, in their survey of 451 professionals (170 returned the survey) who deal with voice disorders, they rely on subjective analysis, a procedure that requires interpretation and experience, more than on instrumentation in the diagnosis of this disorder. Further they prefer descriptive terms such as *strained* and *strangled* (motokinesthetic terms) rather than acoustic terms, such as *hoarse* and *harsh*, in discussing and diagnosing the disorder.

Patients with adductor spastic dysphonia complain about the difficulties they experience fighting the back pressure created by excessive vocal fold adduction. Interestingly, when they are provided with a temporary nerve block to the recurrent laryngeal nerve they are pleased with the extremely breathy voice that accompanies the temporary vocal fold paralysis produced by the nerve block. In patients with a long history, we see symptoms of this disorder in prolonged vowels as well as in connected speech. Most patients with spastic dysphonia experience some normal voice in certain situations. Patients may report that there are some situations in which the voice seems free from shut down. Of interest in this regard are the research findings that, of the intrinsic laryngeal muscles, only the thyroarytenoid muscle has abnormal activation spasms and only then when symptoms are actually occurring (Nash and Ludlow, 1996). During the actual movement of voice disturbance, the thyroarytenoid muscle is overactive, but during the reported moments of normal voice these muscles function normally.

Endoscopic examination (Davis, Boone, Carroll, Darveniza, and Harrison, 1987) shows that the tight voice is indeed produced by hyperadduction (severe approximation) of the true folds, often accompanied by tight closure of the false vocal folds (ventricular folds) with supraglottic constriction of the aryepiglottic folds and contraction of the inferior pharyngeal constrictors. The total laryngeal and lower pharyngeal airway appears to close down (McFarlane, 1988; McFarlane and Lavorato, 1984). No wonder we hear a strangled voice in such patients. In Chapter 4, we will look more closely at SD and its treatment and therapy.

Track
7 & 9

Vocal Fold Paralysis

As presented in Chapter 2, two branches of the vagus (X cranial) nerve, the superior and recurrent laryngeal nerves, have primary motor–sensory functions in the larynx. Laryngeal muscle paralysis can result when either of these two nerves are damaged or severed. The motor component of the superior laryngeal nerve controls the cricothyroid muscles, whose primary role is to change the pitch of the voice by regulating the tension of the vocal folds. The recurrent laryngeal nerve innervates all the other intrinsic muscles of the larynx. Its primary function is the abduction (separation) and adduction (closing) of the vocal folds. If these peripheral nerves (or their central nuclei in the brain stem) are damaged or severed, motor function will be compromised, and the affected muscles will be paralyzed. These nerve functions are discussed more fully in Chapter 4.

Although damage to the superior laryngeal nerve is relatively rare, when it is damaged it produces a paralysis (unilateral or bilateral) of the cricothyroid muscles, so that the patient is unable to elevate or lower voice pitch. In the case of unilateral damage, one vocal fold would be normal (able to adjust its length and tension) while the fold on the side of the paralyzed cricothyroid could not change its length or tension. This unilateral kind of involvement may cause canting (tilting) of the larynx.

Bilateral paralysis of the cricothyroid muscles results in a startling lack of pitch change, and the voice sounds like a monotone. The result is physiologically and acoustically much the same as cricothyroid joint fixation with its lack of pitch-changing ability. The most frequently observed laryngeal paralysis is a unilateral paralysis with the involved fold paralyzed in the paramedian position. The patient is unable to move the paralyzed fold into the midline for normal vocal fold approximation or away from the midline, which can result in stridor on exercise. This type of paralysis is traditionally called *unilateral adductor paralysis:* The patient is unable to adduct the fold to midline. (The name of the paralysis describes what the involved fold is unable to do.) The cause of unilateral adductor paralysis is usually trauma to the recurrent laryngeal nerve from such causes as neck (particularly thyroid) surgery and accidents. Much rarer is bilateral adductor paralysis, in which both folds are paralyzed in the outer, paramedian position. Occasionally, the bilateral positioning is as wide as the glottis can open. Bilateral paralysis is usually caused by a central lesion in the brain stem and is, therefore, a form of dysarthria. The typical voice symptom of adductor paralysis, particularly the bilateral form, is no voice at all, or paralytic aphonia. Unilateral fold paralysis is often temporary because the traumatized nerve can often regenerate. About 50 percent of patients with peripheral injuries to the recurrent laryngeal nerve experience a return of normal function (Casper, Colton, and Brewer, 1986). Regeneration is frequently observed within the first nine months after trauma. Surgical correction of vocal fold paralysis is usually deferred until at least nine months after onset, and is accompanied by hope for some nerve regeneration with a subsequent return of vocal function. McFarlane, Holt-Romeo, Lavorato, and Warner (1991) found that voice therapy produced superior voice quality in patients with unilateral paralysis when compared to patients treated with teflon, and that voice therapy and muscle nerve reinnervation surgery were not significantly different in result. Thus, in the interim period, voice therapy can be effective, helping the patient develop some functional or even near-normal voice.

Voice therapy for this condition is presented in Chapter 4.

Respiration training, the pushing approach, ear training, and promoting hard glottal attack have all been used in helping the patient with unilateral adductor paralysis to develop some voice. We have abandoned the pushing and pulling approach in favor of head-turning, and the lateral digital pressure approach discussed in Chapter 6. Pushing and pulling and the hard glottal attack approach often produce louder voices but the voice they produce is almost always too vocally rough to be acceptable. McFarlane, Watterson, Lewis, and Boone (1998) demonstrate the ability of these voice therapy facilitation techniques (head turning and digital pressure) to reduce the air wastage generally associated with incomplete glottal closure. In Chapter 4, we will discuss more fully the medical–surgical voice therapy management of vocal fold paralyses.

Dysarthria

Many voice disorders are symptoms of some kind of neurological disease or dysfunction. Dysarthria is a motor speech problem that is the result of damage somewhere to the central or peripheral nervous systems. "Dysarthria is the generic name for different motor speech problems that may be caused by a number of nervous-system diseases" (Boone and Plante, 1993, p. 232). Lesions to the recurrent or superior laryngeal nerves involve the peripheral nervous system (the innervating nerves to the larynx) may result in vocal fold paralysis (see Chapter 4). The vocal problems that are classified as dysarthria are usually related to diseases of the central nervous system, such as multiple sclerosis or Parkinson's disease. A description of several CNS diseases that cause symptoms of dysarthria are described in Chapter 4, along with possible medical–voice therapy treatment approaches for each disease.

Voice Disorders Related to Organic Changes of Vocal Mechanisms: Organic Etiology

In Table 3.1, organic disorders of the vocal mechanism that might cause voice problems are listed in the column on the far right. In these disorders, the faulty voice is usually related more to a physical condition than to vocal abuse–misuse per se. We now present each disorder in the order presented in Table 3.1. These are the voice disorders currently considered to have organic etiology.

Sulcus Vocalis

This condition may be either congenital or acquired and of unknown etiology, although vocal abuse may play a role in the acquired form. It may present with a long oval shaped glottal opening during adduction or by a line running longitudinally, parallel to the glottis, down one or both vocal folds. The condition appears to most often be bilateral and is often not noticed until a patient presents with a dysphonia that is low in loudness, breathy, and hoarse. An excessive air wastage may be present so a reduced phonation time may be noted. Incomplete glottal closure is often observed throughout phonation and the mucosal wave may be interrupted as it crosses the vocal fold furrow [the area of the sulcus appears stiff]. We have treated these patients with voice therapy, which seeks to adjust the balance between proper glottal closure, pitch, and loudness. Pitch shifts, loudness changes, lateral digital pressure, and experimentation with firmer glottal closure are productive techniques. While some have suggested teflon injection for the treatment, we find voice therapy is the treatment of choice. Figure 3.6 demonstrates a severe complete sulcus vocalis. The treatment of sulcus vocalis is discussed in Chapter 7.

Contact Ulcers

As we mentioned in Chapter 2, the total length of the glottis can be divided into thirds: the anterior two-thirds is muscular (vocalis portion of the thyroarytenoids) and covered by a membrane; the posterior third is cartilaginous (arytenoids) and covered by a membrane. **Contact ulcers,** which generally form along the posterior third of the glottal margin, seem to result from one of three causes or a combination of these. Figure 3.7 illustrates a moderately large contact ulcer granuloma. The first cause is excessive slamming together of the arytenoid cartilages during production of low-pitched phonation coupled with excessively hard glottal attack and perhaps increased loudness with frequent throat-clearing and coughing. The speaker is usually a hard-driving person who speaks in a loud, controlling low pitch, often with words punctuated with sudden onset. However, Watterson, Hansen-Magorian, and McFarlane (1990) found that hard glottal attack was reported only 26 percent of the time by diagnosing clinicians, while pain was reported in 56 percent of the total of fifty-seven cases studied. Indeed, we now feel that those patients who develop contact ulcer and granuloma due to faulty vocal functioning are in the minority. A far larger group seems to be in the class who develop the disorder due to organic factors. The second etiology for contact ulcer is *gastric reflux*, in which stomach acid is forced up the esophagus and irritates the area between the arytenoids or the vocal fold covering (Koufman, 1991). Koufman feels that this Gastroesophageal Reflux Disease (GERD) may account not only for many contact ulcers but also for many cases of so

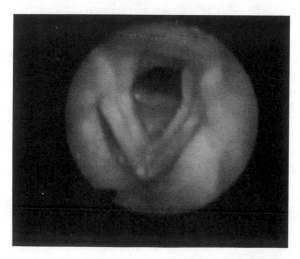

FIGURE 3.6 Sulcus Vocalis *This 68-year-old male represents a complete bilateral sulcus vocalis, appearing as a reduplication of the vocal folds, giving him two sets of vocal cords and two ventricles. The arytenoid cartilages appear to be split as well.*

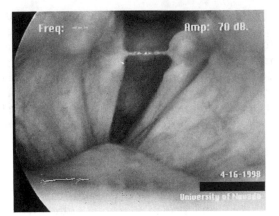

FIGURE 3.7   Left contact ulcer with granuloma, young adult male

called functional dysphonia, and he advocates ambulatory twenty-four-hour pH monitoring for patients suspected of having this disorder. Thirdly, intubation for surgery is a cause of contact ulcer in a small number of cases, especially where bilateral rather large granulomas are the presenting picture following any type of surgery.

The typical symptoms of contact ulcers are deterioration of voice after prolonged vocalization (vocal fatigue), accompanied by pain in the laryngeal area or sometimes pain that lateralizes out to one ear. Watterson, Hansen-Magorian, and McFarlane (1990) also found hoarseness/roughness reported 75 percent of the time and throat clearing in 65 percent of the fifty-seven cases of contact ulcer they studied. Laryngoscopy usually reveals bilateral ulcerations with heavy buildup of granulation tissue along the approximating margins of the posterior glottis. Greene (1980) labeled the toughened membranous tissue changes on the posterior glottis as *pachydermia,* citing the work of Kleinsasser (1979), and wrote that "contact ulcers are not actually ulcers or granulomas but consist of 'craters' with highly thickened squamous epithelium over connective tissue with some inflammation (edema)" (p. 147).

The diffuse irritation of the posterior glottis often associated with contact ulcers may be the result of *esophageal reflux,* sometimes associated with diaphragmatic or hiatal hernia and disease of the lower esophageal sphincter (LES). The patient experiences esophageal reflux while sleeping, which results in the pooling of acid secretions in the vocal process (posterior) end of the glottis (Cherry and Margulies, 1968). In studying the sensitivity of the posterior larynx to gastric juices, Delahunty and Cherry (1968) were able to produce, experimentally, contact ulcers and granulation tissue in dogs by swabbing gastric juices on their vocal folds. Patients with contact ulcers who also demonstrate marked irritation of laryngeal–pharyngeal tissue are candidates for a thorough examination of the gastrointestinal tract (Koufman, 1991). If a hiatal hernia, for example, is found with contact ulcers, the patient may best be treated with antacids, acid-inhibiting agents, diet management, and voice therapy. Other behavioral changes, such as elevating the head of the bed and reducing the size of meals and eating several hours before going to bed, are helpful in reflux management. The focus of voice therapy for patients with contact ulcers is to take the effort out of phonation. The patients must learn to use a voice pitch level that can be produced with relatively little strain (which usually means pitch needs to be elevated), to speak with greater mouth and jaw relaxation, to speak at lower levels of volume, and to eliminate all traces of excessively hard glottal attack. Contact ulcers are rare today, according to Watterson, Hansen-Magorian, and McFarlane (1990); these cases comprise about 1 percent of total voice cases. Those patients who do have contact ulcers, however, seem to respond fairly well to voice therapy that is systematically employed. Surgery is usually not helpful because the ulcers generally return postoperatively.

We have been experiencing some success in a small group of seven patients who have been treated with vitamin C and E therapy. In all these patients we have observed the resolution of the contact granuloma with vitamin therapy without behavioral or other chemical–medical therapy.

Cancer

Cancer or **carcinoma** in the vocal tract is a life-threatening disease that requires serious medical–surgical management. Lip and intraoral cancers rarely contribute to changes in voice, but they may have obvious negative effects on articulation. Extensive oral lesions involving the tongue, perhaps even requiring partial or total surgical removal of the tongue (glossectomy), or palatal and velar cancer can seriously affect articulation and vocal resonance.

The American Cancer Society (1980) reported that about 15,000 new U.S. patients annually develop some form of oral cancer. Some of the identified causes of oral cancer include smoking (particularly pipe smoking), use of smokeless tobacco, chronic infections, herpes, repeated trauma to the irritated site, and *leukoplakia* (whitish plaque). Often patients first experience chronic lesions in the mouth or on the tongue that do not seem to heal. Usually continuous pain near the lesion site brings the patient to the physician. The majority of these oral lesions are treated successfully with microsurgery (removal of small lesions) and radiation therapy. The primary goal of surgery–radiation therapy is to eradicate the primary lesion so that it does not spread (metastasize) to another adjacent or remote body site. Sometimes carcinoma is detected in the nasal sinuses and at sites within the pharynx, although such lesions are relatively rare. The most serious vocal tract malignancies, however, are those that involve the larynx, which by their position in the airway, present a serious potential threat to airway adequacy. According to Case (1991), "laryngeal cancer comprises 2 to 5 percent of all malignancies diagnosed annually in the United States" (229). A cancer of the larynx may be seen in Figure 3.8.

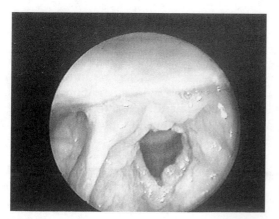

FIGURE 3.8 Cancer of larynx, adult female, 65 years old.

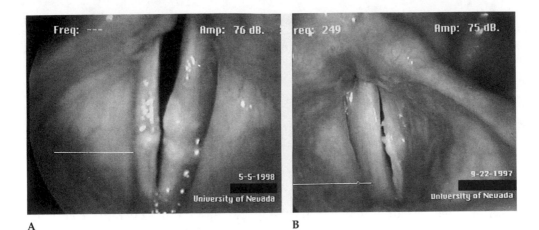

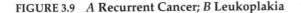

A   B

FIGURE 3.9   *A* Recurrent Cancer; *B* Leukoplakia

In general, there are three classifications of laryngeal cancers, depending on the site of the lesion: **supraglottal,** involving such structures as the ventricular and aryepiglottic folds, the epiglottis, the arytenoid cartilages, and the walls of the hypopharynx; **glottal,** from the anterior commissure to the vocal process ends of the arytenoids; and **subglottal,** involving the cricoid cartilage and trachea. The treatment combines radiation therapy and surgery for small to moderate lesions; extensive cancer requires perhaps a hemilaryngectomy, a supraglottal laryngectomy, or total laryngectomy. We discuss both of these later in this chapter, and we consider laryngeal cancer, rehabilitation after laryngectomy, and the role of the speech–language pathologist in some detail in Chapter 8.

Leukoplakia

Leukoplakia are whitish patches that are additive lesions to the surface membrane of mucosal tissue and that often extend beneath the surface into subepithelial space. Although the lesions are classified as benign tumors, similar to hyperkeratosis, they are considered to be precancerous lesions and must be watched closely. Within the vocal tract, common sites for leukoplakia are under the tongue and on the vocal folds. It is important to note that it is difficult or impossible to distinguish between leukoplakia and cancer of the larynx by visual inspection alone. Figure 3.9 demonstrates the difficulty by comparing photographs A and B. Photograph A is a recurrence of cancer in a twenty-six-year-old female and B is leukoplakia in a fifty-year-old male; both are nonsmokers, nonusers of alcohol, and vegetarians. The primary etiology of these white patches is continuous irritation of membranes. The most common cause is heavy smoking; a heroic effort must be initiated to prevent continued irritation, such as absolute insistence that the patient quit smoking and emotional support for the patient. Continued irritation and subsequent growth of leukoplakia often leads to squamous cell carcinoma.

Although leukoplakia on or under the tongue have only minimal effects on voice, leukoplakia on the vocal folds may dramatically alter voice. The added

Laryngeal Lesions

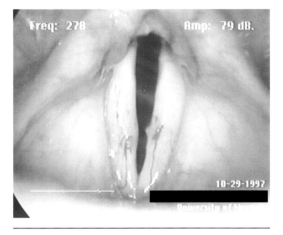

Bilateral vocal fold hemorrhage in 24-year-old male singer

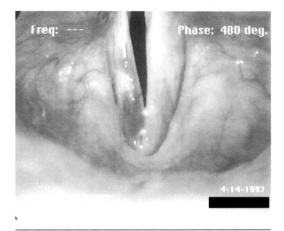

Severe right vocal fold hemorrhage in 29-year-old actor

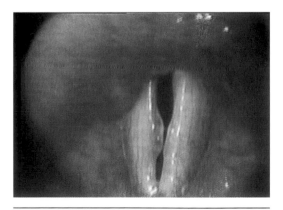

Right vocal fold sessile polyp in 20-year-old female salesperson

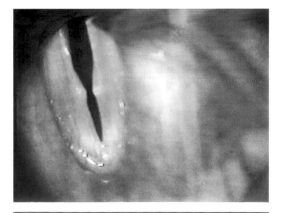

Bilateral vocal nodules in 21-year-old female singer

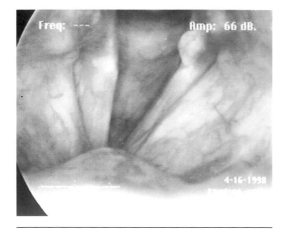

Left vocal fold adductor paralysis with contact granuloma in an adult male

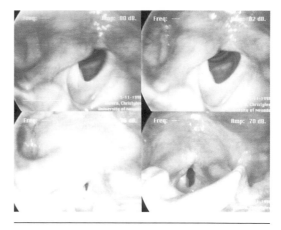

Four views of congenital laryngeal web in a 3-year-old boy

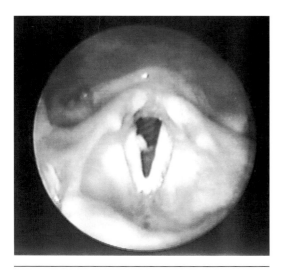

Contact ulcer granuloma in a 46-year-old male

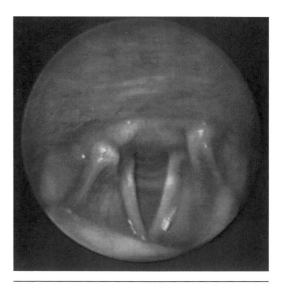

Acute laryngitis in an 8-year-old girl. Note: red swollen vocal folds

lesion mass to the vocal folds lowers voice pitch and frequently causes hoarseness and sometimes weak loudness. Because leukoplakia are also random in size and location, they often cause the vocal folds to be asymmetrical, which may result in diplophonia as each fold vibrates at a different rate because of its different size or mass. Leukoplakia that occupy space on the glottal margin may prevent optimal approximation of the folds, contributing to breathiness, reduced loudness, and overall dysphonia. The treatment of leukoplakia is medical–surgical, and voice therapy only contributes to developing the best voice possible. In spite of lesion effects, a functional aspect of the dysphonia can often be lessened with therapy. These functional aspects may be the only vocal symptoms and thus voice therapy is important to restore normal voice.

Endocrine Changes

Occasionally patients are seen whose voice problems are related to some kind of endocrine dysfunction. Endocrine disorders often have a major impact on developing larynges and cause excesses in fundamental frequency, so that an individual's voice is either too low or too high in pitch. For example, in hypofunction of the pituitary gland, laryngeal growth is retarded. A pubescent child with such a problem will experience a continued high voice pitch. Such a pituitary problem can prevent normal development of progesterone by the ovaries (in girls) and testosterone by the testes (in adolescent males). The resulting lack of secondary sexual characteristics (including a change in voice) is treated by endocrine therapy designed to stimulate normal pituitary function. The opposite problem, caused by some tumors of the pituitary gland, results in a "precocious puberty as well as acromegaly" (Strome, 1982, p. 18). Hypofunctioning of the adrenal glands (Addison's disease) can also contribute to lack of secondary sex characteristics, including a prepubescent voice in males. Sometimes tumors in the adrenal system cause adrenal hormone excesses, causing virilization and a deepening of the voice. McFarlane and Brophy (1992) discuss the effect of various medications on voice. Some birth control medications, for example, can cause virilization of the female voice and vocal huskiness as well. We once treated a middle-aged female who had been mistakenly given massive doses of synthetic testosterone over an eighteen-month period. She grew facial hair, experienced changes in her genitalia, and a lowering of fundamental frequency of the voice before the error in medical treatment was noted. Voice therapy was successful in improving the voice.

Hypothyroidism, insufficient secretion of thyroxin by the thyroid gland, can produce many physical changes over time, including increased mass of the vocal folds, which, in turn, lowers pitch. Aronson (1990) describes the dysphonia of hypothyroidism as "characteristically **hoarse,** sometimes described as **coarse** or **gravelly,** and of **excessively low pitch**" (p. 60). Such symptoms can usually be well controlled by thyroid hormone therapy. In hyperthyroidism (excessive thyroid function), vocal symptoms are less severe, and the patients experience jumpiness and irritability, which result in a breathy voice that may lack sufficient loudness.

Greene (1980) describes the influence of menstruation on the female voice, particularly at premenstruation when estrogen and progesterone levels are at their lowest, resulting in a slight thickening of the vocal folds, which can cause a lowering of pitch and some hoarseness. Some female opera singers avoid heavy singing obligations several days before and after menstruation. The climacteric (menopause) is another time when some women may experience vocal changes, particularly a lowering of fundamental frequency. Because of the secretion of excessive androgenic hormones after the menopause, the glottal membrane becomes thicker, increasing the size–mass of the folds, and producing a lowering of voice pitch (Gould, 1975) and sometimes vocal roughness. It would appear that, in any case in which the larynx is under- or overdeveloped for the age and sex of the patient, some endocrine imbalance might be suspected. If some kind of hormonal imbalance is discovered, the primary treatment, if possible, would be hormonal therapy. Voice therapy can be of help to the patient in developing the best vocal performance possible with the changing (because of hormone therapy) mechanism. Most of the techniques presented in Chapter 6 are appropriate when applied to these patients for direct alteration of voice parameters such as pitch, loudness, and quality.

Granuloma

There are three possible causes of **granulomas,** one resulting from intubation during surgery, another resulting from glottal trauma from abuse–misuse, and a third (larger group) resulting from gastric reflux disease (GERD). Each of these etiologies suggests a different treatment. These were discussed earlier in this chapter under the heading of contact ulcer (see Figure 3.7).

Any patient who is intubated during surgery or for airway preservation risks having a traumatized laryngeal membrane with the subsequent development of granuloma. The risk is particularly greater in children and women, who have smaller airways and are thus more often traumatized by large tubes (Whited, 1979). The physician places a tube down the pharynx into the airway, between the open (it is hoped) vocal folds, and on into the trachea. If the tube is larger than the glottal opening, the patient runs the risk of trauma. Ellis and Bennett (1977) have recommended that, in order to prevent intubation granuloma or hemangioma, patients should be intubated with tubes one size smaller than what would be needed "for a snug fit." Some patients, for example, demonstrate sudden changes in voice after general surgery. If the patient who was intubated shows a persistent hoarseness after surgery, indirect laryngoscopy or endoscopy should be performed to confirm or deny the possible presence of an intubation granuloma. If present, such a granuloma may need to be removed surgically and/or treated with voice therapy. Another form of granuloma may result from vocal fold trauma related to continuous irritation (such as acid reflux) or sudden accident (such as an external injury to the larynx). Other than intubation granuloma, the most common form is associated with contact ulcers. The literature suggests, in fact, that contact ulcer and related vocal fold granuloma are probably the same disorder, related to continuous vocal trauma.

Patients with granuloma may experience severe dysphonia, characterized by hoarseness, breathiness, and the felt need to clear the throat frequently. Voice therapy may play a primary role (McFarlane, 1988; Perkins, 1977) in eradication of some granulomas. After surgical removal of the offending lesion, voice therapy is usually needed to help the patient regain a normal voice.

Hemangioma

Hemangiomas are similar to granulomas, differing only in type of lesion. Whereas a granuloma is usually a firm granulated sac, a hemangioma is a soft, pliable, blood-filled sac. Like granulomas, hemangiomas often occur on the posterior glottis, frequently associated with vocal hyperfunction, hyperacidity, or intubation. This blood-filled lesion, when identified, should be removed surgically (with cold steel or laser). As soon as glottal healing permits, a vocal hygiene program and some voice therapy should be initiated.

Hyperkeratosis

Patients often come to their dentist or otolaryngologist because they are concerned about some oral or pharyngeal lesions they have observed. Once professionally identified, these lesions are often biopsied and found to be either malignant (cancerous) or nonmalignant (benign). Laryngeal examination may also locate and subsequently identify, by biopsy, additive lesions in the pharynx or larynx. Hyperkeratosis, a pinkish, rough lesion, is often the identified lesion, a nonmalignant growth that may be the precursor of malignant tissue change. Hyperkeratotic growths are reactive lesions to continued tissue irritation. Therefore, hyperkeratotic lesions must be watched closely over time for any change in appearance. Favorite sites of hyperkeratosis include under the tongue, on the vocal folds at the anterior commissure, and posteriorly on the arytenoid prominences. Their effect on voice may be negligible or severe, depending on the site and the extent of the lesion. We once had an eight-year-old girl voice patient with hyperkeratosis of the vocal folds who had experienced the secondhand smoke of both parents for those eight years.

It is generally believed that chronic irritation of oral and laryngeal membranes over time—for example, as the result of excessive and continued smoking—is the primary etiology of hyperkeratosis. Consequently, the most effective treatment of the problem is eliminating the source of tissue irritation, possible surgical removal, and voice therapy to improve the voice quality.

Infectious Laryngitis

Some of the same people who experience traumatic laryngitis after only minor abuse misuse of the voice also experience infectious laryngitis when they have a cold. The case histories of such people often contain multiple entries of "**loss of voice,**" aphonia, or laryngitis. In other individuals, infectious laryngitis is a very rare event that occurs as one of the symptoms of a severe head and chest cold. Infectious laryngitis often develops in a patient who has had a fever, headache, running nose, sore throat, and coughing. Although most problems of infectious laryngitis are viral in origin, the more severe problems (often accompanied by high fever and a very sore throat) may be bacterial infections. Bacteria-caused laryngitis can often be dramatically treated, with relatively quick resolution, through antibiotic therapy. Unfortunately, most laryngitis experienced during a cold (viral in origin) does not respond to antibiotics. The standard treatment is "voice rest, humidification, increased fluid intake **(hydration),** reduced physical activity, and analgesics" (Strome, 1982, p. 12).

From a voice conservation point of view, absolute voice rest—no attempts at spoken communication, including voice or whisper—should be initiated by the patient with such a laryngeal infection. Whispering should be discouraged, because most people produce a glottal whisper by placing the vocal folds in close approximation to one another, which, in effect, produces a light voice. The irritated, swollen tissues continue to touch and to vibrate. What infectious laryngitis patients need is total voice rest for a period of two or three days, with the vocal folds in the open, inverted-V position, and increased fluids (hydration).

Laryngectomy

One of the primary functions of the human larynx is to prevent aspiration into the airway. The larynx contains three valve sites: the true folds, the ventricular folds (false folds), and the aryepiglottic folds, each of whose valving action allows them to shut off the airway to prevent the inhalation of liquids, foods, saliva, mucus, and any other stray foreign bodies that may be headed through the larynx into the airway. When the larynx is so compromised by disease (such as advanced cancer) or trauma that it cannot safely perform its valving role, the patient becomes a candidate for a laryngectomy, the total removal of the larynx. Without the larynx to protect the airway, an opening is created in the trachea (tracheostomy) through which the patient breathes all pulmonary (lung) air in and out. The patient must develop a substitute voicing source, such as an artificial larynx or esophageal speech. Recent modifications of the laryngectomy procedure (Singer and Blom, 1980) permit pulmonary air to flow from the trachea through a prosthetic shunt into the esophagus, facilitating the production of esophageal "voice" without extensive special training. We describe the use of and training for other artificial voicing sources and forms of a laryngeal voice in Chapter 8.

Except in cases of traumatic injury to the larynx requiring an emergency laryngectomy, most laryngectomy operations are scheduled only after some counseling has been completed by the surgeon, the speech–language pathologist, and sometimes a laryngectomee (a patient who has had the operation). We describe pre- and postoperative counseling, evaluation, and training of the patient with a total laryngectomy in some detail in Chapter 8. A brief note should be made here of a recent success with total laryngeal transplant, the first successful transplantation of the larynx, performed at the Cleveland Clinic. Dr. Douglas Hicks, a speech–language pathologist, has followed this patient since the operation, and reports the patient has a functional voice. But one should not become overly optimistic about the usefulness of such a procedure with large numbers of patients, such as laryngeal cancer patients.

Papilloma

Papilloma are wartlike growths, viral in origin, that occur in the dark, moist caverns of the airway, frequently in the larynges of young children. They can represent a serious threat to the airway, limiting the needed flow of air through the glottal opening. The majority of papilloma occur in children under the age of six; for this reason, hoarseness and shortness of breath in preschool children should be evaluated promptly. Although the majority of papilloma stop recurring about the time of puberty, Kleinsasser (1979) wrote that 20 percent persist beyond puberty. Papilloma of the airway in adolescents and young adults must be considered a serious laryngeal disease, primarily because of its recurrence and persistent threat to the small airway. We have seen adults who developed papillomatosis in adulthood without ever having it in childhood. When papilloma occur in the larynx, their additive mass often contributes to dysphonia. For this reason, the voice clinician should be particularly alert to any child who demonstrates dysphonia. Any child with continued hoarseness for more than ten days, independent of a cold or allergy, should have the benefit of a laryngeal examination to identify the cause of the hoarseness. If papilloma are identified, the treatment is medical–surgical, and treatment includes laser beam surgery, conventional excision surgery, radiation therapy, and interferon therapy (Lundquist, Haglund, Carlson, Strander, and Lundgren, 1984). The papilloma should only be removed when they impinge on the airway, because repeated surgery can result in postsurgical webbing of the vocal folds. Eventually, when the individual has developed the immunological state needed to resist the virus-inspired papilloma, the papilloma will no longer recur, according to Kleinsasser (1979).

The surgical and radiation therapy approach to papilloma is required whenever the papilloma growths begin to interfere with the airway. If the lesion mass does not interfere with respiration or voicing, it is usually tolerated. According to Wetmore, Key, and Suen (1985), there may be complications from continued surgical procedures for papilloma. These authors followed forty patients (twenty-six children; fourteen adults) who collectively had received a total of one-hundred-twenty-two laser surgeries for papilloma over six and a half years. Eleven of twelve patients who had undergone more than six operations over this time period experienced anterior glottal webs with persistent vocal fold edema as complications, and their vocalization was seriously affected. Dedo and Jackler (1982) report that laser surgery was clearly the superior procedure for removal of recurring papilloma in 109 patients; with the laser approach, they report that almost half of their patients eventually reached remission and had no recurrence of the lesions. Despite the possible complications from continuous surgery from recurring papilloma, the lesions must be removed when they begin to impinge on the airway. Lundquist and colleagues (1984) report a medical approach to the treatment of the viral-caused papilloma: injecting the patients intramuscularly with interferon. In following seventeen juvenile patients receiving interferon therapy over a several-year period, Lundquist and colleagues found that "nine were totally cured, four had no more tumor growth but were still being treated, three experienced diminished tumor growth, and one refused further treatment" (p. 386).

Most recently, interferon drug treatment has been used as a medical treatment for papilloma of the larynx. While this drug has some serious side effects (serious flulike symptoms, etc.), these treatments have produced some good voice results and reduced or eliminated the papilloma. We have seen some patients treated with interferon, have noted significant reduction in the papilloma, and were able to provide effective voice therapy following drug therapy.

In a recent and ongoing study (Rosen, Woodson, Thompson, Hengesteg, and Bradlow, 1998) report preliminary results of a phase 1 trial using Indole-3-carbinol for the treatment of recurrent respiratory papillomatosis. This substance is found in high concentrations in cabbage, brussel sprouts, broccoli, and cauliflower and is an approved FDA nutritional supplement. Eighteen months after treatment with the natural substance (Indole-3-carbinol) one third of the subjects had total cessation of papilloma growth, another one third had reduced growth, and one third had no clinical response to the treatment.

The speech–language pathologist is sometimes asked to see a toddler or young child with obstructive papilloma who has had to have an open tracheostomy to permit adequate respiration. Developing functional communication with such a child and fostering normal language growth are the primary concerns of the clinician. Teaching the child to occlude the open stoma with a finger or fitting the child with a one-way valve that covers the stoma (to permit vocalization without finger occlusion) usually permits some voicing. In older children or adults who are being treated surgically for recurring papilloma, helping them to develop the best voice possible with the compromised laryngeal mechanisms is a realistic goal in voice therapy. Some work on respiration control (such as voicing with larger lung volumes of air) or working on loudness and pitch may improve vocal function.

Pubertal Changes

At about age nine, before the onset of puberty, the larynges of boys and girls are anatomically about the same size, and they produce about the same voice pitch (265 Hz). Pubertal growth changes in girls begin around nine, with the onset of puberty, and gradual pubescent changes occur over a four- to five-year period. In boys, puberty begins around eleven to twelve, and dramatic growth changes occur over the four-to-five-year pubertal period. However, noticeable laryngeal growth and the dramatic change in vocal fundamental frequency occur in the last year of puberty: The "average time from onset to completion of adolescent voice change is three to six months, one year at most" (Aronson 1990, p. 45). By age seventeen, adolescents of both sexes have usually reached their full adult development (Offer, 1980). As we discuss elsewhere (see Chapters 2 and 5), the voice pitch levels of males and females drop dramatically after puberty (the male voice drops at least a full octave; the female voice drops almost half an octave). Laryngeal and airway growth does not happen overnight. Although the changes are gradual, over a four-year period, marked laryngeal growth (particularly in boys) occurs in the last six months of change. During this time of rapid laryngeal growth, boys may experience temporary dysphonia and occasional pitch breaks that are not cause for parental or clinical concern. Because these mass changes in puberty tend to thwart any serious attempts at singing or other vocal arts, junior high school is often a poor environment for choral music. A boy who is a soprano in September may well be the choir baritone by June. Until children experience some stability in laryngeal and airway growth, the demands of singing might well be inappropriate for their rapidly changing mechanisms. Because of such rapid changes, attempting to develop optimum pitch or modal-pitch levels in adolescents should be avoided.

Webbing

A laryngeal web growing across the glottis between the two vocal folds inhibits normal fold vibration, which often produces a high-pitched rough sound as it vibrates, and seriously compromises the open glottis. Webs may be congenital (see

Figure 3.10) or acquired (see Figure 3.11). A congenital web, which is detected at the time of birth, is the result of the glottal membrane failing to separate in embryonic development. Depending on the size of the web, the baby will produce stridor (inhalation noises), shortness of breath, and often a different high-pitched (squeal) cry. Approximately three fourths of all laryngeal webs cross the glottis (Strome, 1982). The presence of a congenital web requires immediate surgery, often followed by a temporary tracheostomy; usually, an infant larynx will recover over a period of four to six weeks.

Acquired webs result from some kind of bilateral trauma of the medial edges of the vocal folds. Anything that might serve as an irritant to the mucosal surface of the folds may be the initial cause of the webbing. Because the two vocal folds are so close together at the anterior commissure, any surface irritation due to prolonged infection or trauma may cause the inner margins of the two fold surfaces to grow together. To explain further, one principle of plastic surgery is that, when approximated together, offended tissue surfaces will tend to grow and fuse together. This same principle explains why webbing occurs. The offended surface of the two approximated folds tends to grow together, in this case forming a thin membrane across the glottis. Webbing grows across the glottis in an anterior to posterior fashion, usually ceasing about one third of the distance from the anterior commissure, where the distance between the two folds becomes too great. Severe laryngeal infections sometimes cause enough glottal irritation to precipitate web formation. Bilateral surgery of the folds, perhaps for papilloma or nodules, can also be followed by a web (Wetmore, Key, and Sven, 1985). External trauma to the folds, such as a direct hit on the thyroid cartilage that causes it to fracture, may damage the folds behind it, thus creating enough glottal irritation for a web to develop. Laryngeal surgery is the most frequent event which produces the postsurgical acquired web. Whatever causes the original bilateral irritation, as a part of healing, both folds grow together anteriorly, forming a glottal web sometimes called a *synechia*.

Laryngeal web may cause severe dysphonia as well as shortness of breath, depending on how extensively the webbing crosses the glottis. The treatment for the formation of a web is surgery. The webbing is cut, freeing the two folds. To prevent the surgically removed web from growing again, a vertical keel is placed

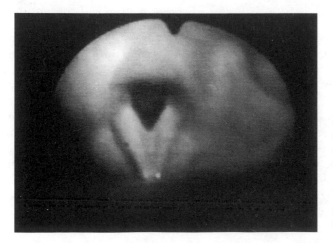

FIGURE 3.10 Webbing *This congenital laryngeal web was discovered in a 36-year-old woman who complained of a "lifetime with a lousy voice." The web was surgically removed, followed by successful voice therapy.*

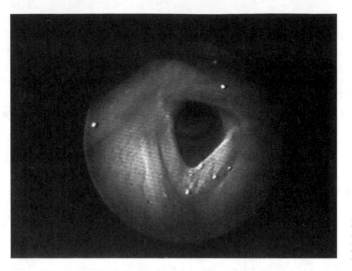

FIGURE 3.11 Acquired postsurgical web, 36-year-old female

between the two folds and kept there until complete healing has been achieved. The laryngologist fixates the keel, which is shaped very much like a boat rudder and is about the size of a fingernail, between the folds, preventing them from approximating together. The patient is then on voice rest as long as the keel is in place, because its presence inhibits normal fold vibration. When the keel is removed, often in six to eight weeks, the patient generally requires some voice therapy to restore normal phonation. If there was extensive damage to the larynx from the trauma, it may well be impossible after healing and voice therapy to ever develop the same kind of normal voice the patient had before the accident. The prognosis for voice recovery after webbing and its surgical treatment is highly individualized, depending on the extent of the trauma and the size of the resulting web. We have had patients who were able to speak and sing with a normal voice following surgical reduction of the web and a course of voice therapy.

Summary

The majority of voice disorders are related to vocal hyperfunction. Vocal excesses, such as voicing too loud and too long and excessive throat-clearing, are examples of causal factors of symptoms of aphonia or dysphonia. These we classify as functional disorders, perhaps resulting in vocal fold thickening, nodules, or polyps. We then looked at the neurologic factors of voice disorders, such as vocal fold paralysis and spasmodic dysphonia. These neurogenic voice disorders and their management are presented more fully in Chapter 4. Organic voice problems may result from various laryngeal disorders, such as cancer (discussed in Chapter 8), papilloma, granuloma, webbing, and other disorders. For each of the various organic voice disorders, we discussed medical management and the role of the speech–language pathologist in evaluation and therapy.

CHAPTER

4

Neurogenic Voice Disorders

In previous chapters, we have talked about the normal anatomy and physiology required for voice (Chapter 2), and we have considered the causes and treatment of a number of voice disorders (Chapter 3). In this chapter, we will take a brief look at the neurological structures and processes that must function in coordinated balance to produce what we perceptually consider as normal voice. Neurogenic voice disorders occur when there is some interruption to this balance. This neuro-balance may be disturbed by faulty innervation of respiratory components (such as in bulbar polio), or in adductory incompetence of the two vocal folds (as in vocal fold paralysis), or in the incoordination of vocal tract components (as heard in cerebral palsy dysarthria), or in velopharyngeal incompetence (when caused by faulty velar innervation).

By keeping our focus on voice disorders (consistent with the scope of this text), we will not take a detailed look at the central and peripheral nervous systems and their function. Rather, we will take a schematic look at the neural aspects of voice, developing an understanding of the neural coordination and innervations required for normal voice. We will then place our emphasis on adductory voice problems and the typical voice symptoms that are experienced by children and adults with various neurological disorders. Descriptions will be given of each neurogenic voice disorder, its voice symptoms, and its medical–voice therapy management.

In Table 4.1, we outline this chapter. Although the reader already knowledgeable about normal neuroanatomy and physiology may wish to skip ahead to the presentation on adductory voice problems and voice disorders, we invite you to look at our simplified neural function summary. The sophisticated reader can appreciate the omissions and simplifications we have made here in our quest to keep the textual focus on voice disorders and avoid getting into neuroanatomical/ neurophysiologic detail and controversy.

The scheme presented in Table 4.1 will guide the reader to the three primary sections of this chapter: a working view of the nervous system; adductory voice disorders and their medical–surgical–voice therapy management; and neurological diseases that affect voice with their medical–voice therapy management.

A Working View of the Nervous System

Both the central nervous system (CNS) and the peripheral nervous system (PNS) participate heavily in all laryngeal operations: from the delicate nuance sung by

TABLE 4.1   A Scheme for Understanding Neurogenic Voice Problems

A Working View of the Nervous System

The Central Nervous System (CNS), the Cortex, and Its Projections
    Pyramidal Tract
    Extrapyramidal Tract
CNS, the Thalamus, Internal Capsule, and the Basal Ganglia
CNS, the Brainstem, Cerebellum, and Medulla
The Peripheral Nervous System (PNS)
    Cranial Nerve Nuclei (IX, X, XI, XII)
    Superior and Recurrent Laryngeal Nerves

Neurogenic Problems of Vocal Fold Adduction

Vocal Fold Paralysis
Spasmodic Dysphonia

Voice Problems in Neurological Diseases

Amyotrophic Lateral Sclerosis
Cerebral Vascular Accident
Essential Tremor
Huntington's Disease (Chorea)
Multiple Sclerosis
Myasthenia Gravis
Parkinson's Disease

the operatic lyric soprano to the elevation of the total larynx for swallowing to the triple-valving folds that protect the airway by coughing. We know far less about the neural controls required for human singing and talking than we do about the neural governing in all mammals (including the human) of such laryngeal vegetative functions as breathing, coughing, or swallowing. The human not only has all the sensory–motor structures and functions of most mammal species, but has added abilities to subdue or augment response (for example, suppress crying when the situation is not appropriate), and the ability to use phonatory functions for expression of emotions, or in verbal and nonverbal communication or artistic expression. The expanded cerebral cortex unique to the human species has much to do with the enabling of the human to use voice in a controlled sequential pattern as heard or said in spoken language, or in the exact pitch and loudness requirements of singing, or in the voicing cues (inflection, loudness changes, etc.) we use in spoken communication.

The Central Nervous System (CNS), the Cortex, and Its Projections

The central nervous system is composed of the brain and spinal cord and is housed in the bony structures of the cranium and vertebral column. Below the midbrain, beginning with the medulla, is the peripheral nervous system. It collects either sensory information from the periphery or carries motor impulses to the muscles of the body. The highest functions (such as thinking or voicing) of the human brain appear to be directed by the cerebral cortex, a six-layered composite of millions of neurons, interconnected by their dendrites and axons. The outer bark of the cerebrum is the cerebral cortex, which contains gray matter (colored by the density of neurons) that is about ¼ of an inch thick, with some specification of function related to where the cortex is located within the brain. For example, there are four major cortical divisions of each cerebral hemisphere, each in a distinct anatomical site with markedly different functions:

> frontal—cognitive function, motor function
> parietal—associative, sensory function
> temporal—associative, auditory function
> occipital—visual function

It would appear that, at the cortical level, both the frontal and temporal lobes have the most to do with voice. As we will see shortly, both the pyramidal and extrapyramidal nerve tracts carry sensory impulses back (afferents) to the cortex and carry motor impulses from (efferents) cortical areas. The third frontal convolution (Brodmann 44, Broca's area) in each hemisphere has much to do with preplanning a motor speech–voice response. For example, in regional cerebral blood flow studies, Broca's area shows greater density of blood just before something is said. The actual saying of the utterance at the cortical level activates bilaterally (both left and right cerebral hemispheres) a specific location on the precentral gyrus (Brodmann 4, motor strip). It should be mentioned at this point that both laryngeal and pharyngeal innervation appears to be bilaterally innervated in the basal ganglia and below; therefore, there is very little area 4 cortex devoted to vocal fold function. For example, we do not see unilateral vocal fold paralysis resulting from a contralateral area 4 lesion. The unilateral vocal fold paralysis is more often related to brain stem or lower lesions. It appears that the insula (older cortex buried medial to the temporal lobe) plays an active role during vocalization. The temporal lobe plays an obvious role in speaking and singing, providing the cortical inputs of audition. Heschl's gyrus (Brodmann 41, primary auditory cortex) has tonotopic frequency input coming from the medial geniculate bodies of the thalamus. The understanding of what is said appears to be from cortex adjacent to Heschl's gyrus that is more posteriorly on the sylvian surface of the temporal lobe (Wernicke's area, 42) and, also, from the more posterior temporale planum. Wernicke's area of the temporal lobe connects directly with Broca's convolution via the bundle of fibers known as the arcuate fasciculus. The actual execution of voice may be dependent on temporal cortical connections to lower brain centers, such as from the temporale planum of the cortex to the pulvinar body of the thalamus (Minckler, 1972). It would appear that the temporal lobes play a much more active role in execution of voicing than has been previously acknowledged (Boone, 1998).

The typical unilateral pyramidal tract damage experienced by a patient with a cerebral vascular accident (CVA) produces pharyngeal or laryngeal symptoms in some, but not all, patients. High cortical lesions or lesions in the ascending–descending projection system are classified as upper motor neuron lesions. Such high lesions do not account for many voice problems. However, patients who experience bilateral damage from two or more CVAs will often show some laryngeal–pharyngeal symptoms (harshness, nasality, dysarthria) but will not have vocal fold paralysis. Such patients with bilateral pyramidal tract lesions are often classified as having pseudobulbar palsy displaying moderate to severe dysarthria and emotional lability (crying or laughing inappropriate to the stimulus).

Pyramidal Tract.   The pyramidal tract is composed of long axons that extend from cortical neurons and project uninterrupted until they reach the brainstem or medulla. The pyramidal tract is composed of white matter nerve fibers that pass in a bundle between the basal ganglia and the thalamus, which is called the internal capsule, as shown in Figure 4.1. One way to think of the pyramidal tract is that it functions like a neural turnpike, permitting the transmission of impulse from cortex to final pathway without interruption of local neural traffic. In contrast is

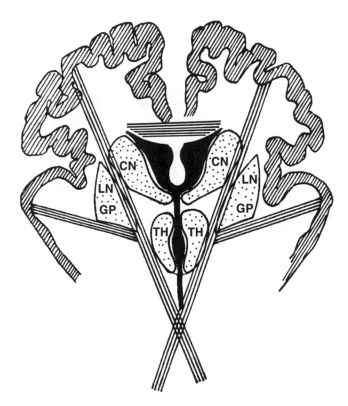

FIGURE 4.1   A Schematic View of the Pyramidal Tract

The pyramidal tract is like a neural turnpike with fibers descending uninterrupted via the internal capsule from their cortical origins to their decussation in the medulla. This line drawing shows basal ganglia (including CN, caudate nucleus; LN, lenticular nucleus; GP, globus pallidus) and TH, thalamus. Pyramidal fibers are depicted as ≡≡≡.

the extrapyramidal tract, which is more like a country road, stopping at multiple neural stations along the way. Phylogenetically, the pyramidal tract represents a newer bundle of fibers, developed most extensively in the human nervous system. It enables cortical voicing controls. For example, one might wish to cry out in anguish at a frightening event but protocol of some kind discourages it. Lower centers of the brain are ready to activate the "cry" but the human cortex enables the individual to suppress or delay the cry. Another example of the use of cortex via the pyramidal tract can be seen in our waiting to sing a note until the choir director points at us to sing. Instantly (near 100 msec), we can sing (thanks to uninterrupted cortical transmission via the pyramidal tract).

Extrapyramidal Tract.   The extrapyramidal tract (Figure 4.2) has most of its cortical origins in Brodmann 6 (superior frontal lobe). The axonal bundles carrying both afferent and efferent fibers extend to and from area 6 and go to many subcortical neural stations where they interconnect. Using the "country road" model, these extrapyramidal fibers stop everywhere, bringing neural transmission to areas of the basal ganglia (like the caudate and lenticular nuclei) across to the thalamus and subthalamus and then via the reticular system to the cerebellum, pons, and medulla. The extrapyramidal tract enables extensive checking and balancing between sensory information and motor response with its many interconnections between the thalamus and the basal ganglia. The examples of extrapyramidal function are numerous. For example, dribbling a basketball down the court is an example of coordinating a lot of visual, tactual, kinesthetic, proprioceptive, and auditory information into instantly changing motor responses. The act of just speaking will require a tremendous amount of sensory information. Or, when a singer is asked to sing an A3 note with "a little louder voice" when directed requires a great amount of sensory feedback to do so without being sharp or flat.

CNS, the Thalamus, Internal Capsule, and the Basal Ganglia.   The subcortical areas occupied by the thalamus, which is medial in the hemisphere, the internal capsule that runs laterally adjacent to it, and the more lateral basal ganglia are known collectively as the corpus striatum. It gets its name from the contrast of the gray matter nuclei and the white matter projections between them. The corpus striatum is the site of most of the sensory–motor integrations of the cerebrum. The thalamus is to sensation what the basal ganglia are to motor behavior. The thalamus lies more posteriorly within the cerebrum than the basal ganglia following the same anterior (motor function) and posterior (sensory function) pattern that represents the nervous system at all levels (cortex down to spinal cord).

Even the thalamus has its posterior (pure sensory) and anterior (sensory influenced motor) divisions. The posterior thalamus is known as the pulvinar body, which receives neural impulses from the auditory tract via the medial geniculates, the most inferior–posterior of the pulvinar. From the medial geniculates, after some central "mixing" within the thalamus, the auditory fibers radiate in a bundle superiorly to the primary auditory cortex, Heschl's gyrus. Similarly, the visual fibers come into the lateral geniculate bodies of the pulvinar section of the thalamus, undergo central "mixing," and exit in a bundle from the lateral geniculates and go directly to primary visual cortex (Brodmann 17) in the occipital lobes.

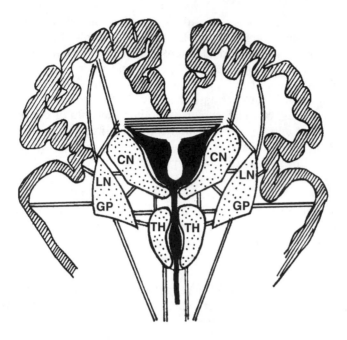

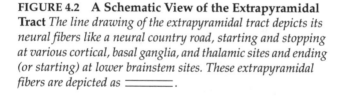

FIGURE 4.2   A Schematic View of the Extrapyramidal Tract *The line drawing of the extrapyramidal tract depicts its neural fibers like a neural country road, starting and stopping at various cortical, basal ganglia, and thalamic sites and ending (or starting) at lower brainstem sites. These extrapyramidal fibers are depicted as* ═══════ .

There is also some speculation (Boone, 1996, 1998; Minckler, 1972) that afferent–efferent fibers between the lateral wall of the pulvinar body and the temporale planum play an important role in auditory comprehension of the spoken word and some control in producing vocal response. Within the main thalamic body there appears to be much integration of sensory information occurring, getting organized for some kind of motor response via the anterior nuclei and ventral anterior nuclei of the thalamus. From the anterior thalamus, sensory projections go either directly to the sensory cerebral cortex or to nuclei within the basal ganglia.

It should be acknowledged at this point that the transmission of neural impulse between various nuclei via white matter nerves is facilitated by several enzymes, known as *neurotransmitters*. At the termination of nerves within the cerebrum, where neural synapses occur, serotonin functions as a nervous system neurotransmitter. The autonomic or sympathetic nervous system employs epinephrine and norepinephrine to aid in the transmission of neural impulses for innervation of smooth muscle, glands, and viscera. The basal ganglia are dependent on dopamine as the primary neurotransmitter. The facial, neck, and skeletal muscles are dependent on acetylcholine as the chemical mediator between the muscle's nerve nucleus and the muscle body itself. While neural transmission can be altered or stopped by isolated lesions to the gray body or its nerve connections, many of the diseases of the CNS cause inhibition or overproduction of neurotransmitter solutions. For example, in Parkinson's disease (described later in this chapter), situated close to the basal ganglia is gray matter known as the *substantia nigra,* which does not produce enough of the neurotransmitter dopamine to permit normal nervous system function. The symptoms of Parkinsonism result, but are vastly improved by a medication known as *L-dopa,* which artificially stimulates the production of needed dopamine, often resulting in a marked reduction of symptoms.

While there are some basal ganglia–thalamic connections crossing within the internal capsule, the main body of the internal capsule is largely composed of the descending–ascending neural projections of the pyramidal tract. The internal capsule area of the brain is highly susceptible to CVA, primarily because much of its blood supply is furnished by an artery known as the *lenticular striata* (often called the *artery of apoplexy*), which for some reason seems to be blocked by thrombosis more than other cerebral arteries. Such blockage of blood would cause white matter projections to die, resulting in contra-unilateral symptoms of paralysis (note: such a high-level lesion would not cause contralateral vocal fold paralysis). Any lesion (disease, CVA, or trauma) to the internal capsule could cause contralateral sensory–motor symptoms of skeletal muscles, classified as upper motor neuron lesions. Sensory loss could include hypesthesias and motor loss would be seen in hemiparesis or hemiplegia (paralysis with spasticity).

The basal ganglia utilizes the sensory information provided by the thalamus. The main nuclei of the basal ganglia are the caudate nuclei and the lenticular nuclei, which includes the putamen and globus pallidus. Bilateral innervations of both smooth and striated muscle occur within both the caudate and lenticular nuclei, and, at this level, we first see bilateral innervation of velar, pharyngeal, and laryngeal muscles. The basal ganglia utilize the continuous, multiple sensory information from the thalamus in organizing appropriate motor responses (including vocalization).

CNS, the Brain Stem and the Cerebellum. The projection fibers from both the pyramidal and extrapyramidal extend anteriorly into the pons and posteriorly via the cerebral peduncle terminating into the medulla oblongata. This cortical to lower center tract includes both afferent and efferent fibers. There are neural connections from the midbrain to the pons and on to the cerebellum and connections from the peduncle area into the cerebellum. The medial hypothalamus is the lowest structure of the midbrain, under which are the lesser (in number) gray bodies and myelinated nerve tracts (innumerable) that compromise the brain stem. The hypothalamus forms the lateral walls of the central third ventricle and connected to it are some gray bodies hugging the third ventricle acqueduct, containing important vegetative respiratory areas known as the periacqueductal gray (Davis, Zhang, Winkworth, and Bandler, 1996). Hypothalamic fibers, pyramidal, and extrapyramidal projections communicate anteriorly in the brain stem to the pons, while posterior fibers form the cerebral peduncle, which extends down, forming the medulla. The medulla extends from the lowermost portion of the pons with its upper portion forming the floor of the fourth ventricle.

The cerebellum wraps around the pons and cerebral peduncle and has many interconnections with the pons, cerebral peduncle, medulla, and spinal cord. The cerebellum functions as the great regulator of the extrapyramidal tract, coordinating sensory information (proprioceptive, kinesthetic, tactile, auditory, visual) with coordinated motor response. Lesions to the cerebellum from trauma or disease cause symptoms of incoordination. The voice–speech symptoms of cerebellar lesions are prosodic slowdown (scanning speech), changes in resonance, and inarticulate speech—all sounding like the speech of someone highly intoxicated.

Eighty percent of the descending projection fibers coming from the cerebral peduncle cross over (decussate) to the other side in the medulla just below the brain stem; 20 percent remain ipsilateral. Of great importance to voice is the nucleus ambiguus in the superior medulla, located just below the pyramidal decussation. As the medulla extends downward, it begins to narrow into the spinal column. The same posterior-sensory/anterior–motor organization continues in the medulla and down into the spinal cord. Posterior nerve tracts and gray nuclei (left and right) are sensory in nature while the anterior white matter tracts and anterior horn nuclei (left and right) execute motor function.

Let us consider briefly at this point what constitutes an upper motor neuron lesion or a lower motor neuron lesion. Functionally, an upper motor lesion produces symptoms of spasticity, such as in a CVA in which the patient may experience hemiplegia (one-sided spastic paralysis of extremities). A lower motor lesion, such as the cutting of the recurrent laryngeal nerve, causes unilateral vocal fold flaccid paralysis. Upper motor neuron function begins at the cerebral cortex and ends at the nucleus ambiguus; lower motor neuron function begins at the nucleus ambiguus and travels down the spinal cord, ending at the lowest spinal nucleus. Also included as lower motor neuron structures are the nerves exiting from the pons and medulla (such as the cranial nerves) and the nerves that carry sensory and motor impulses to and from the various spinal nuclei for their particular muscles. The autonomic motor system and these cerebrospinal nerves, including their associated sensory receptors, constitute what is known as the peripheral nervous system (PNS).

The Peripheral Nervous System (PNS)

We will limit our discussion of the peripheral nervous system primarily to those cranial nerves that have direct impact on voice, and, in particular, two branches of cranial nerve X, the Vagus, that innervate the larynx, the superior and recurrent laryngeal nerves.

While cranial nerves V, VII, and VIII have direct impact on speech, they do not appear primary in the production of voice. Cranial nerve V, Trigeminal, emerges from the pons with its primary motor fibers innervating the muscles of mastication; the sensory components that might influence voice are the tactile sensations of the nose and oral mucosa. Cranial nerve VII, Facial, leaves the lower portion of the pons and terminates in its motor innervation of facial muscles; its sensory components include taste in the anterior two thirds of the tongue and sensation to the soft palate. Cranial nerve VIII, Acoustic, has its cochlear division ending in the dorsal and ventral cochlear nuclei in the superior medulla; leaving the cochlear nuclei, the auditory pathways begin and continue to various neural stations, ending in Heschl's gyrus in the temporal lobe. As mentioned earlier in this chapter and throughout the text, the auditory system appears to play a primary role in voice production and control.

Cranial Nerves (IX, X, XI, XII).   We will give special attention to cranial nerves IX, X, XI, and XII as each has some role in phonation and/or voice resonance. For each nerve, we will look at origin and insertion with a brief statement relative to nerve function, especially as it relates to voice.

Cranial Nerve IX, Glossopharyngeal.   Originating laterally in the medulla, the nerve passes through the jugular foramen coursing between the internal carotid artery and the external jugular vein and subdivides into its numerous branches that go to various innervation sites. Its functions include taste in the posterior third of the tongue, sensation to the fauces, tonsils, pharynx, and soft palate. Its primary motor innervation is to the superior pharyngeal constrictor in the pharynx and to the stylopharyngeus muscle.

Cranial Nerve X, Vagus.   The vagus nerve, in addition to its many functions of control of the autonomic nervous system involving thoracic and abdominal viscera, has two important branches that innervate the larynx, the superior laryngeal nerve (SLN), and the recurrent laryngeal nerve (RLN). In the next section of this chapter, we will present in greater detail the origins and functions of the SLN and the RLN. The vagus nerve originates in the nucleus ambiguus in the medulla from which it emerges laterally and courses its way, with continuous branching along the way, with particular branches terminating at the various innervation sites from the pharynx to the abdominal viscera. Affecting voice are the sensory components of the vagus with sensory innervation of the pharynx and larynx; motor aspects affecting voice include innervation of the base of tongue, middle-inferior pharyngeal constrictors, larynx, and autonomic ganglia of the thorax (affecting the respiratory aspects of phonation).

Cranial Nerve XI, Spinal Accessory.   Cranial nerve 11 is a motor nerve that has innervation of the neck accessory muscles as its primary function. It is composed of two sections, the cranial portion and spinal portion. The cranial branch originates in the nucleus ambiguus and emerges from the side of the medulla with five successive small rootlets. Some fibers are distributed to the superior branches of the vagus nerve, innervating the levator veli palatini and uvula. Fibers from the spinal portion of the nerve originate from the anterior horn of the spinal cord and merge with lower spinal portion fibers to innervate the major muscles of the neck, such as the sternocliedo mastold and the trapezius muscles. Lesions to cranial XI can cause obvious problems of resonance and in the contribution of neck accessory muscles to respiration.

Cranial Nerve XII, Hypoglossal.   The hypoglossal nerve is a motor nerve innervating (as the name suggests) the extrinsic and intrinsic muscles of the tongue as well as some of the neck strap muscles. The nerve originates in its own nucleus, the hypoglossus nucleus, in the lower medulla, exiting laterally and entering the hypoglossal canal in the occipital bone, descending and then moving laterally into its many innervation sites. The muscles it innervates are the omohyoid, sternothyroid, styloglossus, hyoglosus, genioglossus, geniohyoid, sternohyoid, and all of the intrinisc muscles of the tongue. Cranial XII has much to do with positioning of the larynx, i.e., depression or elevation of the total laryngeal body, and is essential for all intrinsic movements of the tongue. Its primary impact on voice is on resonance and quality.

Superior and Recurrent Laryngeal Nerves.   As the vagus nerve leaves the nucleus ambiguus and exits laterally from the superior medulla and descends down the neck, it soon begins a series of branches. The first and most superior nerve branch off the vagus is the pharyngeal branch that contains both sensory and motor branches that supply the mucous membrane and selected muscles of the pharynx and soft palate. The next branch off the vagus bilaterally is the superior laryngeal nerve.

The superior laryngeal nerve branches off the vagus at about the level of the carotid sinuses in the neck (above which begins the carotid artery bifurcation) and angles medially toward the superior larynx. The superior laryngeal nerve divides into two branches (internal and external). The internal branch provides sensory innervation to the mucous membrane at the base of the tongue and to the mucous membrane of the supraglottal larynx. The external branch provides motor innervation to part of the lower pharyngeal constrictor and to the cricothyroid muscles. Although presented briefly in Chapter 2, let us consider the function (and symptoms of disorder) of the cricothyroid muscle:

> *Cricothyroid (CT).* Like all intrinsic laryngeal muscles (except the transverse arytenoids), the cricothyroid muscles are paired (L and R). The muscle is divided into two parts, the recta and the obliqua. Contraction of the cricothyroid muscles increases the distance between the cricoid and thyroid cartilages, increasing the length of the vocal folds, which decreases their cross-sectional mass. This action results in an increase of vibratory frequency and is heard as a rise in pitch. This stretching action also contributes to an adducting action of the vocal folds. Lesions to the CT are relatively rare and are seldom due to trauma but more often are related to some form of viral neuropathy (Tucker and Lavertu, 1992). Inability to elevate vocal pitch is the primary symptom of CT disease or trauma; in the case of unilateral CT paralysis, there may also be extreme hoarseness and occasional diplophonia (because of the disparate tension between the two vocal folds).

The next nerve branching off the descending vagus nerve is the recurrent laryngeal nerve (RLN). The RLN branches off the vagus considerably below the level of the larynx, almost at the level of the middle of the trachea. The right RLN loops "behind the right common carotid and subclavian arteries at their junction and courses vertically to the larynx" (Zemlin, 1988, p. 370). The left RLN leaves the vagus at a lower level than the right RLN, looping under and behind the aortic arch before making its vertical ascent to the larynx. Of some relevance to its frequent accidental cutting during surgery is its precarious location in the neck, ascending to the larynx in a groove between the trachea and the esophagus; the RLN then divides into three branches that enter the larynx through the cricothyroid membrane. The RLN is vital to the abductory–adductory function of the larynx as it innervates the five intrinsic muscles of the larynx, as first introduced to the reader of this text in Chapter 2. At this point, however, we will reintroduce the five intrinsic muscles of the larynx that are innervated by the RLN, with a brief description of their function and voice symptoms if they do not receive their innervations:

Thyroarytenoid (TA). The thyroarytenoid muscle is the main mass of the vocal fold. The muscle originates on the posterior side of the thyroid cartilage, which is known as the *anterior commissure.* The medial portion of the muscle is often described as the *vocalis muscle,* inserting posteriorly in the vocal process of the arytenoid. The larger muscle portion of the TA, known as the *thyromuscularis,* leaves the inner thyroid cartilage wall and extends posteriorly to the anterior surface of the arytenoid muscular process. The TA muscle mass, its ligament, and its cover (known collectively as the *vocal fold*) when adducted serves as the primary protective valve of the airway. Airway protection appears to be the primary role of the larynx and the TA is certainly a primary valve in this protection. Secondly, the vibrating mass of the vocal fold produces phonation. Changes in pitch are related to changes in tension of the thyroarytenoid muscle, either from its internal muscle contraction or stretching from external causes. TA contraction also contributes to medial vocal fold adduction. Flaccid paralysis of this muscle resulting from cutting or trauma to the RLN will in time lead to vocal fold atrophy resulting in weakness in vocal fold approximation, midfold bowing, and dysphonia. Subtle changes of pitch variation required in normal talking and singing will also be compromised with lack of TA innervation.

Posterior Cricoarytenoid (PCA). The paired PCA is the lone abductor muscle of the vocal folds. Originating on the posterior surface of the cricoid cartilage, the muscle rises laterally and obliquely to the posterior muscular process of the arytenoid. When the muscle contracts, it rocks and slides the arytenoid on its cricoid mount, parting the arytenoids and abducting the vocal folds. The primary symptom of PCA paralysis is the inability to open the glottis on the involved side, creating a unilateral abductor paralysis.

Lateral Cricoarytenoid (LCA). The paired LCA is the primary adductor muscle of the vocal folds. The LCA originates on the superior, lateral surface of the cricoid arch and rises to the lateral muscular process of the arytenoids. When the LCA contracts, it slides the arytenoids together, which adducts the vocal folds. The LCA is an antagonist to the PCA: LCA relaxation facilitates PCA action and, conversely, relaxation of the PCA makes LCA adductory action easier. The primary symptom of LCA paralysis is vocal fold paralysis in the fixed, abducted, paramedian position.

Transverse Arytenoids. The transverse arytenoid muscles are the only unpaired muscles among the laryngeal intrinsic muscles. They are bilaterally innervated, crossing over the surfaces and space between the two arytenoid cartilages. When they contract, they have the effect of sliding the arytenoid cartilages together, contributing to vocal fold adduction. An RLN lesion may produce weakness or paralysis not only in transverse arytenoid function but in other adductory muscles as well.

Oblique Arytenoids. The oblique arytenoids are paired muscles, originating from the base of one arytenoid cartilage and rising obliquely to the apex of the opposite arytenoid. When they contract, they assist in bringing the arytenoids together, contributing to vocal fold adduction. It appears that, among those few people who can, with intent, produce ventricular phonation, differential contraction of the oblique arytenoids enables the more superior-lateral surfaces (the insertion points of the false folds) to approximate, resulting in ventricular voice. If a unilateral oblique arytenoid is paralyzed from lack of RLN innervation, this further contributes to unilateral adductor paralysis.

Having had a quick but somewhat intense look at the central and peripheral nervous system and the innervations of muscles responsible for voice, let us now consider neurogenic problems in vocal fold adduction and voice problems that typically appear in certain neurological diseases.

Neurogenic Problems of Vocal Fold Adduction

There are basically two distinctly different neurogenic voice problems related to faulty vocal fold adduction: (1) aphonia and hypophonia related to vocal fold paralyses, and (2) the hyperphonia that we find in spasmodic dysphonia. We will look at each disorder separately.

Track
7 & 9

Vocal Fold Paralysis

As we saw in Figure 4.1, the lower the lesion in the brain the greater the likelihood of vocal fold paralysis. In the medulla, below the point of tract decussation, lesions of nerve fibers may produce unilateral (ipsilateral) paralysis of the vocal folds. A lesion in the medullary nucleus ambiguus from which the vagus nerve exits or of the superior laryngeal nerve (SLN) or recurrent laryngeal nerve (RLN) after they have branched out of the vagus will produce a lower motor neuron, unilateral paralysis.

Cricothyroid Muscle Paralysis.   The SLN branches first or higher than the RLN from the descending vagus nerve and soon branches again into its internal and external branches that insert directly into the larynx. Because of its relatively direct course after it has branched out of the vagus down to the larynx, the SLN is rarely injured by trauma. Although other etiologies may be considered, viral infection appears to be the most common cause of SLN involvement, unilateral or bilateral, causing paralysis of left or right (or both) cricothyroid muscles (Dursun et al., 1996). Cricothyroid function is primarily in the tensing of the vocal fold, essential for elevation of pitch as well as contributing to vocal fold adduction. On examination, the patient displays a slight rotation of the involved vocal fold to the normal side as well as a slight bowing of the vocal fold on the involved side (Tanaka, Hirano, and Umeno, 1994). The patient's primary voice symptoms are an inability to elevate pitch and some breathiness (due to the bowing). The virally-caused cricothyroid paralysis is usually temporary, with the patient responding well to corticosteroids and antiviral agents; voice therapy has been found helpful in correcting the effects of the anterior glottal rotation (Dursun et al., 1996).

Bilateral Vocal Fold Paralysis.   Bilateral paralysis of the vocal folds is usually the result of central brain stem impairment of nuclei and descending tracts, and *not* the result of bilateral destruction of the recurrent laryngeal nerves. The patient is aphonic and has a vulnerable open airway. Bilateral vocal fold paralysis is usually accompanied by other symptoms, such as weakness or paralysis of the tongue, pharynx, or velum. Voice per se is of secondary concern to respiratory survival and feeding. Medical–surgical treatment is often needed to improve the efficiency of the airway by creating a tracheostomy. Andrews (1995) offers specific procedures for the SLP to use in working with young children with bilateral vocal fold paralyses, i.e., how to manage the tracheostomy, the use of tracheal valves, and the need for minimizing the negative effects of the vocal fold dysfunction on the child's expressive language and speech development.

Continued bilateral vocal fold paralyses may require surgery to improve greater airway competence in both children and adults. Surgical reinnervation of the muscles of the vocal folds has been successfully reported by Crumley and Izdebski (1986). Perhaps used more often is the unilateral removal of one arytenoid with cauterization of muscular attachments to stimulate eventual contracture, resulting in more anterior glottal closure with posterior airway dilation (Tucker and Lavertu, 1992).

Track
7 & 9

Unilateral Vocal Fold Paralysis. Disease or trauma to the recurrent laryngeal nerve (RLN) on one side is the most common form of laryngeal paralysis. The most common causes of unilateral trauma to the RLN is penetrating gunshot or stab wounds, surgical approaches to the neck and upper thorax, and accidental neck trauma (Shindo, Zaretsky, and Rice, 1996). Because of the extended course of the left RLN, traveling down the neck and looping around the aorta arch in the chest and then traveling up again to the larynx, the left RLN appears to be more prone to traumatic or surgical injury than the right RLN. When the RLN is compromised on one side, the laryngeal adductor muscles (particularly the lateral cricoarytenoid) are not able to perform their adductory role. This keeps the paralyzed fold fixed in the paramedian position for both inspiration and expiration (including attempts at phonation).

On endoscopy, we see the paralyzed fold remaining abducted as the normal vocal fold moves to midline. Because of the proximity of the folds at the anterior commissure, there is usually some anterior approximation, which helps to set the two folds into vibration during phonation attempts. Colton and Casper (1996) discount that there is any slight crossover of the normal fold to meet the paralyzed fold, and, generally, what we observe on phonation attempts is the vibration of the paralyzed fold set in motion by the outgoing airflow passing between the two folds, particularly at the anterior one-third. Also, the Bernoulli effect, described in Chapter 2, plays a role here in drawing the two folds together.

The voice in unilateral paralysis is markedly dysphonic or aphonic. Because many traumatic vocal fold paralyses have spontaneous recovery during the first eight months postonset, permanent corrective procedures should be delayed until, at least, nine months after onset. The SLP can help the patient develop temporarily a better-sounding, more functional voice. First, if the patient has normal cricothyroid muscle function, having the patient speak at a higher pitch will often contribute to better fold adduction and a better-sounding voice. Other facilitating approaches that are helpful are the half-swallow boom (McFarlane et al., 1998), masking, digital manipulation, and head positioning. It should be remembered that voice therapy attempts at this time are temporary, reserved for developing a more functional voice, and will not have any long-term effect in restoring neural innervation. Similarly, there is a temporary surgical procedure that can "fatten" the paralyzed fold sufficiently to produce better voice, the injection of autologous fat into the paralyzed fold, which has been found to increase functional medialization for a period of "at least 2 to 3 months" before the fat is absorbed away (Shindo, Zaretsky, and Rice, 1996).

During the eight months postonset period, while waiting for spontaneous recovery of the paralyzed vocal fold to occur, the patient should be offered several treatment options. McFarlane and others (1991), in comparing voice therapy as a treatment option to several forms of surgery for continued unilateral vocal fold paralysis, found voice therapy to be significantly more effective using these therapy approaches: elevation of pitch, fewer words per breath segment, digital manipulation, half-swallow boom (McFarlane et al., 1998), and head positioning. Another option is to offer the patient some kind of voice amplifier to use permanently.

Since Arnold (1962) introduced the injection of Teflon as a surgical approach for promoting better medialization, there are numerous reports (Dedo and Carlsöö, 1982; Lewy, 1983) in the literature citing advantages, problems, and precautions. In general, Teflon injection no longer appears to be the procedure of choice for unilateral vocal fold paralysis. In greater use today is collagen, reported to be successfully used in 119 patients with glottic insufficiency (Ford, Bless, and Loftus, 1992) who were injected with soluble bovine collagen. A distinct advantage of the collagen injection is that it can be custom contoured or recontoured to fit the glottal deficit without appreciable damage to surrounding tissues. Gelfoam (another often-used injection compound), Teflon, and collagen have been compared with thyroplasty in the treatment of unilateral paralysis (D'Antonio, Wigley, and Zimmerman, 1995); one disadvantage of injection approaches is that the vocal cover is often violated, resulting in increased stiffness.

Thyroplasty I is a surgical approach to medialization of the paralyzed fold, using a free-moving cartilage wedge to move the paralyzed fold to midline (Blaugrund, Isshiki, and Taira 1992). The surgeon cuts a rectangular window (4 by 12 mm) out of the thyroid cartilage on the side of involvement. The patient is conscious during the procedure and produces voice when the surgeon places the wedge at various sites against the paralyzed fold. When it is confirmed that a certain site produces the best phonation, the cartilage wedge is fixed surgically at that point. Thyroplasty in the hands of a competent surgeon produces excellent results (Lu, Casiano, Lundy, and Xue, 1996), and patients should expect "voice improvement as early as 1 month postoperatively and should remain stable with slight fluctuations for at least 6 months" (p. 576). Although there are few reports following thyroplasty patients and their voices over many years, it would appear anecdotally by these text authors (DB, SMF) that the vocal gains after thyroplasty appear to last for several years. Some patients, after injection or surgery, continue to display the hyperfunctional vocal behaviors they were using before treatment. Direct symptom modification can usually reduce such problems as squeezing the words out, using pushing behaviors, and using excessive glottal attack. Following injection or surgical forms of medialization, the SLP may help the patient reestablish a normal voice, giving some attention to adequate breath support, phonation free of effort, with some attention given to voice focus and adequate loudness.

Another procedure for unilateral paralysis, reported by Crumley and Izdebski (1986), involves reinnervating the paralyzed muscles by nerve grafts from the phrenic nerve, or by grafting a section of the superior laryngeal nerve with a portion of the hypoglossus nerve into the vocal fold adductor muscles. Laser surgery has been successful in decreasing open glottal space (Prasad, 1985) for bilateral adductor fold paralysis, and laser arytenoidectomy for bilateral abductor paralysis has successfully opened the glottis (Lim, 1985). Most surgical attempts at reducing the symptoms of unilateral or bilateral vocal fold paralysis need to be supplemented by voice therapy designed to produce optimum phonation with whatever glottal configuration is found after surgery.

Spasmodic Dysphonia

Spasmodic dysphonia is the most severe form of vocal hyperfunction, with the patient exhibiting a strangled harsh voice with observable effort in pushing the air out during most voicing attempts. Patients' voices sound strained, choked off with the attempts to voice, as if they are trying to push the outgoing airstream through a tightly adducted laryngeal opening. Endoscopic examination (Davis, Boone, Carroll, Darveniza, & Harrison, 1988) shows that the tight voice is indeed produced by hyperadduction (severe approximation) of the true folds, often accompanied by tight closure of the false vocal folds (ventricular folds) with supraglottal constriction of the aryepiglottic folds and contraction of the lower pharyngeal constrictors. The total laryngeal and lower pharyngeal airway appears to close down (McFarlane, 1988; McFarlane and Lavorato, 1984). No wonder we hear a strained, "strangled" voice in such patients.

In addition to the problem of voicing, patients with spasmodic dysphonia complain about the difficulties they experience trying to force expiratory air out whenever they desire to phonate. Aronson (1990) comments that the tight voice during adductor spasmodic dysphonia "occurs only during voluntary phonation for communication purposes and not during singing, vowel prolongation, laughing, or crying" (p. 161). However, in patients who have carried the diagnosis of spasmodic dysphonia for some period of time and who are more severe, we see symptoms of this disorder in prolonged vowels as well. The patients soon learn to expect phonation difficulties whenever they attempt to speak. In this sense, spasmodic dysphonia resembles stuttering. In European writings, in fact, the condition is sometimes called the *laryngeal stutter*. McFarlane and Shipley (1979) make a case for spasmodic dysphonia *not* being considered as laryngeal stuttering based on there being a greater number of important dissimilarities than important similarities between the two disorders. Most patients with spasmodic dysphonia experience some normal voice in certain situations. Case histories of these patients reveal that such situations as "talking to my cat" or "speaking to others in a pool while I tread water" are times when patients have experienced normal voice.

The most common type of spasmodic dysphonia appears to be related to tight laryngeal adduction (known as adductor spasmodic dysphonia). Aronson (1990), however, also describes a second form of the disorder, known as abductor spastic dysphonia. Patients with this disorder exhibit normal or dysphonic voices that are suddenly interrupted by temporary abduction of the vocal folds, resulting in fleeting aphonia. After such momentary aphonia, the patients' voice patterns are restored again (until the next aphonic break). Endoscopy shows that the vocal folds of such patients abduct suddenly, "exposing an extremely wide glottic chink" (Aronson, 1990, p. 185). More often than not, the abductor spasms appear to be triggered by unvoiced consonant sounds. The abductor-type disorder is a much rarer form of spasmodic dysphonia. For example, Davis and others. (1988) reported that of 25 successive cases of spasmodic dysphonia observed in a Sydney, Australia, hospital, 24 were adductor type and one was an abductor type. The abductor spasm can often be treated successfully as a phonation break. Watterson and McFarlane (1992) make a strong case for considering the abductor type as a different disorder altogether and not a subtype of spasmodic dysphonia. Colton and Casper (1990) also seem to indicate that the two are different in pathophysiology and require different treatments. The symptoms and the treatment between adductor and abductor spasmodic dysphonia are so different, the authors of this text will confine our further comments about spasmodic dysphonia to the adductor type. Symptoms and treatment for the sudden abductory spasms described by Aronson (1990) may be found in Chapter 7 under abductor spasms.

Spasmodic dysphonia (SD) today is classified as a form of focal dystonia. Dystonia is a neurological dysfunction of motor movements, either more generalized to major body movements or seen in focal disorders, such as in the eyelids (blepharospasm), in the neck (torticollis), or in the larynx (spasmodic dysphonia). The site in the brain where a lesion might occur that would cause spasmodic dysphonia is still not definitively known. One of the first studies using MRI, SPECT, and BEAM for identifying possible SD lesion sites was reported by Finitzo and Freeman (1989) who concluded that "SD is a supranuclear movement disorder primarily, but not exclusively, affecting the larynx. Fully half of our subjects evidence isolated functional cortical lesions" (p. 553). While there is increasing consensus among medical and voice pathologists that SD is a neurological problem (Blitzer and Brin, 1991), the treatment of SD has not embraced symptom-modifying medication or intracerebral neurosurgery treatments. Of all the intrinsic laryngeal muscles (except the important adductor, the lateral cricoarytenoid, which was not studied), it has been clearly demonstrated using simultaneous EMG recordings that only the thyroarytenoid (the vocal fold) has abnormal muscle activation during SD-voicing (Nash and Ludlow, 1996). What are the treatment options available today for reducing the hypertonic approximation of the vocal folds during SD-voicing attempts?

Let us consider separately several treatment options that can be offered to the SD patient: voice therapy, surgical cutting of the recurrent laryngeal nerve, BOTOX injection, and surgical modification of the vocal folds.

Track 8

Voice Therapy for SD.   For a clinical lifetime, this writer (DB) encountered each new SD patient with the optimism that the strangled-sounding, harsh voice could be modified by voice therapy, only to find repeatedly with each new patient that apparent success in producing an easy normal voice temporarily in the voice clinic seemed to have no carryover out of the clinic. Case (1996) writes of similar failure with the SD patient, adding "Historically, the poor prognosis is one of the most significant symptoms of this disorder and has been pathognomonic and diagnostic to it" (p. 199). There have been a few reported positive outcomes for SD patients who have received voice therapy, such as Cooper's (1990) "direct voice rehabilitation" and the more conventional voice therapy reported by Shulman (1991). For the typical speech–language pathologist, our role with the SD patient is careful, meticulous assessment to permit evaluation of treatment outcomes and to combine voice therapy efforts with surgical treatment, before and after surgery (Murry and Woodson, 1995).

The description and quantification of the symptoms of spasmodic dysphonia require administration of perceptual judgment scales and instrumental measures. An excellent judgment scale was developed (Stewart et al., 1997) for assessing the SD patient, known as the Unified Spasmodic Dysphonia Rating Scale (USDRS). The Scale offers the SLP a standardized way of asking for speech–voice responses and a seven-point rating scale for evaluating such SD-voice parameters as overall severity, aspects of voice quality, abrupt voice initiation, voice arrests, loudness variations, tremor, expiratory effort, speech rate, speech intelligibility, and related movements and grimaces (Stewart et al., 1997, p. 100). The administration of the perceptual rating scale should precede such instrumental assessments as airflow/pressure data, fundamental frequency values, perturbation measures, and intensity documentation (see Chapter 5).

Some trial voice therapy should follow assessment, used at least as diagnostic probes. Many SD patients experience an easier voice with less effort "pushing voice out" through working on an easy breath cycle, employing the yawn-sigh, relaxation methods, coupled with hierarchy analysis. Boone (1998) has found both real-time amplification, auditory feedback, and masking (so patients cannot hear their own voicing) are facilitative for some SD patients. Speaking on inhalation is reported as less likely to reduce the symptoms of "long-standing adductor spasmodic dysphonia" (Harrison, Davis, Troughear, and Winkworth, 1992). Roy, Ford, and Bless (1996) have employed the musculoskeletal tension reduction techniques recommended by Aronson (1990) with over 150 cases of "muscle tension dysphonia," described under "massage" in Chapter 6 of this text. Included in the group of muscle tension dysphonia patients were some SD patients (the number was not specified in the article) who received the manual lowering of their larynx but experienced only "transient improvements in voice that could not be stabilized or generalized" (Roy, Ford, and Bless, 1996, p. 855). In summary, from long clinical experience and in reviewing the literature, there appear to be few SD patients whose difficulty getting air out while voicing with continued strained, harsh voice is resolved solely by voice therapy. It would appear that voice therapy coupled with laryngologic surgery offers the best therapeutic management of spasmodic dysphonia.

Recurrent Laryngeal Nerve (RLN) Sectioning. Introduced by Dedo (1976), the RLN section (Izdebski, Dedo, and Boles, 1984) was the first surgical procedure for SD that was widely used. Patients are selected for RLN section after a thorough diagnostic evaluation by both the surgeon and the SLP, which includes an injection of Xylocaine into the RLN, which produces a temporary unilateral adductor paralysis. The patient's airflow, relative ease of phonation, and change of voice quality are assessed. If there is marked improvement in airflow (greater flow rates with less glottal resistance) and in both ease and quality of phonation, the decision may be made to cut the RLN permanently. Postoperatively, then, the patient usually has an easily produced but breathy voice, similar in sound to the patient with unilateral adductor paralysis. Voice therapy focusing on a slight elevation of pitch, some ear training, head positioning and digital manipulation have all been effective in developing a better-sounding voice.

The long-term results of RLN resection have been mixed. Wilson, Oldring, and Mueller (1980) reported a woman who had received RLN cut 13 months previously who then experienced a regeneration of the severed RLN and a return of spasmodic dysphonia; a second RLN resection again produced immediate relief from her phonatory struggle. Over three years Aronson and DeSanto (1983) followed thirty-three patients with spasmodic dysphonia who had each received RLN cut. Although all experienced improved voice and ease of airflow immediately after surgery, three years later twenty-one of them, or 64 percent, had failed to maintain their gains and were considered failures. Much different results were reported by Dedo and Izdebski (1983) on over 306 patients who had received RLN cut for spasmodic dysphonia; they reported that 92 percent of the patients maintained voice improvement and required less effort to phonate.

The arguments over the long-term effectiveness of RLN section as posed by Aronson and DeSanto (1983) versus Dedo and Izdebski (1983) contributed to a significant reduction in the use of RLN sectioning as a treatment for SD. Regeneration of the severed RLN appears to be the primary factor in symptoms of tight voice coming back a few months or years after RLN section. To meet this regeneration problem, Weed and others (1996) recommended the use of avulsion (tearing out or entire removal) of as much of the recurrent laryngeal nerve as is surgically possible. In the Weed study, long-term follow-up of RLN avulsion patients revealed that "72 to 78 percent of patients retained clear benefit from the procedure beyond 3 years..." (p. 600).

The present authors combined treatment efforts with the surgeon, offering voice therapy after RLN section, primarily assisting the patient to take the struggle out of phonating. Even though higher airflow rates and lower pressures were noted after the RLN cut, some patients persisted in the habit-set of many hyperfunctional postures, such as pushing and working hard to produce outgoing expiration, grimacing, and continuing to experience a marked reduction in normal prosody. Most of these hyperfunctional postures were "unlearned" with voice therapy, allowing us to agree with Dedo and Izdebski (1983) that the vast majority (92 percent in their study) of patients continue for years to enjoy improved voices with ease of airflow after RLN section.

Botulinum Toxin (BOTOX) Injections.   The primary surgical method today for treating SD appears to be the injection of botulinum toxin (BOTOX) in one or both vocal folds (Miller, Woodson, and Jankovic, 1987). For many years, injection of BOTOX into muscles in spasm has been found effective for eyelid spasms (blepharospasm) and for severe neck muscle spasms (torticollis). One of the early reports of successful use of BOTOX injections for SD patients (Blitzer and Brin, 1991) found that BOTOX injection into the thyroarytenoid (TA) experienced by 210 SD patients was "a relatively safe and effective mode of therapy for laryngeal dystonia" (p. 88). BOTOX is injected into the TA, unilaterally or bilaterally in very low dosages (1 to 3 U). While the typical site of injection for SD is on the vocalis section of the TA, there is strong research (Inagi, Ford, Bless, and Heisey, 1996) that found the best postinjection voice and the voice that lasted the longest was the result of unilateral injection toward the posterior end of the TA with some absorption occurring in the lateral cricoarytenoid (LCA). These authors concluded that BOTOX appears to have the best effect with a single "unilateral injection placed strategically at the posterior portion of the TA and directed toward the LCA so that both muscle groups are affected" (p. 306). Other BOTOX teams continue to use bilateral injections with slightly lower BOTOX dosages injected into each TA (*Advance*, 1998). The amount of BOTOX required and the site(s) of injection vary according to the experience of the individual team members and the patient's response to the drug.

It is commonly observed in patients who have received BOTOX injection in the TA that they experience for a short time (two to three weeks) some mild symptoms of aspiration, coughing, and breathiness. Instead of tight phonation with low airflow rates with high subglottal pressures, the SD patient now displays temporarily the symptoms of a patient with unilateral vocal fold paralysis, i.e., high flow rate, low pressure, and a breathy voice. The patient at this time requires counsel from the SLP that the aspiration and breathiness are temporary. About three weeks after injection, the patient should return to the SLP for voice therapy. Murry and Woodson (1995) found in twenty-seven patients that those who received both injection plus voice therapy had significantly better flowrates and acoustic improvement than those patients who received only BOTOX without follow-up voice therapy. Typically, those patients who received both BOTOX and follow-up voice therapy will maintain good, functional voice from four to six months. As the patient experiences increasing adductory tightness while phonating, reinjection of BOTOX will be required. Although there is no definitive information available specific to long-range effects of continued BOTOX injection, the authors have contact with patients who have had in excess of a dozen BOTOX injections with no known measurable negative effects.

Murry and Woodson (1995) usually begin with "five voice-therapy sessions planned for each patient" (p. 462). Some patients may require less therapy and some may need more. Beginning therapy is designed to reduce continued vocal hyperfunction. The typical SD patient has used for many years hyperfunctional behaviors in an attempt to "push voice out." Even though such excessive effort is no longer needed after injection, the patient's habit-set of vocal hyperfunction continues. Counseling, showing the patient differential airflow rates, and listening to pre- and postinjection recordings can be used to help the patient cognitively recognize that effort for voicing is no longer required. A useful task is to model in front of a mirror or on videotape the saying of "ah" with no discernible effort, no visible neck muscle activity, resulting in a slightly easy, breathy voice. Stay with this task until the patient can demonstrate taking the "work" out of voicing. Therapy then follows with learning to find the optimal breath for saying a series of syllables on one expiration, perhaps reducing voice production in the beginning to saying only six to eight syllables per breath. If the patient is observed to squeeze out the last syllable or two, the syllable target per breath should be reduced further. Practice should be given to developing the number of syllables that can be comfortably voiced on one expiration. When breath volume gets low, the patient should pause; during the pause breath will renew without the patient doing anything consciously but pausing (Boone, 1997).

A voice therapy practice plan should be individualized for each postinjection SD patient. Telephone follow-up, with the SLP hearing the patient talk, can provide several things: (1) quality of voice can be observed (compromised of course by the telephone), which might signal that the patient should return for several therapy sessions; and (2) the need for possible reinjection can be determined by patient report and the sound of his or her voice. The patient with spasmodic dysphonia requires the long-term observation and treatment of both the speech–language pathologist and the laryngologist.

Surgical Modification of the Vocal Folds. The primary treatment options for spasmodic dysphonia are voice therapy, recurrent laryngeal nerve section, and BOTOX injection. Of the three, BOTOX appears to be the most successful and widely used. Medications, such as primidone, an anticonvulsant used primarily for control of generalized and psychomotor seizures, has been tried to relieve the tight, struggle phonation of SD patients and patients with essential tremor with relatively little success (Hartman and Vishwanat,1984). Beyond the use of primidone, there are very few reports of trial medication for reducing the breath struggle and voice symptoms of SD patients. There have been far more attempts at surgical modification of the tight airway closure at the level of the glottis.

Attempts at reducing the thickness of the vocal folds to reduce medialization tightness by application of CO2 laser was first introduced by Strong and Jako (1972) and later advanced by Abitbol (1994). Abitbol (1998) further presented the utilization of laser surgery for assisting in medialization of the vocal folds in paralysis as well as the opposite application of opening the airway in problems of excessive vocal fold approximation. Dedo (1997) reports that he occasionally combines laser surgery in SD to reduce vocal fold mass in combination with RLN sectioning. Various thyroplasty approaches have been attempted to improve vocal fold function in SD including unilateral arytenoidectomy to increase posterior glottal width (Hirano, 1989; Tucker and Lavertu, 1992), which then permits greater airflow. Another surgical attempt in SD was to slacken the vocal folds through surgical excision near the anterior commissure (Isshiki, 1989), reducing the glottal tension experienced by some SD patients. Of all the surgical attempts for treating the symptoms of spasmodic dysphonia reported in the literature, only RLN cuts and BOTOX injections continue to be used with relative success. The authors' prefer treatment with BOTOX injection followed by voice therapy.

Voice Problems in Neurological Diseases

The dysarthria that characterizes many neurological diseases (Kent, Weismer, and Kent, 1994) often includes many alterations of voice. In this section, we will consider several neurological diseases, presented alphabetically, that include changes in voice among their symptoms. Typical voice symptoms for each listed disease will be identified along with management steps that may aid in improving vocal function.

Amyotrophic Lateral Sclerosis (ALS)

ALS is a progressive degenerative disease of unknown etiology involving the motor neurons of the cortex and the gray bodies within the brain stem and spinal cord. Involving both upper and lower motor neurons, the disease is often called *motor neuron disease.* The speech–language pathologist often sees these patients initially relative to their early complaints of difficulty in articulating rapid speech, experiencing occasional hoarseness, and complaining of occasional swallowing problems. On peripheral oral examination, on extension of the tongue, fasiculations (traveling, wavelike muscle tremors) on the surface of the tongue may be observed. The diagnosis of ALS often requires a muscle biopsy to identify lack of innervation to particular muscle groups; the diagnosis is often related to exclusion of other identifiable etiologies. As ALS progresses, the patient experiences proximal atrophy of extremities rather than distal (for example, shoulder atrophy before hand involvement or back tongue impairment more than anterior involvement). The ALS patient may develop voice harshness, hypernasality, back-pharyngeal resonance focus, breathiness, and monopitch (Silbergleit, Johnson, and Jacobson, 1997). In addition to these voice symptoms, these authors also report an articulatory deterioration and increasing dysphagia.

Of life-threatening concern is the patient's growing inability to clear the throat and to cough. Because most ALS patients are experiencing continuing bulbar involvement, more clinical focus needs to be given to swallowing/coughing, rather than to speech and voice per se. Yorkston, Strand, Miller, Hillel, and Smith (1993) present the speech scale from their Amyotrophic Lateral Sclerosis Severity Scale, which rates the patient's speech–voice function. In the early course of the disease, some voice improvement may occur by helping the patient renew breath more often, develop a high front voice focus, with some attention given to increasing speaking rate (we have found metronomic pacing to be helpful). Negative changes in the patient's voice performance by comparing such values as mean phonation time, frequency and intensity range, and jitter and shimmer ratios (Leeper, Millard, Bandur, and Hudson, 1996) usually correspond to progression of the disease.

As the disease progresses, the SLP must help the patient work on diet modification and swallowing (trying different head positions with good mouth closure). These patients have good cognitive function and follow suggestions well if the suggestions are within their motor ability to execute them. As the Yorkston scale suggests, eventually the patient may require some kind of augmentative communication aid. Before a communication aid is selected, the SLP must determine the patient's hand function and mobility. At about this time, the SLP should help the patient manage excessive pharyngeal–oral secretions by using syringe suction evacuation devices increased swallowing and medications.

Despite the relatively rapid progression of ALS, the SLP plays a vital role in the early management of the ALS patient. As the patient becomes more physically dependent, there is a greater need for verbal communication, requiring that the patient use maximally all voice and speech functions that are still available. With some SLP encouragement and practice by the patient on voice and speech intelligibility, within the motor limits imposed by the disease, better functional communication can be maintained but only for a relatively short time.

Cerebral Vascular Accident (CVA)

A CVA, known more commonly as a *stroke*, is a temporary impairment of blood flow to the brain. There are generally recognized three types of CVA: thrombosis (the most common obstruction, a clot forms within an artery obstructing the flow of blood); embolus (a traveling blood clot that lodges within an artery preventing the flow of blood); or hemorrhage (blood flows out of a break in an arterial wall).

Because the distribution of blood for most of the higher areas of the brain (cortex through thalamus–basal ganglia) is distributed superior to the Circle of Willis, the blood supply to each of the two cerebral hemispheres is unilateral. That is, each hemisphere has its own blood supply. This is why most strokes appear to involve motor and sensory function on one side of the body. A CVA in the left hemisphere will produce a right-sided weakness or paralysis; a right hemisphere stroke will involve the left side of the body.

Voice is seldom affected by a single, unilateral cerebral lesion. Rather, lower bilateral lesions are much more likely to produce voice problems as part of a motor speech disorder (dysarthria). We can generalize this observation by this statement: The lower the lesion in the brain, the greater the probability of a voice problem. From the basal ganglia downward to the nucleus ambiguus in the medulla (Larson, 1988), laryngeal innervations are bilateral. Therefore, a unilateral lesion above the basal ganglia will not produce a unilateral paralysis of one of the two vocal folds. Figure 4.1 shows the separation of the left hemisphere from the right hemisphere. High unilateral lesions are likely to produce more isolated symptoms, such as aphasia or a one-sided paralysis (hemiplegia). As the fibers project downward connecting to many lower neuronal stations, we reach the "handle of the fan," where there are innumerable bilateral interconnections. At this low brain stem or medullary level, the patient may experience devastating motor and sensory losses, such as complete loss of speech and voice (anarthria).

Several successive strokes that produce bilateral cerebral lesions may produce severe voice symptoms, producing what is known as pseudobulbar palsy (Aronson, 1990). The voice symptoms are part of a severe dysarthria, which may include a strained/strangled voice quality, low pitch, monopitch, and reduced loudness with hypernasality (Murdoch and Chenery, 1997). Symptomatic of patients with bilateral pyramidal and extrapyramidal tract damage is emotional lability, which may severely influence voice quality and resonance. The patient will laugh or cry easily, inappropriately to the intensity of the stimulus. For example, we remember a fifty-five-year-old patient with pseudobulbar palsy who, when meeting an old friend, would appear to be crying on inhalation and laughing on exhalation. His lability-influenced voice would have severe posterior focus with extreme hypernasality. He had so much massive escape of airflow through his nasal passages that his oral articulation was severely compromised. When he cried or laughed, his speech was unintelligible. Management of his voice was best helped by attempting to reduce his lability.

Voice therapy for patients with voice problems caused by strokes is highly individualized, depending on the site and extent of the cerebral damage. The patient with a single, unilateral CVA may not have a voice problem. Lower and/or bilateral cerebral lesions may produce moderate to severe voice symptoms. For a voice problem that is part of a dysarthria, the SLP is advised both in assessment and possible therapy to determine the amount of involvement for each of the parameters of respiration, phonation, quality, and resonance; management of the problem will require working closely with medical and other rehabilitation therapies.

Essential Tremor. Patients with essential tremor may only produce tremor during voicing. When not speaking, there is no tremor observed; in essential tremor, there is no tremor at rest. When there are active muscle movements involved, there is tremor (known as intention tremor). The tremor appears present in tongue, velar, pharyngeal, and laryngeal structures, producing a vocal tremor in the 4 to 7 per sec range. Other patients with voice tremor may show similar tremorous movements in the hands, arms, neck, and face (Aronson, 1991). A common form of essential tremor is familial tremor, which may begin in early adulthood, in which the patient shows exaggerated tremorous behavior, showing more than the normal tremor that may be observed in people who are "overworking" particular muscles, such as may be felt or seen while carrying a heavy weight, "like carrying a case of twenty-four quarts of milk." Another form of essential tremor appears to be related to aging, although Colton and Casper (1996) and Greene and Mathieson (1991) report the senile form of tremor begins generally in the patients' late fifties.

Vocal tremor may also be heard in other neurogenic voice disorders, such as in spasmodic dysphonia and in Parkinson's disease. Such tremors must be differentiated from a diagnosis of essential tremor, which is basically intention tremor that appears to exist independently of other neurogenic conditions. The diagnosis of essential tremor is best made by eliminating contextual speech, asking the patient to sustain the production of vowels in isolation. The longer duration of the vowel, the more severe the tremor. On prolonged vowel production, the tremor is well isolated, permitting the frequency count and an acoustic evaluation of the tremorous voice. Endoscopic examination of the vocal folds while prolonging the vowel will show a structurally normal larynx with the vocal folds producing the alternate tension changes that are part of the overall tremor production. Flexible endoscopy can also reveal velar, pharyngeal, and tongue movements in absolute tremorous synchrony with one another, all contributing to the acoustic observation of voice tremor.

There is little in the literature to suggest adequate management of essential tremor, either medically or by voice therapy. The speech–language pathologist who first encounters an essential tremor patient, either of the familial or aging type, should make a referral to a consulting neurologist who might offer some medication control, reducing the severity of the tremor (but not its frequency). Professional meeting papers and anecdotal reports by voice clinicians offer three therapy approaches that seem to minimize voice symptoms: (1) reducing voice intensity levels appears to minimize tremor identification; (2) elevating voice pitch a half-note seems to change the tension level of the vocal folds sufficiently to reduce severity of the tremor; and (3) attempting to shorten vowel duration while speaking minimizes the identification of voice tremor (we are less likely to hear it). Aronson (1990) also writes that reducing "emotional stress and fatigue" seems to reduce the severity of the tremor.

Huntington's Disease (HD, or Huntington's Chorea)

The speech–language pathologist who encounters a Huntington's patient for the first time will be startled by the novelty and severity of speech and voice disorders. While the patient with mild beginning symptoms of HD will display prosody and voice changes that can be helped temporarily (the disease is rapidly progressive), the moderate to severe patient will show sudden, jerky prosodic changes with extreme changes in voice duration and loudness (Yorkston, Miller, and Strand, 1994).

Huntington's Disease is an inherited autosomal dominant degenerative, neurological disease in which the first symptoms begin to emerge in middle age (forty to fifty years). Each child of an affected parent has an even 50 percent chance of inheriting the disease, with the onset of symptoms delayed until middle age. The disease is an extrapyramidal disorder of the basal ganglia, characterized by an overabundance of dopamine. This results in the onset of the disease beginning with occasional jerks or spasms in either the extremities or more centrally in speech and voice, "progressing rapidly into chorea, athetosis, and mental deterioration" (Berkow, Beers, and Fletcher, 1997). The typical voice symptoms include strained/strangled voice quality, monopitch, excessive loudness variations, equal stress on ordinarily unstressed words, with sudden forced changes in breath control (Aronson, 1985). Among the most prominent symptoms are the jerky, irregular bursts of loud voice (Colton and Casper, 1996) and obvious interruptions of prosody.

In the early stages of HD, the SLP can guide the patient into maintaining better speech and voice, permitting good, functional communication. Voice seems to remain more normal when the patient works on easy, forward prosody, maintaining a rate near 150 syllables per minute. Both the DAF and metronomic pacer of the Facilitator can help the patient develop and maintain a slower controlled speaking rate. The slower rate seems to smooth out some of the unacceptable jerkiness. The yawn–sigh has been found a useful technique for opening up the vocal tract and developing ease of voice production. Similar to the patient with Parkinson's disease (another disease of the extrapyramidal tract), speaking with greater intention often enhances the patient's speech and voice behavior (Boone and Plante, 1993).

As HD progresses, with death occurring fifteen to twenty years after onset (Yorkston, Miller, and Strand, 1994), the patient usually begins experiencing some cognitive decline. At about this time, attempts at modification of speech and voice are no longer successful. Extreme choreic interruptions of airflow and flailing athetoid movements make speech intelligibility impossible. Because of both cognitive decline and severe motor control limitations, "there are no reports in the literature of successful application of augmentative communication technology in Huntington's disease" (Yorkston, Miller, and Strand, 1994, p. 158). Therefore, improving speech, voice, and functional communication in the HD patient is usually possible only in the first few years after onset of the disease.

Multiple Sclerosis (MS)

Among various demyelinating diseases, multiple sclerosis is the most common, affecting about 400,000 people in the United States (Berkow, Beers, and Fletcher, 1997). Although the cause of MS is believed to be viral, specific causes are unknown. This slowly progressive disease attacks the myelin sheath covering of nerves, literally causing breaks in transmitting axons, within the white matter of the CNS and PNS. The symptoms of the disease depend on the site of involvement. The patient may experience either sensory deficits (tingling, numbness, visual changes) or motor deficits (weakness, spasms, lack of coordination); more commonly both sensory–motor systems are involved. Citing the early work of Darley, Aronson, and Brown (1975), nearly 60 percent of 168 MS patients studied were judged to be normal in speech adequacy (Yorkston, Miller, and Strand, 1994).

The increasing presence of dysarthria with problems of voice in MS is generally related to multiple neural system involvement associated "with cerebral, brain stem, and cerebellar involvement" (Yorkston, Miller, and Strand, 1994, p. 192). The voice problems experienced by MS patients were earlier described (Darley, Aronson, and Brown, 1975; Farmakides and Boone, 1960); they are listed here in descending order of most common to least common: impaired loudness control, harsh voice quality, a scanning sameness of prosody and voice pitch control, decreased breath control, and hypernasality. If the MS patient is experiencing some or all of these symptoms, direct voice therapy can often minimize symptom effects, improving the patient's communicative effectiveness. Considering the progressive nature of the disease, communication between caregiver and the patient is increasingly needed.

Changing the patient's speaking rate (slightly slower or faster) will often have positive effects on loudness and harshness. The patient learns to pace speech (Yorkston, Beukelman, and Bell, 1988) or uses the metronome pacing program developed for use with the Facilitator (Boone, 1998). Improving rate control is also consistent with developing better coordinated breath support. MS patients may profit from reducing the number of words they say on one expiratory breath. Baseline measures of expiratory breath control can serve as a starting place. The SLP then instructs the patient to cut in half the number of words he or she has been saying. This reduces vocal fold tension, the tendency to squeeze out the last words of an utterance. Developing good vertical postural habits with the patient, keeping the chin down, and minimizing mouth opening (while at rest) all seem to afford the MS patient a neutral postural-set before initiating speech–voice responses. This postural control and attempt to pace an even spoken response seems to inhibit the sudden jerkiness and loud voice excesses that interfere with effective communication.

In the advanced stages of the disease, natural speech–voice may not be possible. Setting up alternative means of communication, also, may have many obstacles, as the patient's hand control for using keyboards, pointing, or pressing switches may be seriously compromised by ataxia, spasticity, and excessive tremor. Also, in advanced stages of multiple sclerosis, the patient may have severe visual problems and even blindness.

Myasthenia Gravis (MG)

Some patients with myasthenia gravis experience problems of severe voice fatigue with associated problems in adequate breath support. MG is an autoimmune disease in which the neuromuscular junction becomes impaired as the patient uses that particular muscle or muscle group, resulting in extreme muscle fatigue. Muscles innervated by the cranial nerves in the head and neck are particularly vulnerable to the disease. In MG, the immune system (for reasons unknown) produces antibodies that attack the receptors that lie on the muscle side of the neuromuscular junction (Berkow, Beers, and Fletcher, 1997). Symptoms occur because there is damage to the receptors at the neuromuscular junction, preventing the normal transfer of impulse from the nerve into the particular muscle. The disease occurs twice as often in women over men with females reporting the onset in their thirties and men reporting onsets in their sixties.

Typically, sustained repetitive performance of a particular muscle group will lead to a complete performance fatigue: Tapping two alternate notes repeatedly on a piano will result in a progressively slower tapping rate with eventually an inability to continue the task. For the mysathenia gravis patient with voice problems, the patient experiences a vocal change with voice usage from a normal voice to a breathy, weak, barely audible voice. With a few minutes of complete voice rest, the voice will be restored, but after a few minutes of usage, the weak voice will return. In severe cases, the patient will report difficulty swallowing with occasional nasal regurgitation (Hopkins, 1994).

The diagnosis of myasthenia gravis should always be suspected in patients who experience weakness after usage of the muscles of the eye, face, and throat, but with some recovery after rest. Because acetylcholine receptors are blocked, drugs that increase the amount of acetylcholine are useful in helping to confirm the diagnosis. "Edrophonium is most commonly used as the test drug; when injected intravenously, it temporarily improves muscle strength in people with myasthenia gravis" (Berkow, Beers, and Fletcher, 1997, p. 333). Accordingly, the treatment of MG is primarily medical, giving medications that increase levels of acetylcholine.

The speech–language pathologist often plays the primary role in discovery of the disease. Patient complaints of deteriorating voice after usage, particularly when coupled with other visual symptoms, such as a drooping eyelid (ptosis), or new problems in swallowing, should be referred through the patient's primary care physician to a neurologist. At the time of the evaluation, the SLP should give the patient sustained oral reading tasks; a determination should be made of how long oral reading must continue before vocal–speech deterioration is heard. From the onset of voice change, time measurements should be made of continued oral reading until further voicing is almost impossible. Then determine the amount of time required before there is some restoration of vocal strength. Beyond oral reading, the SLP might take measures of airflow/pressure, spirometric determination of air volumes, test diadochokinetic rates for various oral tasks, make glottographic determinations of vocal fold approximation, and administer articulation tests. Once the patient is receiving treatment with some form of drug regimen, the SLP should select any of these measures for comparison over time, giving objective evidence of medication effectiveness. The SLP's role is one of discovery and comparison of motor response data over time, and not one of providing voice therapy. With appropriate acetylcholine levels achieved through medication, MG patients will usually experience the levels of speech and voice competence they had before the onset of symptoms.

Parkinson's Disease (PD)

There is probably no neurogenic speech–voice disorder that has had more written about it than the descriptions of Parkinson's disease (Lieberman, 1992; Ramig, Bonitati, Lemke, and Horii, 1994). Parkinson's disease is a degenerative, progressive disease of the basal ganglia, manifesting itself in a hypokinetic dysarthria, nonintention tremor (at-rest tremor), with sluggish initiation of motor movements (such as gait). PD affects "about 1 out of every 250 people over 40 years old and about 1 in every 100 people over 65 years old" (Berkow, Beers, and Fletcher, 1997, p. 315). The disease is caused by a lack of sufficient dopamine (from several different causes) in the substantia nigra of the basal ganglia, which seriously limits neurotransmission within the basal ganglia and to and from the thalamus. This interruption of normal neurotransmitter activity causes severe slowness of motor movements or hypokinesia.

The Parkinson patient exhibits a hypokinetic dysarthria characterized by reduced loudness, breathy voice, monotony of pitch, intermittent rapid rushes of speech, and soft production of consonants. Some investigators of PD have found diminished function in one or more components of speech–voice; for example, Solomon and Hixon (1993) found significant respiratory difficulties as possibly contributing to the PD patient's voice symptoms; Ramig and others (1994) found that thirty-five of forty PD subjects had bowed vocal folds. It would appear that isolation of any one speech component for study in the PD patient will find a deficit in function. Fortunately, the most effective voice therapy approach is a holistic one, finding that to exaggerate one component helps improve function in all other components.

When patients attempt to speak in a quick conversational pattern, speech is often unintelligible. When they speak with intent, however, their speech can be slower, louder, have better voice quality, and better articulation. Following the model of intention used in physical therapy for gait training (thinking where you are going to place each foot as you walk makes walking easier), the same model of intent works to improve speech. Using intention with these patients, the writers have asked PD patients to speak with an accent, or use a different pitch, or speak slower, or speak louder (Boone and Plante, 1993). Taking the automatic motor-set out of speaking by speaking intentionally different seems to help the patient's speech in all parameters: loudness, voice quality, appropriate pitch, and rate. Ramig and others (1994) have demonstrated the effectiveness of using the intention model with Parkinson's patients by asking the patient to speak louder, thinking "shout."

Ramig's observations have been formalized into a therapy program for the Parkinson's patient, known as the Lee Silverman Voice Treatment (LSVT) (Ramig and others, 1994). One study of LSVT effectiveness had forty PD patients receive one hour of voice therapy four times a week for one month, receiving thirteen to sixteen hours of individual voice therapy. There were three general therapy tasks: increasing vocal fold adduction, increasing respiratory support, and increasing maximum fundamental frequency range. Of all the therapy tasks, speaking "louder shout" seemed to be the most unique and beneficial part of the Silverman therapy approach. There was significant improvement in all variables studied between pre- and posttherapy treatment. It would appear that voice therapy, as outlined in the Ramig-designed program, is the only voice–speech therapy program that has been documented at this time to be of help to these patients.

The diagnosis of Parkinson's disease and its medical management belongs to the neurologist. Besides speech and voicing problems, the PD patient begins to develop problems of gait, difficulty initiating the sequential movements required for dressing, feeding, and overall self-care. In mild to moderate cases, Lieberman (1992) recommends that the low levels of dopamine in the PD patient be raised by placing the patient on a regimen of levodopa, "the single most effective antiparkinson drug" (p. 558). Over time, the period of relief from continued levodopa administration becomes shorter, requiring new medication protocols and possible neurosurgical approaches, such as anterior thalamotomies (Stacy and Jankovic, 1992).

Summary

We looked earlier in the chapter to a schematic model that showed the pyramidal tracts moving from the cortex nonstop to their final terminus in the medulla or further to spinal cord stations. We then looked (with a bias toward understanding voice) at the many stops and intraneuronal connections of the extrapyramidal tract, interconnecting the basal ganglia, the thalamus, the brain stem, and the cerebellum. At the level of the pons and below, we looked at the cranial nerves, which in particular play primary roles in voicing. Vocal fold adductory problems were seen in vocal fold paralysis and in spasmodic dysphonia, with management and therapy hints for the speech–language pathologist. Six more common neurological diseases, often seen by the SLP, were presented from the perspective of the SLP in his or her management and voice therapy.

CHAPTER

5

Voice Evaluation

When confronted with a patient presenting with a voice disorder the speech–language pathologist begins a systematic process of assessment, evaluation, and diagnosis. This is indeed a process and is ongoing rather than being accomplished in the first meeting of the SLP and the patient. Also, voice evaluation is the first step in the treatment process of a voice disorder. Although identification of a deviant voice may come from several sources (parents, teachers, school nurse, physician, employer, or coworker), the voice evaluation must be a carefully and scientifically conducted procedure performed by a competent speech–language pathologist. Voice evaluation may either precede or follow a complete examination of the patient by the laryngologist. However, the laryngological results must be considered with the rest of the findings of the voice evaluation in order for the voice clinician to make a tentative voice diagnosis and a treatment plan. While it is the province of the ENT physician to make a medical diagnosis of the larynx, it is the province of the voice clinician to make the voice diagnosis (analysis of the acoustic, perceptual, and physiological factors) and to plan voice treatment. These two diagnoses (laryngeal diagnosis by the laryngologist and voice diagnosis by the speech–language pathologist) are combined to guide in the best management of the patient's voice disorder.

Successful voice therapy is highly dependent on how well the voice clinician can identify what the patient is doing vocally. The typical voice evaluation is completed after someone else, such as the laryngologist, has already diagnosed the presence or absence of laryngeal pathology that may be contributing to a voice disorder. The speech–language pathologist must make a detailed analysis of what the patient is doing relative to respiration, phonation, and resonance. To do this, he or she makes good use of whatever medical descriptions of the problem may be available, takes a detailed case history, observes the patient closely, uses those testing tools and instrumentation (to include visualization of the larynx via videoendoscopy and stroboscopy by the speech–voice pathologist, (ASHA 1992b; McFarlane, 1990; Watterson, 1991) necessary to make an accurate assessment, and introduces to the patient various therapeutic probes (clinical stimulation) to obtain clues about what direction the voice therapy should take. Two important points need to be made here. First, the joint statement of the American Academy of Otolaryngology, voice and swallow committee, and the American Speech, Language, and Hearing Association Special Interest Division on Voice and Voice Disorders (1998) confirms the role and scope of practice of the speech pathologist to include visualization of the larynx by strobovideolaryngoscopy. Second, both the

ENT and the SLP need to combine their information and expertise to best serve the needs of the patient with a voice disorder.

Although we present the voice evaluation here in a separate chapter, it is important for the reader to appreciate that voice evaluation and voice therapy cannot be separated. Effective voice therapy requires continuous, ongoing assessment. Evaluation and therapy overlap. What is found at the evaluation and given back to the patient as a form of feedback may also have great therapeutic value. Indeed Weiss and McFarlane (1998) reported an investigation that demonstrated that the response to clinical stimulation during the initial diagnostic session can be both a guide to voice therapy and a preview to the outcome response to voice therapy. They found that a comparison of pretreatment jitter values in unstimulated and stimulated conditions during the diagnostic session provides some indication of a patient's response to voice therapy (Weiss and McFarlane, 1998). Further, McFarlane, Watterson, Lewis, and Boone (1998) demonstrated that clinical facilitation techniques can be used in the initial diagnostic session with unilateral vocal fold patients to indicate the airflow wastage, which may be reduced by various techniques. This aids the voice clinician to select among various clinical techniques in the planning of voice therapy. Using various therapy approaches as diagnostic probes in an attempt to identify a patient's best possible voice can be an important part of every therapy session. Many of the evaluation procedures and tools described in this evaluation chapter are also used by clinicians in voice therapy. Finally, while we believe in the value of using appropriate instrumentation to evaluate and diagnose voice disorders, the best instrument remains the scientific and clinically trained mind, followed closely by the trained ear and trained eye.

We will discuss two major areas in this chapter: voice screening and voice evaluation.

Voice Screening

Speech–language pathologists in the public schools are in an excellent position to develop voice screening procedures for the early identification of children with voice problems. Most public and private schools have speech screening programs for new children and for all children in certain grades at specified times of the year. For example, in the fall, clinicians may screen all children in kindergarten and third grades. By using some kind of voice screening form, clinicians are able to make better judgments about the parameters of voice. With very little additional testing time per child (perhaps 60 to 90 seconds), a voice screening program can be added to existing speech- and language-screening measures.

Different clinicians in various settings have developed various screening forms. The items on the form usually represent the aspects of voice that the clinician considers important for identifying children who may be having voice problems. The screening form helps clinicians focus and organize their listening observations. Wilson (1987) recommends that clinicians use the following tasks in voice screening: counting from one to ten; giving a connected speech sample (one minute); reading a sample (one minute); and prolonging for five seconds each of five selected vowels (high to low). Previous screening forms published by Boone (1973, 1977) have included observations specific to rating the parameters of pitch, loudness, quality, and resonance. These forms have generally been modified as they are field-tested and used in various settings. We have found, over time, for example, that the rating task must be as focused as possible to be useful. The more parameters to be rated and the more gradations of the rating, the poorer the reliability in using the form. Nonetheless, McFarlane, Holt, and Lavorato (1985) and McFarlane and others (1991) have reported that even lay listeners can be nearly as accurate as speech pathologists or ENT physicians in rating voice disorders if the vocal parameters are well defined and limited in number. These authors used a ten-point scale for each of six vocal parameters (pitch, loudness, hoarseness, breathiness, roughness, and overall vocal quality).

The form in Figure 5.1 offers clinicians the information they need for a screening test (Boone, 1993). The single criterion for each of the scale judgments (pitch, loudness, quality, nasal resonance, oral resonance) is whether or not the child's voice on that particular parameter sounds like the voices of peers of the same age and sex. If a child's voice appears lower in pitch than that of peers, the minus sign (–) is circled on the form; if pitch appears normal, the neutral symbol (N) is circled; if the pitch level is higher than the child's peers, the plus sign (+) is circled. This simple three-point scale is especially useful for rating the parameter of pitch because, as McFarlane and others (1985, 1991) point out, all of their listeners (speech pathologists, lay, and ENT) had the most difficulty making consistent and accurate judgments of the pitch parameter.

Inadequate loudness is specified as minus (–); normal loudness as neutral (N); and excessive loudness as +. Any deviation of quality is represented by – or +; a breathy, hoarse voice is marked as –, and a tight, harsh voice as +. If denasality (insufficient nasal resonance) is noted, the form is checked –; normal nasal resonance is marked N, and hypernasality is characterized by +. Oral resonance deviations do not occur as often as other problems; however, excessive posterior tongue carriage that produces inadequate oral resonance is marked as –, no problem in oral resonance is N, and excessive front-of-the-mouth resonance characterized by a baby voice (thin vocal quality) is marked as +. If the child receives either – or + on any of the five clinical parameters, he or she should be rechecked. If problem areas are again identified, a complete voice evaluation (McFarlane, 1990; Watterson, 1991) would be recommended (Boone, 1993).

Most screening forms allow a brief space for comments examiners may want to add to the screening data. For example, the notation "she had a bad cold" would be helpful information for a follow-up visit with someone previously noted as exhibiting "denasality." At the second visit, screening data are compared with present observations. Arrangements should be made for full voice evaluations for those individuals who on follow-up continue to show some departures in voice from their age–sex peers.

The Voice Evaluation and Medical Information

Voice patients evaluated by speech–language pathologists have either been "discovered" in voice screening programs, or referred by teachers and other professionals in the schools, referred by physicians (usually laryngologists), or self-referred. Regardless of the referral source, in early contacts with the patient the

FIGURE 5.1 A Voice Screening Form

VOICE SCREENING FORM
The Boone Voice Program for Children

Name ______________________ Sex M F Grade ____________
School______________________ Teacher ______________________
Examiner ____________________ Date_________________________

VOICE RATING SCALE

Circle the appropriate symbol(s)

Pitch	– N +	Describe:
Loudness	– N +	Describe:
Quality	– N +	Describe:
Nasal Resonance	– N +	Describe:
Oral Resonance	– N +	Describe:

S/Z RATIO

Record 2 trials of [s] and 2 trials fo [z] expirations

s = _______seconds
s = _______seconds

Longest s ÷ by Longest z = S/Z Ratio: _______

z = _______seconds
z = _______seconds

DISPOSITION:

❑ Complete voice evaluation required
(one or more rating of + or – or an S/Z ratio of greater than 1.2)
❑ No further evaluation required
❑ Second screening required _______
(Date)

Comments:

10 9 8 7 6 5 4 3

Additional copies of this form may be purchased from PRO-ED, 8700 Shoal Creek Blvd., Austin, Texas 78758 512/892-3142

(*The Boone Voice Program for Children*, Austin, Texas. Copyright © 1993 by PRO-ED, Inc.)

speech–language pathologist will arrange for a full voice evaluation. For those patients not referred by laryngologists, part of the evaluation process may include a medical evaluation. Occasional voice patients, such as those who do not talk loudly enough or those who use aberrant pitch levels for what appear to be functional reasons, may not require medical evaluation. Patients with voice quality and resonance problems generally require some medical evaluation of the ears, nose, and throat as part of the total voice evaluation.

The most effective voice rehabilitation programs seem to have close team cooperation between the speech–language pathologist and the laryngologist (McFarlane, 1990; Watterson, 1991). Unfortunately, some rural areas of the country still have no laryngologists, and it is not uncommon for speech–language pathologists in these areas to report that there are no medical doctors available who can perform **indirect laryngoscopy** (mirror view of the vocal folds). The speech pathologist in such a situation should confer with the patient's local physician, saying, for example, "Tom seems to be hoarse every day. Could you please see that his vocal folds are examined?" Rarely will a physician not appreciate such a request. Physicians who feel that they do not possess the skills required for indirect laryngoscopy will refer the patient to a laryngologist. It is not unusual for patients living in remote areas of the United States to travel several hundred miles for an examination by a laryngologist.

A laryngeal examination must be completed before a patient can begin voice therapy for problems related to quality or resonance. As part of the diagnostic process the speech–language pathologist may wish to use therapy approaches as diagnostic probes. Indeed, Weiss and McFarlane (1998) demonstrated, in a recent empirical study, that responses to clinical facilitation techniques may be used as an indication of the outcome from voice therapy, and McFarlane, Watterson, Lewis, and Boone (1998) found that the response of sixteen patients with unilateral vocal fold paralysis to voice facilitation techniques applied during the initial diagnostic session was helpful in designing voice therapy. For example, asking a patient to turn the head, or receive digital manipulation, may provide important diagnostic information about how tighter vocal fold approximation (due to the application of these techniques) affects voice quality (see Chapter 6). The technique that improves the voice the most is initially used in voice therapy. Voice therapy efforts should be deferred until after the medical examination (which would include laryngoscopy) is concluded, because there are occasional laryngeal pathologies, such as papilloma or carcinoma, for which voice therapy would be strongly contraindicated, because these diseases require medical attention. In such cases, the delay of accurate diagnosis of these pathologies and the appropriate treatment could be life-threatening.

The laryngologist's examination includes an assessment of the larynx and related structures. The vocal folds are assessed by indirect mirror, or, more commonly now, by endoscopic laryngoscopy, and their color, configuration, movement, and position are noted. During the patient's quiet respiration, the laryngologist looks for the normal inverted-V position of the cords. For phonation, the patient is often asked to phonate a relatively high pitch, perhaps by extending an e-e-e (/i/) for several seconds. The higher the pitch, the further the epiglottis and root of the tongue are extended upward and forward, permitting a relatively unobstructed full-length view of the vocal folds from the anterior commissure to the arytenoids. A judgment is made on the adequacy of fold approximation during phonation. Other structures that may be examined include the ventricular folds, laryngeal ventricle, pharynx, tonsils–adenoids, nasal cavities, velopharyngeal mechanism, glands and muscles of the neck, and so on. The laryngologist's examination is directed at finding the cause of the patient's presenting voice problem and evaluating the overall status of the larynx and related mechanisms. If the laryngologist wants additional information about how the patient uses his or her voice, or if the laryngologist feels voice therapy may be needed, the patient will be referred directly to the speech–language pathologist. Such referral usually requires a written statement by the laryngologist describing the patient's problem. In actual practice, the written referral may be supplemented by a brief telephone conversation further describing the problem. The laryngologist's referral usually includes an abbreviated statement of the patient's history, a descriptive statement of the presenting problem, what was told to the patient, and a statement describing the results of evaluation and treatment direction, what medications were given (if any), and probable prognosis. It should also request an evaluation and voice diagnosis by the speech–voice pathologist and his or her suggested course of treatment.

The following letter of referral from a local laryngologist who placed strong and continued emphasis on voice therapy for most of his patients with hyperfunctional voice problems was taken from a clinic file:

> I have asked Pearl to see you for your voice evaluation at the earliest opportunity. This 44-year-old woman works as a secretary to an insurance executive, a position that requires much talking on the telephone. In the past six months she reports continued hoarseness, usually worse at the end of the day, and she complains of occasional pain in the general hyoid region after prolonged speaking. She is married, the mother of three young adult sons. Until six months ago, there was no history of vocal distress. On mirror laryngoscopy, I found the patient to have small bilateral nodes at the anterior one-third junction. Areas immediately adjacent to the nodes were characterized by increased vascularization, suggesting much irritation at this site. On cord adduction, there is noticeable open chinking on each side of the approximated nodes. Her voice, as you might suspect, is quite breathy with an audible escape of air, probably escaping through the open chinking. Inadequate voice loudness, also, appears to be a problem for her.
>
> I am referring her to you for your ideas on what she may be doing wrong with her voice. If you feel she would benefit from voice therapy, please schedule her. I told her that if you felt voice therapy were indicated, we would begin there. She appears strongly motivated to improve her voice and will, I'm sure, gladly accept whatever you recommend.

Physicians develop different methods of describing their findings for the speech–language pathologist. Their descriptions may range from a brief "normal vocal folds" to a multipage written evaluation. Typically, the speech–language pathologist may receive statements from the laryngologist similar to these:

> Large tonsils and adenoids; no need to remove at this time. Larynx normal. Bilateral thickening runs for the total AP distance on both folds. Could well be related to voice abuse. Could you take her on for voice therapy? No physical basis for the tight voice. Cords show good mobility and normal function. No cord lesions. Do you think she'd be a good candidate for nerve resection? A short, relatively immobile velum. Good symmetry. VP distance looks too excessive for normal closure. Recommend a pharyngeal flap. Could you do pressure–flow study and endoscopic photography? We'll staff her next month.

The laryngologist and the speech–language pathologist work together in planning both the evaluative procedures and remediation steps to be followed. Other professionals sometimes included in the evaluation, which we outline in

Chapter 9 when we discuss problems of nasal resonance, may include a pediatrician, plastic surgeon, a neurologist, an orthodontist, a prosthodontist, and a psychologist. Specialization today requires a team of professionals for the effective management of some patients with voice disorders.

We firmly believe in the advantages of a team approach; for example, we very rarely recommend surgical removal of nodules even in adults because voice therapy is generally effective for complete reduction of the nodules (McFarlane and Watterson, 1990). Even in cases of long-standing vocal nodules, we have been able to eliminate the nodules or, in some cases, normalize the voice with some residual (nonsymptomatic) nodules left. Note that it is possible to have normal vocal quality with some small remaining nodule tissue. In such cases, however, the ENT physician should be advised not to remove the remaining nodule tissue when the voice is normal in quality. Surgical removal of this small remnant is unnecessary and may actually jeopardize the newly established normal vocal quality, due to scarring. Similarly, we do not recommend surgical removal of contact granulomas or surgical removal of excessive benign polypoid vocal fold tissue. Finally, we do recommend voice therapy for unilateral vocal fold paralysis as soon as it is diagnosed because we can usually help patients obtain a much improved or even near normal voice with voice therapy while they are waiting to see if the nerve recovers (McFarlane, et al., 1998). Such treatment philosophies and observations are best shared when there is a good team relationship between the laryngologist and the voice clinician. McFarlane, Fujiki, and Brinton (1984) have discussed this team relationship from the view of the speech–language pathologist:

> The most desired goal is to be regarded by these professional practitioners as peer professionals. This means that we must be able to talk intelligently about their field (be "bilingual," using our jargon and theirs) and their clients, provide a valuable and effective treatment service to their patients, and possess a knowledge and skill base somewhat unique from these other specialties (pp. 133–134).

Some laryngologists prefer an evaluation form containing a glottal figure. This allows them to quickly make their statements and accompany them with a line sketch of the pathology (if present) specific to its site and size. Figure 5.2 shows part of such a form (Boone, 1980a) that would be completed by the examining physician and returned to the speech–language pathologist.

Community health centers and university clinics routinely obtain medical information and some case history data from patients when the initial appointment is made, and, if a voice problem is indicated, schedule the patient first for a medical diagnostic evaluation. Sometimes, however, a voice patient will make the initial appointment without identifying the problem as one of voice. If, for whatever reason, a patient arrives to be treated for some form of dysphonia but has not had a previous medical examination, the speech–language pathologist will want to defer final disposition of the patient until the medical information is obtained. The voice evaluation by the speech clinician may begin, however, even in the absence of the medical information. The case history can be taken, and respiration–phonatory–resonance observations and test data can be obtained; only the decision about whether to begin voice therapy need be deferred until the database is complete with the ENT exam results.

FIGURE 5.2   A Voice Referral to Physician Form

VOICE REFERRAL TO PHYSICIAN
The Boone Voice Program for Children

To the Physician: This child was recently seen for a voice evaluation. Voice therapy has been deferred until a medical diagnosis has been made. Please complete Section 2 of this form and return it with your recommendations.

Name_____   Sex   M   F   Birth Date_____   Age _____

School _____   Referring Clinican _____ Telephone_____

SECTION 1
Voice Evaluation Summary
(to be completed by Speech–Lanuguage Pathologist)

SECTION 2
Summary of Medical Findings
(to be completed by examining Physician)

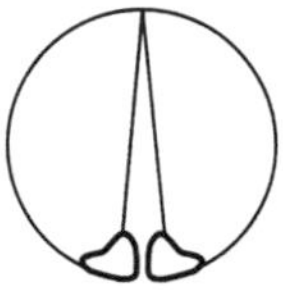

Indicate site and
extent of lesion

Recommendations:

_____ Voice therapy recommended

_____ Voice therapy not recommended

Comments:

Return this form to:

_____

_____

_____   Physician's Signature

_____
                                       _____

                                       Date

Additional copies of this form (#2353) may be purchased from PRO-ED, 8700 Shoal Creek Blvd., Austin, Texas, 512/451/3246.

The ethics and efficacy of speech–language pathologists themselves doing indirect laryngoscopy are worth discussing at this point (ASHA, 1998; Watterson and McFarlane, 1991; Watterson, McFarlane, and Brophy, 1990). Some speech–language pathologists are trained to perform endoscopy or mirror laryngoscopy, procedures that are not difficult to master; these persons use indirect laryngoscopy primarily to teach students laryngeal function and to observe the folds directly to determine any changes during therapy. As speech–voice pathologists, we use videolaryngoscopy and stroboscopy for research, for teaching purposes, for voice evaluation and voice diagnosis, and to develop new and more effective voice therapy treatment techniques. Appropriately trained speech–voice pathologists may employ laryngeal visualization techniques in accordance with ASHA (1992b) Guidelines for Vocal Tract Visualization and Imaging and scope of practice outlined in The Roles of Otolaryngologists and Speech–Language Pathologists in the Performance and Interpretation of strobovideolaryngoscopy ASHA (1998). Primary identification of laryngeal pathology is the clear responsibility of the laryngologist, who is also equipped with the medical techniques required to treat the pathology once it is identified. For the ethical and legal protection of the speech–language pathologist, the voice patient who comes in for evaluation without prior medical examination should be given an ENT laryngeal examination before beginning treatment by the speech–language pathologist. A diagnostic examination of the vocal cords must be done by the laryngologist. The speech–language pathologist trained in videolaryngoscopy may also use mirror laryngoscopy or endoscopy to view the folds for voice diagnosis; this will facilitate the voice therapy treatment of the patient by allowing the clinician to make judgments about vocal fold response to voice therapy techniques. Because the ENT physician is looking for laryngeal disease and the speech–voice pathologist is looking for function related to clinical stimulation, this is not a duplicate procedure and is wholly justified and necessary. While on the surface these examinations may seem redundant, they are proper because both specialties have different concerns and goals. Both the ENT physician and the speech–voice pathologist, for example, have the patient phonate but with different goals in mind and with different procedures or vocal maneuvers for the patient to perform. Further, detailed discussion of the ethics of the speech–language pathologist performing videolaryngealendoscopy is presented by Watterson, McFarlane, and Brophy (1990) and in ASHA Guidelines (1992, 1998).

The Voice Evaluation

Voice evaluation may be done either instrumentally or noninstrumentally. This means that one can use instruments to measure various aspects of voice or the evaluation may be done without instruments (Blakeley, 1991; Lavorato, 1991). There are advantages to each approach but there are some similarities between them. Time and cost factors may differ with the two approaches. In the area of voice evaluation, a true expert can do a very good evaluation of voice with or without instrumentation. The use of instrumentation does not assure better results. In the hands of an expert, the use of instrumentation adds important elements of documentation and quantification, which are not available without instrumentation. In the noninstrumental approach one relies on perception (pitch judgment, loudness, quality, etc.), while in the instrumental approach the emphasis may be on the physical measures (frequency, intensity, wave complexity, airflow rate, etc.). One should not rely on instrumentation to strengthen weak powers of observation, modest clinical skills, or lack of knowledge about diagnosis or of voice production. If one has mediocre skills, instrumentation alone will not make up for this weakness. The most important skills are to be able to listen critically and carefully, and to think objectively. It is more important to know how to ask a proper question during the case history or to be able to elicit a change in vocal behavior than it is to know how to operate a clinical instrument. Having said this, we do feel that instrumentation is important and knowing how to use it and how to interpret results of instrumental measures will be presented against a backdrop of normative data and diagnostic processes.

Among the most important elements of a voice evaluation are:

1. Case History

2. Evaluation of the pitch/frequency of the voice

3. Evaluation of the loudness/intensity of the voice

4. Analysis of the quality/wave complexity of the voice

5. Analysis of ENT report and other medical information

6. Ability to select and present appropriate clinical facilitation techniques (probes)

7. Judgments of air wastage or measurement of airflow rate

8. Ability to analyze videoendoscopic data (we will say more about the SLP's role)

9. Ability to observe the patient's behavior

10. Ability to analyze electroglottographic data

To understand patients with voice disorders and to understand their problems, it is necessary for clinicians to assemble a case history. Most texts and manuals dealing with diagnosis and appraisal of communicative disorders present general strategies for history-taking. Recent texts on management of voice disorders that offer suggestions for history-taking include Aronson, 1990, Boone, 1993, Case, 1996, Greene, 1980, and Wilson, 1987.

Many individualized voice evaluation forms are available for clinicians. Most history forms include major headings that include description of problem, signs and symptoms of the problem, cause of problem, consistency or variability of problem, and voice usage. The form shown in Figure 5.3 is typical.

Case History

During the case history the clinician must establish rapport with the patient so that information will be freely and honestly shared. The questions asked and the tone of this interview must be well thought-out. A question that is too specific may cause patients to think they are expected to answer in a certain way. For

FIGURE 5.3   A Voice Evaluation Form *This type of form helps to organize the case history according to each informant.*

VOICE EVALUATION FORM

The Boone Voice Program for Children by Daniel R. Boone, Ph.D.

Name _____ Sex M   F Date of Birth_____ Age _____

School _____ Teacher _____ Grade _____

Referral Source: Screening_____ Teacher _____ Physician _____ Self _____Other _____

Examiner _____ Date of Evaluation _____

SECTION 1
History of the Voice Problem

	Child's Report	*Parent's Report* (Informant_____)	*Teacher's Report*
Description of Problem			
Cause of Problem			
Onset of Problem			
Prior Voice Therapy			
Variability through Day			
Voice Usage			

Abuses: _____

_____

Misuses: _____

_____

Comments:_____

_____

_____

---

example, "You don't drink alcohol in the late evening do you?" may well bring forth a response that the patient thinks you want rather than the truth. A question that might be better would be, "Describe your typical use of alcohol to include times, amounts, and types used."

It is also good to ask questions in different ways. For example, one may ask "What medications do you take?" Later in the interview you may ask about certain medical problems such as, "You mentioned a heart problem. What do you take for that?" "Also, you said you have some problems with acid reflux." "What do you take for that and how do you manage it?"

When one asks "How much water or other fluids do you take in a day?" the answer is usually. "Not enough." A better approach is to say, "Estimate how much water and other fluids you drink in a typical day." This should be followed up with another question, "How do you take this fluid, from a water bottle, drinking fountain, or in coffee and sodas?"

Description of the Problem and Cause.   It is valuable for understanding patients to ask directly what they feel are the problems and what might have caused them. It is often effective to ask the same questions of family members, a spouse, or teachers. The different views about what the problem may be and the various guesses about probable causation may offer tips for management. Patients' descriptions often reveal much about their own conceptualization of the problem. What a patient feels the problem is may not be consistent with the opinions of the referring physician or the speech–language pathologist, a discrepancy that may be due to what we call "the patient's reality distance." This distance may be the result of the patient's lay background and inability to understand adequately what had been explained. Often we hear highly discrepant reports of "what the doctor said" as a patient recounts the diagnoses of previous clinicians. More often this distance is primarily the result of the inability to accept and cope with the real problem. An individual's defenses may force him or her to describe the problem in a way that is not consistent with the perceptions of others. What a patient says about a problem may, however, provide the clinician with insights that no amount of observation or testing can match. This sort of reality distance is well illustrated by excerpts from the clinic records of a twenty-eight-year-old computer programmer:

> *Physician's Examination Statement:* George was an extremely hard man to examine with indirect laryngoscopy. He was very fearful during our exam and gagged with the slightest touch to the posterior tongue. His vocal folds show broad-based bilateral polyps, about 4 mm wide along the anterior–middle third junction. Trial voice therapy is indicated.
> *Speech–Language Pathologist's Statement:* Patient voices with much audible strain, characterized by diplophonia, hoarseness, and severe glottal attack. Patient participated in all phases of our evaluation with a fixed smile on his face, contrasted with tight, clenched fists. We may well need here a combined voice therapy–counseling approach.
> *Patient's Statement of the Problem:* Now that I have recently found the Lord, I want to serve him. Whenever I go to teach at the church, I seem to lose my voice. My computer work presents no problem, because I don't need the voice much there. It's a problem of going hoarse and even losing the voice when I work with the groups at the church.

Consistently from these descriptions we view a patient who was showing some tension signs when relating to other people. He was hypersensitive during laryngoscopy attempts, his vocal patterns and facial–hand mannerisms suggested tension, and his description of his problem voicing with other people all suggested psychological tension as a possible contributing factor to his dysphonia. Aronson (1990) has written, "If the dysphonia is of greater severity or different in character than warranted by the lesion, a psychogenic component is strongly suspected" (p. 120). The bilateral polyps alone should not have caused the complete voice breakdown the patient experienced while teaching groups at the church. Successful management of this man's problem necessitated a combined voice therapy and psychological counseling approach, similar to what was suggested initially by the speech–language pathologist.

Onset and Duration of the Problem.   How long patients believe they have had the voice problem is important. A problem of acute and sudden onset usually poses a severe threat to a patient. That is, it keeps the patient from carrying out his or her customary activities (playing, singing, acting, selling, preaching, teaching, campaigning, or whatever). Sudden onset of aphonia or dysphonia deserves thorough exploration by both the laryngologist and the speech–language pathologist. Some dysphonias develop very gradually. Such gradual, fluctuating dysphonias are often related to varying situations in which patients may find themselves; sometimes they only occur during moments of stress or after fatigue. A history of slow onset sometimes suggests a gradually developing pathology, such as the development of bilateral polypoid degeneration of the vocal folds or dysphonia that is but an early developing symptom of some kind of progressive neurological disease. Long-term chronic dysphonia usually exists for so long because the patient has never been particularly disturbed by the voice problem. Voice therapy, like other forms of remedial therapy, is usually more successful with those patients who are motivated to overcome their problems. Patients with a long history of indifference toward their dysphonia usually present an additional challenge to the voice clinician and a more unfavorable prognosis than the ones who have recently acquired the disorder, depending, of course, on the type and etiology and relative extent of the pathology involved.

Variability of the Problem.   Most voice patients can provide rather accurate time tables of the consistency of their problem. If the severity of a voice problem is variable, a clinician may be able to identify those vocal situations in which the patient experiences the best voice and the worst voice. The typical patient with vocal hyperfunction reports a better voice earlier in the day, with increasing dysphonia later in the day as the voice is used more. For example, a high school social studies teacher reported a normal-sounding voice at the beginning of the day; toward the end of a day, after six hours of lecturing, he reported increasing hoarseness and a feeling of "fullness and dryness in the throat." Voice rest and then dinner at the end of the day usually restored his voice to its normal level. Obviously, such fluctuations in the daily quality of the voice enables the clinician to identify easily the situations contributing to the patient's vocal abuse. Another patient, whose dysphonia was closely related to allergy and postnasal drip experienced during sleep, presented this variation in hoarseness: severity in the morning on awakening, decrease in severity with usage of the voice, complete disappearance by late afternoon, and severity again the next morning. In cases of dysphonia related to GERD, we may also see a poor voice quality in the morning and some improvement by midday.

The variation of the voice problem can provide even more specific clues as to what situations most aggravate the disorder. A nightclub singer reported that she had no voice problem during the day in conversational situations or while practicing her repertoire. She developed hoarseness only at night and only on those nights she sang. Further investigation of her singing act revealed that the adverse factors were the cigarette smoke around her, to which she was unusually sensitive, and the noise of the crowd, above which she had to increase her volume to be heard. Her singing methods were found to be satisfactory. A change of jobs to a summer tent theater provided her with immediate relief. Variability of situation also affected a housewife allergic to a specific brand of meat tenderizer. This patient lost her voice completely shortly after using the tenderizer during meal preparation. When she discontinued the use of this product, she did not lose her voice; when the product was reintroduced, the aphonia followed. Inhaling only a small amount of this substance rendered her almost completely aphonic for fifteen minutes or more with a longer period of dysphonia following the aphonic period.

Description of Vocal Use (Daily Use/Misuse).   **Abuse, misuse,** and **overuse** of the voice cause most functional voice problems. It is important for clinicians to determine how voice patients are using their larynges in most life situations. The voice a child or adult exhibits in the speech–language pathologist's office may in no way represent the voice used on the playground, in the classroom, or in other settings. Sometimes patients can recreate some of their aversive laryngeal behaviors as a demonstration for the clinician, but more often a valid search for aversive vocal behaviors requires the clinician to visit the environment where the abuse–misuse occurs. Successful voice clinicians must thus build into their schedules actual visits to playgrounds, theaters, churches, courtrooms, or offices. In reducing one child's vocal abuse (and vocal nodules), a major factor was our visiting the school lunchroom and changing his manner of repeating the phrase "Do you want white or chocolate milk?" 300 times each day as he passed out the milk during the noisy lunch period. Similarly, we were able to make major vocal gains with a dysphonic attorney only after attending the courtroom trial where we observed his excessively loud and effortful legal objections and jury addresses and modified them firsthand. Apparently, only a little voice abuse–misuse in whatever setting is all that may be needed to keep a glottal membrane inflamed or a pair of vocal nodules irritated and fibrotic. Case (1996), for instance, has demonstrated the effects of cheerleading on the larynges of teenagers, comparing them with laryngoscopy before and after two weeks of attendance at a cheerleading camp. His data strongly suggest that continued cheerleading has a direct adverse effect on the larynges of the majority of the adolescents studied. It is obviously important for the clinician to identify the vocal use pattern of the patient.

Special attention must be given to the identification of playground screaming and yelling in children. One only has to listen to the noise level of the typical primary school playground to realize that yelling at play appears to be a normal childhood behavior. A child with a voice problem, however, often has a history of yelling a little louder and a bit more often than normal-voiced peers. Sometimes public school clinicians must enlist the help of teachers, friends, and the family to determine the everyday vocalization history of the child. Perhaps the most important part of voice therapy for children is identifying vocal abuse and developing strategies to reduce its occurrence. The voice clinician must get parents, teachers, and even the child's peers involved in the search for abuse and the plan for abuse reduction.

Additional Case History Information.   It is important to determine at the time of the voice evaluation if the patient has ever had previous voice therapy. If so, what type of past therapy would have obvious relevance to present management? When previous voice therapy attempts have failed to improve the vocal quality or have been unsuccessful in reducing a vocal pathology, the knowledge of previous therapy is important. We must, however, make every effort to present the appearance of a fresh and different approach to the patient who has experienced failure in previous voice therapy; even if we use the same goals of therapy as before, we must **redirect** (McFarlane and Lavorato, 1983) the new approach to voice therapy in a manner that appears to the patient to be headed down a completely different road. Determining whether other members of the family have similar voice problems is helpful. We have had particular patients present a certain voice problem, only to interview members of the family and find that all or many of them have the same voicing patterns. Deviations in resonance are often the most commonly observed family patterns. We recently observed a mother and her middle-aged daughter and a second younger daughter who all three presented with different degrees of essential tremor. On questioning, the mother noted that her mother (the grandmother of the two girls) had a similar shaky voice, which developed in midlife and persisted until her death.

Voice evaluations should also include some kind of health history. An example of a health history taken from a child evaluation form (Boone, 1993) is shown is Figure 5.4. Certainly for adult patients it is important to determine such conditions as allergies, medication or hormone therapy, smoking, use of alcohol, and of drugs (over-the-counter, prescribed, and illegal). It is also very important to check the level of hydration by asking about daily fluid intake. Once a patient is comfortable with an examiner, or perhaps after voice therapy has begun, a social history should be taken to provide the clinician with useful information about the patient as a person. One patient spoke with two completely different voices, constantly shifting between one voice and the other. When we asked why she used these two voices, she said her first voice was "My voice before I died." Further case history questioning revealed that she had been a patient in a mental hospital on two occasions. It became clear as the interview progressed that she was still having psychological problems and her voice disorder was a symptom of a more serious unresolved disorder. She was convinced that she had died and that she was now a channel for another person who had also died. The different voices represented different people.

Observation of the Patient

Observations of our patients often tell us more about them than their histories and test data. Speech–language pathologists must become critical observers, attempting

FIGURE 5.4   A Health History Form *This type of form helps to organize a health history.*

SECTION 2
Health History

Informant: _____
_____

Birth History
_____

Feeding Problems
_____

Illnesses and Allergies
_____

Accidents
_____

Surgery
_____

Medications
_____

Voice Change
_____

Family Voice Problems
_____

Previous Voice Therapy

(*The Boone Voice Program for Children*, Austin, Texas. Copyright © 1993 by PRO-ED, Inc.)

to describe behavior they see rather than merely labeling it. Writing observations about a patient is one of the few ways clinicians can note what they observe (audio and videotape recordings are two other means). Even here, however, it is important for clinicians to minimize any subjectivity by describing only what they see and hear, and not adding interpretation to the observation. For example, an adult laryngectomy patient was seen preoperatively and gave this report:

> I work as a hod carrier. I have done this kind of work for years. A question I have is how will this operation go along with my work? My Mom and I live together and she needs my help and my paycheck. If I have a hole in my neck what about the cement dust? Can I still work? My boss likes my work and I have done it for a long time. And what about my girlfriend, will she be able to understand me? I go to a bar and have a beer and sandwich sometimes and it is loud in there. Will they hear me?

By watching the patient during his interview he gave "little cues" about his doubts concerning his skills and his ability to work at other jobs. We asked him if he could read or write. He said "How did you know? Only one other doctor ever knew in all my thirty-eight years." He was fearful that he might never be able to return to work and, without the ability to read and write, he was likely to not be able to find another job, which meant that he and his mother would be without an income. He became not only a good alaryngeal speaker using the Tokyo Larynx (see Chapter 8) and somewhat of a celebrity in his community (the bar), but he also learned to read and write when we referred him to an adult literacy program. He also went back to his hod-carrying work. It was important to notice the clue that gave important information about the patient. He would never have told us that he was unable to read or write. His mother or girlfriend would fill out papers for him. He had picked up our clinic form and brought it in at his visit, completed by his mother.

Because voice difficulties are often symptomatic of the inability to have satisfactory interpersonal relationships, it is imperative that the clinician consider the patient's degree of adequacy as a social being. Patients who exhibit extremely sweaty palms, who avoid eye contact with people to whom they are speaking, who speak through clenched teeth, who use excessive postural changes or demonstrate facial tics, or sit with a masked, nonaffective facial expression, or who exhibit obvious shortness of breath may be displaying behaviors frequently considered as symptomatic of anxiety. Their struggle to maintain a conversational relationship may be accompanied by much struggle to phonate. Such observed behavior in the voice patient may be highly significant to the voice clinician planning a course of voice remediation. The decision about whether to treat a problem symptomatically (that is, by voice therapy) or by improving the patient's potential for interpersonal adjustment (perhaps by psychotherapy) is often aided by a review of the observations of the patient. A patient who demonstrates friendly, normal affect is telling the clinician, at least superficially, that he or she functions well in a two-person relationship; such information may well have clinical relevance. Such observations are extremely valuable to voice clinicians planning treatment approaches. Note, however, that in our experience very few voice patients require referral for psychotherapy.

Testing of the Patient

A voice rating scale of some kind aids the clinician in separating the various processes contributing to voice into separate components. A children's voice rating scale is shown in Figure 5.5. This particular scale permits clinicians to observe each of seven parameters: pitch, loudness, quality, nasal resonance, oral resonance, speaking rate, and variability of inflection. Each of the parameters is judged for voice production in three settings: in conversation, in play, and in reading. This particular scale is basically a seven-point rating scale with normal production checked in the middle. To the left of normal are the rating slots for insufficient performance of the parameter to be rated; for example, a voice pitch that appears too low would be rated on the pitch scale to the left of normal. The individual's pitch level is compared with the pitch levels of age peers. The mild, moderate, and severe boxes are checked according to the clinician's judgment. The rating scale is not a test per se but provides clinicians with a structure for systematizing their observations. Actual measurements of frequency, intensity, quality, and resonance are made separately, and these data can often help clinicians make the summary judgments placed on the voice rating scale. Because rating scales force clinicians to focus their measurements and observations into some kind of

FIGURE 5.5   A Voice Rating Scale *This seven-point rating scale allows clinicians to rate various aspects of voice during conversation, play, and oral reading.*

SECTION 8
Voice Rating Scale

	–			N			+
Breathing	1	2	3	4	5	6	7
(words per breath)	too few			normal			too many
	–			N			+
Loudness	1	2	3	4	5	6	7
	soft			normal			too loud
	–			N			+
Pitch	1	2	3	4	5	6	7
	low			normal			high
	–			N			+
Pitch Inflections	1	2	3	4	5	6	7
	none			normal			excessive
	–			N			+
Quality	1	2	3	4	5	6	7
	breathy			normal			harsh
	–			N			+
Horizontal Focus	1	2	3	4	5	6	7
	front			normal			back
	–			N			+
Vertical Focus	1	2	3	4	5	6	7
	throat			normal			nasal
	–			N			+
Nasal Resonance	1	2	3	4	5	6	7
	denasal			normal			hypernasal

(*The Boone Voice Program for Children,* Austin, Texas. Copyright © 1993 by PRO-ED, Inc.)

summary, many voice clinicians have developed scales and found them useful. Wilson (1987) describes several equal-appearing interval scales having ratings from 1 to 7, with interjudge reliability in excess of .90.

   If we consider that, as we said earlier, one can do a noninstrumental voice evaluation by using perceptions and recording our observations of various forms, such as those presented, useful perceptual data can be gathered. We can observe pitch use and note pitch as too high or too low when compared to one's peers. We can also make similar observations of loudness. These can be entered on a form for later analysis and interpretation. It is very helpful to note important quality differences that may be perceived without instrumentation. At the very least one could note qualities such as breathiness, hoarseness, thinness, vocal tightness, or strained/strangled quality, and tremor. These perceptions of vocal characteristics such as pitch, loudness, quality are very helpful in the diagnostic process and in selecting which clinical facilitation techniques to try during the initial diagnostic session. When these perceptions are recorded on a form and combined with the response to clinical stimulation and the history and ENT examination one can come to a good tentative voice diagnosis. It is the speech–language pathologist's province to make the voice diagnosis; it is the ENT physician's province to make a physical diagnosis of disease. We find the form in Figure 5.6 to be helpful for recording both perceptions and physical measures of voice. The resultant profile helps with the diagnostic process and with planning voice therapy. If one uses instruments as well as perceptual judgments the form is very helpful in integrating the two evaluative approaches.

The Oral Evaluation.　Careful assessment of the oral mechanisms is part of the voice evaluation. Although we focus on evaluation of the larynx and respiratory systems, some examination of facial structures, mouth, dentition, tongue, teeth, hard and soft palate, pharynx, and nasal cavities is required. In our evaluation of the oral mechanisms of the voice patient, we must pay particular attention to possible signs of neural innervation problems. Every now and then, when we evaluate a patient with "functional dysphonia," we find some subtle neurological signs of fasciculation and atrophy of the tongue, or asymmetries of the velum related to neural innervation changes, and so on. Subsequent medical–neurological evaluations may find that the early dysphonia is simply the beginning symptomatology of a serious neurological disease such as multiple sclerosis (MS), muscular dystrophy (MD), amyotrophic lateral sclerosis (ALS), or myasthenia gravis (MG). It is important to evaluate the voice patient specific to structural and functional adequacy for all parts of the oral mechanisms. In Chapter 2, we presented sites of possible hyperfunction where voice patients may experience some difficulty. Let us now review some of these sites of hyperfunction and look at them closely as part of our total peripheral mechanism evaluation. Beyond observing obvious problems in breathing, some attention should be given to the amount of neck tension. The accessory neck muscles and the supralaryngeal strap muscles in some patients literally stick out like bands as the patient speaks (this is also observed in untrained singers). Often, mandibular restriction is closely associated with neck tension; affected patients speak with clenched teeth, with little or no mandibular movement. Such restricted jaw movement places most of the burden of speech articulation on the tongue, which, to produce the various vowels and diphthongs in connected speech, must make fantastic adjustments if no cavity-shaping assistance from the mandible is forthcoming. Another externally observable hyperfunction of the vocal tract is unusual downward or upward excursion of the larynx during the production of various pitches. Any unusual movement upward while phonating higher pitches, or unusual movement downward while phonating lower ones, should be noted. The angle of the thyroid cartilage may be felt digitally as the patient sings a number of varying pitches; typically the fingertips will feel little discernible change in thyroid angle as the patient sings up and down the scale. Sometimes, however, the thyroid cartilage can be felt to rock forward slightly in the production of high pitches, as it sweeps upward to a higher position toward the hyoid bone. It is helpful to gently move the larynx manually from side to side to note the degree of tension with which the strap muscles of the neck hold the larynx in place. We also ask patients to move their larynx manually from side to side and to observe how fixed it appears compared to our own larynx. Any really noticeable amount of lifting or lowering of the larynx, as

Pitch (children)	Low	Mid	High

F_o Hz (children)	196 220 245 262	294	330

Keyboard (children)	G_3 A_3 B_3 C_4	D_4	E_4

Pitch (women)	Low	Mid	High

F_o Hz (women)	147 164 175 196 220 245 262 294

Keyboard (women)	D_3 E_3 F_3 G_3 A_3 B_3 C_4 D_4

Pitch (men)	Low	Mid	High

F_o Hz (men)	65 73 82 87 98 110 123 131 147 164 175

Keyboard (men)	C_2 D_2 E_2 F_2 G_2 A_2 B_2 C_3 D_3 E_3 F_3

Loudness	Soft	Comfortable	Loud

dB SPL	20 30 40 50 60 70 80 90

Breathiness	Strained	Normal	Breathy

Airflow ml/sec	50 70 90 110 130 150 170 190 210 230 250

MPT secs	high to low	30 28 26 24 22 20 18 16 14 12 10 8 6 4 2
MPT secs	low to high	2 4 6 8 10 12 14 16 18 20 22 24 26 28 30

	F_o Hz	MPT	Airflow ml/sec	dB SPL
Children 5-10 yrs:	270-340	12-15	15-128	45-65
Children 10-14 yrs:	240-270	15-20	15-128	45-65
Males 20-80 yrs:	85-155	15-25	100-200	45-65
Females 20-80 yrs:	190-250	10-22	100-200	45-65

Name:_____ Age:_____ Gender:_____ Dx:_____

Date:_____

FIGURE 5.6   A clinic form that combines acoustic-air measurements with perceptual ratings. For explanation, see page 162.

well as the tipping forward of the thyroid cartilage in the production of high pitches, should be noted as possible hyperfunctional behavior. The majority of hyperfunctional behaviors associated with voice problems are probably not directly observable from examination of the peripheral mechanism. For example, to determine the extent of the tongue's impinging on the oropharyngeal space we would need to rely on oral or nasal endoscopy or videoendoscopy. Let us now consider some of the measurement instruments used by speech–language pathologists in the voice evaluation and diagnostic process.

Endoscopy.   The endoscope may be introduced intraorally or intranasally; the light at the tip of the scope (which comes fiber-optically from an external light source) illuminates the nasal and oral pharynx, which is viewed through a window lens on the other end of the endoscope. Of relevance to voice evaluation is that the tip lens of the oral endoscope can be directed up at the velopharyngeal closure mechanism or down at the larynx below. A nasal endoscopic voice evaluation (flexible examination) is pictured in Figure 5.7.

When the oral or nasal endoscope is attached to a small video camera, the examination is termed a videoendoscopic evaluation. It provides a permanent video record of the observations. Using a stop-frame feature of the video recorder and a video printer, we can make a hard-copy picture of the observation to include in the patient's file of voice evaluation. When we use a stroboscopic (flashing) light source instead of a steady-state light source, we can produce what appears as a slow motion observation of the vocal physiology (video stroboscopic endoscopy). With

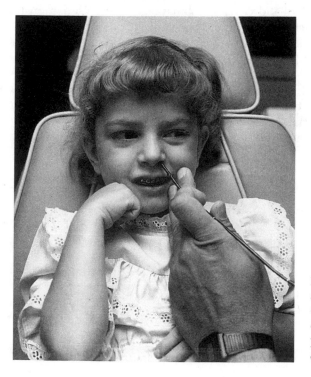

FIGURE 5.7   Nasoendoscopy in a child with a voice disorder. (When this examination was done the use of gloves was not part of the universal precautions as it *now* is.)

such instrumentation we are able to make valuable observations of deviations in both vocal tract anatomy and, more importantly, physiology (McFarlane, 1990; McFarlane, Watterson, and Brophy, 1990). The mucosal wave, which changes for production of normal or abnormal voice, can only be studied with stroboscopy. The mucosal wave movement represents the vibratory pattern that is responsible for the normal or abnormal voice produced. In Chapter 2, Figure 2.15 demonstrated normal mucosal wave movement. Abnormal voice production is the product of abnormal physiology by using the vocal mechanism in deviant ways. With most voice patients, these deviations are subtle, inappropriate vocal adjustments in glottal approximation of the vocal folds, overtensing of the vocal folds, in tongue position or in pharyngeal constriction, rather than the result of laryngeal or neurological lesions. When performing observations and measures of intraoral phenomena contributing to normal and faulty voice, we are forced to use various measuring instruments that help quantify aspects of respiratory, phonatory, and resonance function. Videolaryngealstroboscopy is an extremely valuable tool for the speech–language pathologist interested in voice disorders. Indeed, its use by the speech–language pathologist is now considered as part of the SLP's scope of practice. The conduct of the videostroboscopic visualization of the larynx and the interpretation of the results for the purpose of assessing voice production and vocal function are part of the well-trained speech–language pathologist's role (ASHA, 1998). Many inappropriate laryngeal adjustments produce vibratory abnormalities leading to abnormal mucosal wave production and disordered voice. These adjustments usually cannot be seen without videostroboscopy. Oral videostroboscopy (rigid examination) is performed with the oral scope in place during production of sustained vowels and the production of bilabial and vowel combinations. Figure 9.4 demonstrates visualization of the larynx using oral videostroboscopy. This produces an excellent picture of the larynx due to the fact that the oral scope is a solid glass rod rather than bundles of smaller fiberoptic cables. Because the oral scope is rigid it cannot bend and thus can be used only in the mouth. The flexible nasal endoscope may be placed through the nose and used to view connected speech. Many disorders are better observed under conditions of connected speech. This is a distinct advantage of the nasal scoping versus the oral scoping.

Some of the advantages of videostroboscopy of the larynx for the voice clinician are:

1. A permanent record (hard picture and video) is made;

2. A study of the function of the larynx is made during both typical voice production and during clinical stimulation (McFarlane, 1988; McFarlane, 1990);

3. The picture of the larynx aids in patient counseling;

4. The picture helps to get patient compliance with therapy tasks;

5. Pictures can be shared with the referral source;

6. The picture can be retained for comparison with later results to observe progress;

7. A frame-by-frame analysis can be helpful in understanding abnormal physiology;

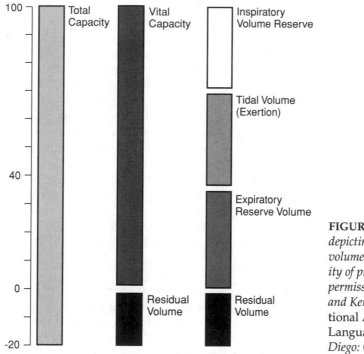

FIGURE 5.8   *A bar graft depicting relative respiratory volumes as part of total capacity of pulmonary air. (Used by permission of Perkins, W. H. and Kent, R. D. (1986).* Functional Anatomy of Speech, Language, and Hearing. *San Diego: College Hill.)*

8. Responses to clinical stimulation can be reviewed in planning therapy;

9. The video and picture record provides for research and teaching;

10. The mucosal wave activity can be studied by no other means (except high-speed photography).

Videoendoscopy of the larynx has been a tremendous asset to the accurate diagnosis of voice disorders and has led to many valuable research studies of dysphonia and its successful treatment. We have performed thousands of videoendoscopic evaluations of voice disordered patients and have benefited in our teaching and research by the enhanced understanding of voice production and the effects of voice facilitation techniques. Many times the information gained from videostroboscopic visualization of the larynx has been the most important information gained during the diagnostic process. When coupled with the other information gathered during the diagnostic process we have greatly improved our chances of an accurate diagnosis and for designing a successful voice therapy plan.

Respiration Testing.   Because the vocal folds are activated for phonation by the outflowing airstream passing through the closed glottis, some observation and measurement of respiratory adequacy is a necessary part of the voice evaluation. Early phoniatrists placed much emphasis on breathing adequacy, particularly with regard to adequacy for singing; such a view was prominently advocated by Tarneud and frequently cited by Luchsinger and Arnold (1965). Many speech–language pathologists, but certainly not all, continue to show interest in how well voice patients breathe, and particularly in how well patients are able to extend and use their exhalations for phonation. Breathing exercises are not usually helpful for voice therapy. Airflow control is helpful especially in singers and for those with neurological disorders (this was discussed in Chapter 4). It is commonly recognized, for example, that shortness of breath or speaking after too much breath is already expired will noticeably affect phonation. For these reasons respiration testing is important. Because lung capacities are generally far greater than the amount of air required for typical speaking situations, patients' *use* of air supply is usually more important than their lung volumes. This is true even for patients who present with severe breathing disorders such as emphysema or chronic obstructive pulmonary disease, or even with patients who have only one lung. Large lung volumes are more important for singing than for speaking. We shall consider separately those instruments that can be used for measuring various aspects of respiratory movement and, finally, those observations and tests that we can use to assess the patient's use of respiration as it applies to phonation. Specifically, we shall consider separately four types of information: lung volume, air pressure, airflow, measures and motions of the torso.

Lung Volume.   It is important to determine how much of the total lung volume a patient uses in phonation. We can easily observe the patient speak or sing, and make a judgment about the overall adequacy of respiration while the patient is performing the task. Does she run out of her air supply before finishing the planned utterance? Is he forced to renew air intake more often than is desirable? Part of evaluating respiratory adequacy is measuring the patient's lung volume. Specific dimensions of volume that can be measured include vital capacity (maximum amount of air that can be expelled from the lungs following a maximum inspiration), tidal volume (amount of air inspired and expired in a normal breathing cycle), inspiratory reserve (maximum amount of additional air inspired after a tidal inhalation is completed), and expiratory reserve (maximum volume of air expired after a tidal expiration). Normal speakers use only a small amount of their total vital capacity when speaking. Hixon, Goldman, and Mead (1973) have written that normal speakers use only about twice the air volume for speech that they use for quiet, easy normal (or tidal) breaths. Does the typical patient use greater or lesser volumes than this?

The capacities and volumes we need to measure can be determined by using wet or dry spirometers. In the wet spirometer, a container floats in water placed in a larger container. As air is introduced to the smaller floating container, it floats higher in proportion to the volume of air introduced. The distance or rise of displacement is measured in terms of cubic centimeters or liters. The values for lung volumes given in Chapter 2 (in the lung volumes section) were: Vital capacity 3500–5000 cc, Tidal volume 750 cc, Inspiratory reserve 1500–2500 cc, and Expiratory reserve 1500–2000 cc. (See Figure 5.8.)

Some spirometers are of the dry type. A flexible container enlarges on inspiratory tasks and decreases in volume on expiratory tasks, in both instances measuring the volume of displacement. The wet spirometer appears to have greater clinical usage and also to provide greater volume accuracy. Again, we should point out, however, that volume data do not have the same clinical relevance as measures of expiration (pressure and flow) and data specific to neck, thoracic, and abdominal movements.

Airflow Pressures.   One can hear the effects of air pressure on the perceived loudness of the voice. Greater vocal intensities require higher airflow volume and pressures passing through the glottis for a shorter time, producing greater excursions of the vibrating vocal folds. In the ensuing section on loudness we further describe the measurement of voice intensities by several methods, such as using a sound-level meter. We often hear symptoms of inadequate airflow volume and pressure in voice patients who experience varying and inadequate loudness; we may also hear quality disturbances related to inadequate pressure for normal fold vibration.

Relatively inexpensive pressure measuring gauges and manometers are available for the measurement of airflow pressures. In measuring air-pressure adequacy for voice, we are interested in finding an individual's oral pressures. One way of doing this is to ask the patient to produce a series of /pa/ sounds. In the production of /pa/ the glottis is open, and the pressure peaks during the production of the /p/-phase of the /pa/. Netsell and Hixon (1978) have found that the oral pressures obtained in the pa production or in a blowing task (when the mouthpiece has a small air leak) correspond to the pressures found in the lungs and at the glottis. They have concluded that, if patients can produce 5 to 10 cm of pressure over a period of five seconds in a sustained blowing task, they probably have sufficient expiratory pressures to produce normal voice.

Pressure measurements are used diagnostically more often when attempts are made to measure velopharyngeal adequacy (described in more detail in Chapter 9). Using some kind of manometric device, the patient is asked to produce a consonant such as /p/ or /k/; oral pressures are taken and nasal pressures (a nasal olive is inserted in the nares attached to the flow tube) are also determined. Sometimes the oral and nasal measurements are taken sequentially back-to-back, but such measures are perhaps more meaningful when taken simultaneously. For simultaneous oral–nasal pressures, the patient wears a face mask that is divided into oral and nasal sections, which provides separate oral–nasal pressure ratings. Oral speech should have little or no nasal pressure flow; as puffs of air escape through an inadequately closed velopharyngeal port, the sensitivity of the pressure gauge would detect such inappropriate escape.

Airflow Measures.   An important diagnostic measure in voice evaluation is a measurement of airflow, which indicates the volume of air passed through the glottis in a fixed period of time. For example, the normal production of a vowel requires about 100 cc (80–200 cc or ml) of air passage through the glottis in one second. A patient with large bilateral nodules who cannot effect adequate glottal closure will exhibit much higher airflow rates and perhaps will use 100 cc in far less than a second. His or her voice would be characterized by much breathiness, and the leakage of air caused by the lack of normal glottal resistance would actually be audible. Poor glottal resistance to the airflow, as would be caused by the formation of nodules on the glottal margin, results in elevated airflow measures. In unilateral vocal fold paralysis the airflow rate or air wastage may be much greater. We have seen patients who have air flow rates as high as 1000 ml per second in the case of unilateral vocal fold paralysis with the paralyzed fold in the paramedian or even the lateral position. This can produce a huge glottal gap during phonation. An opposite kind of problem, in which the glottis is highly constricted, such as is observed in adductor spasmodic dysphonia, results in markedly reduced flow rates. We generally will monitor airflow rates in our SD patients and when the airflow rate is near 50 ml per second will reinject them with BOTOX (BOTOX treatment is discussed in Chapters 4 and 7) to increase the rate to 250 to 300 ml per second.

The rate of flow, particularly when combined with pressure ratings, thus gives much diagnostic information about what is happening to the outgoing air at the level of the glottis. Measurements of airflow are usually substantiated by critical listening to the voice. We also can note the duration of phonation. If one has a high airflow rate the phonation time is reduced while in restricted airflow rate the duration of phonation can be longer. If a voice appears to be produced by a relatively lax glottal closure as observed in breathiness, the flow rates are high and the duration of phonation is short; if the voice appears harsh and sounds constricted, flow rates are often markedly diminished and duration of phonation can be longer, as long as the phonation is not cut off altogether by too much constriction. Not only is flow rate information of diagnostic importance, it also helps us measure the effects of therapy. For example, as we attempt to move patients into more optimal phonatory behaviors, we see flow rates shift toward normal values (such as 100–200 ml per second).

An extremely useful instrument is the Phonatory Function Analyzer (see Figure 5.9). We have used this to great advantage in clinical situations (McFarlane et al., 1998). This device makes five simultaneous measures of phonation that demonstrate the efficiency of the larynx during phonation. It also demonstrates the interaction of these five measures (phonation time, frequency, intensity, airflow rate, and total volume of expired air) with one another. When one parameter, such as pitch, is altered during clinical stimulation the effect on another parameter, such as airflow rate, is easily demonstrated. The tracing (see Figure 5.10) from the Phonatory Function Analyzer demonstrates that a slight elevation in pitch during the production of a vowel can reduce the excessive airflow rate that gives rise to the perception of extreme breathiness in this adult patient with bowed folds. An improved vocal quality, with reduced breathiness, is correlated with the tracing of reduced airflow. The airflow measurement, as mentioned earlier, is made in milliliters per second (ml/sec), which is the equivalent of cubic centimeters (cc/sec).

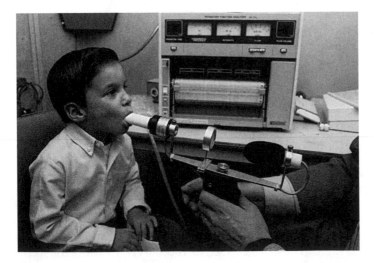

FIGURE 5.9 **Phonatory Function Analyzer** *The phonatory function analyzer is used here to evaluate phonation time (in seconds), fundamental frequency (Hz), vocal intensity (dB SPL), airflow rate (ml/sec), and total volume of air (ml) during each phonation attempt.*

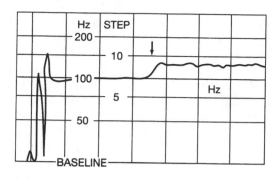

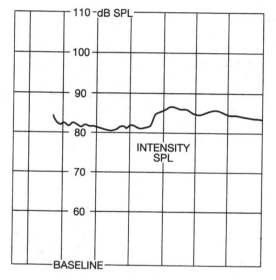

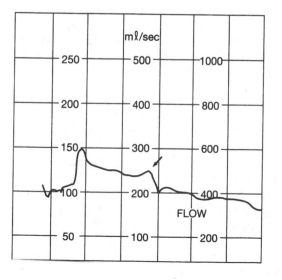

FIGURE 5.10   Tracing from a Phonatory Function Analyzer

These tracings from the phonatory function analyzer demonstrate how a change in one vocal parameter (pitch, for example) can make a significant change in another parameter (such as rate of airflow). As the pitch level is raised from 100 Hz to a level of 130 Hz, the airflow rate is reduced from 260 ml/sec to a level of 180 ml/sec. Intensity is also increased from 83 to 88 dB SPL.

Another useful device for measuring airflow is the pneumotachometer. The patient produces vowel prolongations with airflow captured in the oral mask, and the flow rate is measured by the pneumotachometer. Much data is available for normal flow rates both in children (Leeper, 1976) and adults (Yanagihara and von Leden, 1967), as are many references examining changes in flow for various voice disorder groups (Gordon, Morton, and Simpson, 1978; Isshiki and von Leden, 1964). Somewhat related to a measure of flow are the various duration studies that determine how long the individual can sustain a voiced or voiceless expiration (Bless and Saxman, 1970; Eckel and Boone, 1981; Ptacek and Sander, 1963; Tait, Michel, and Carpenter, 1980). One measure of differential duration measures that is used diagnostically in the voice evaluation is the s/z ratio. The patient is asked first to sustain the /s/ as long as possible, and then to sustain the /z/. The typical s/z ratios of normal subjects approximate 1.0, indicating that the voiceless expiration time (the /s/) closely matches maximum phonation time (the /z/) (Tait et al., 1980). In 95 percent of their patients with glottal margin pathologies (nodules, polyps, thickening), Eckel and Boone (1981) found elevated s/z ratios in excess of 1.4, indicating marked reduction in voiced duration values. It should be cautioned that the s/z ratio is a crude, quick appraisal technique based on the "possibility of air wastage due to a possible vocal fold lesion." It may be helpful for those clinicians without the benefit of instrumentation. Elevated s/z ratios may be a red flag to check the glottal edge of the vocal folds for a lesion. The clinical value of the s/z ratio is illustrated in this clinical case:

> A nineteen-year-old university singer was self-referred to the University Speech and Hearing Clinic for her continuing "breathiness and hoarseness." Initial voice evaluation techniques included a pneumotachic evaluation, which found airflow measurements of 240 cc/sec with oral pressure readings of 5.5 cm H 20; her initial /s/ duration was 18 sec, her /z/ duration was 11 sec, and her s/z ratio was computed at 1.64. Initially, she resisted having a medical evaluation that included indirect laryngoscopy. The clinician, however, knowing that her high s/z value may well have been predictive of laryngeal disease, insisted that she have laryngoscopy. A subsequent examination found her to have bilateral vocal nodules that occupied almost a third of her total anterior–posterior glottal length. Following laryngoscopy, she was enrolled in individual voice therapy. Repeated testing after nine weeks of voice therapy revealed a lower airflow measure of 219 cc/sec and higher oral pressure readings of 7.3 cm H20; her s/z ratios had decreased to 1.28.

These improved scores all suggested better laryngeal function. Subsequent laryngeal examination confirmed some decrease in the size of the nodules, although small bilateral nodes were still present. Her voice quality had improved. The s/z ratio as used here provided one additional, noninstrumental, check (requiring no instrumentation other than a stopwatch) and observation for the clinician in conducting the overall voice management of the patient. A newer instrument that combines both airflow and air pressure measures is the Aerophone by Kay Elemetrics. Figure 5.11 shows the configuration of the Aerophone, which may be used for clinical or research purposes. It can provide motivation and feedback to patients as well as quantify diagnostic measures for the clinician.

A simple but useful clinical maneuver, for the clinician without instrumentation, which can be employed to demonstrate the degree of laryngeal tension, is the

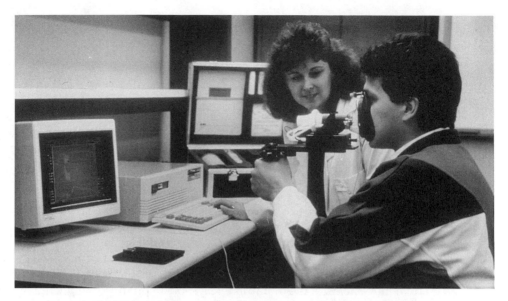

FIGURE 5.11 *The KAY Aerophone II with face mask for measuring simultaneous airflow, air pressure, intensity, and fundamental frequency of same utterance.*

application of hand pressure to the patient's abdomen during phonation of the sustained /i/ vowel. The palm of the hand is placed firmly over the middle of the abdomen just above the level of the belt (Figure 5.12). The hand is pulsed as the phonation is sustained. The more hyperfunction present during the voice production, the less the voice will pulse; conversely, the more relaxed the vocal folds and the larynx are, the more the voice will pulse in response to the hand pressure. When the clinician applies the technique to patients who are producing their typical voice,

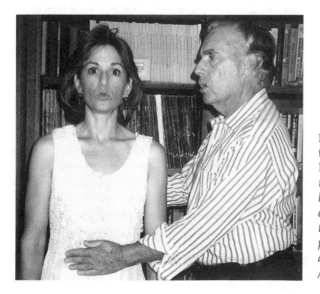

FIGURE 5.12 Demonstrating the Presence of Excessive Laryngeal Tension *A simple but useful clinical maneuver that can be used to demonstrate the presence of excessive laryngeal tension is the application of pulsing hand pressure to the patient's abdomen during phonation of the sustained /i/ vowel.*

and then reapplies the technique after using a facilitating approach such as glottal fry, the dramatic difference in vocal pulsing becomes obvious to the patient. Patients can be taught to perform this maneuver for themselves to check for inappropriate laryngeal tension.

Motions of the Torso.   For many years students of voice have been able to use the pneumograph to track and record thoracic and abdominal movements during inhalation and exhalation. The pneumograph is usually connected to a recording device, of which there are two main types, the kymograph and the polygraph, both of which provide graphic measurement writeouts. The pneumograph provides straps, which are placed around the thorax or abdomen; at the ends of the straps are rubber tubes. As the tubes are stretched, a partial vacuum is created within them, and the amount of vacuum is communicated to the recording instrument. The pneumographic recordings help speech–language pathologists study the frequency of the respiration cycle, focusing on the regularity of the inhalation–exhalation ratio. How well a patient can sustain an exhalation can be determined very well by using the pneumograph with a kymographic or polygraphic writeout. For the study of differential movements of the thorax in inspiration–expiration, the pneumograph is used less today in favor of newer methodologies. Today, for study of the movements of the thorax the respiratrace is used. It has applications in the areas of both voice and stuttering.

To study the relative coordination between abdominal movements and thoracic movements, Hixon, Mead, and Goldman (1976) have used magnetometers to examine the relative "anteroposterior diameters" of both the abdomen and thorax, particularly as the two areas relate to one another. When using the magnetometers, the clinician can determine the synchrony of movements of the rib cage and the abdomen during speech breathing. Some clinical voice disorders related to such problems as cerebral palsy or other motor–speech disorders produce severe problems in this synchrony between the different parts involved in breathing. Small magnets are placed on the back, on the front chest wall, and on the lower back and abdominal wall; the anterior–posterior distance varies between the magnets in each area (chest or abdomen), and this information can be traced either on an oscilloscope or on some kind of graphic printout.

The experimental use of the electromyograph (EMG) in investigating the use of particular muscles in breathing during speech has been explored in several studies reported by Hoshiko (1962), but there has been little regular use of the electromyograph as a clinical tool for respiration assessment. Which muscle is doing what may be determined by the clinical EMG, whereby recordings are made of the variations in electrical potential as detected by needle or surface electrodes inserted into or placed over a muscle. Whenever that muscle becomes active (contracts), its electrical activity is displayed on a graphic writeout.

Movement of the thorax and the downward excursion of the diaphragm can be identified very well by various X-rays techniques. The degree of inflatability, as seen by thoracic expansion and downward movement of the diaphragm, has been evaluated with convenience by still X-ray. Still X-rays taken at moments of maximum inhalation and exhalation have been helpful in identifying those sites of respiration (apical versus base of lungs) that show the most deflation or inflation and have provided knowledge about the type of breathing the patient employs: abdominal–diaphragmatic, midthoracic, or clavicular. Similar information can be obtained by viewing the respiratory mechanism in action, assessing actual movement by the use of other X-ray techniques, namely, fluoroscopy and videofluorography.

Other Aspects of Respiration Testing.   The type of breathing the patient uses can often be accurately determined by visual observation. The most inefficient type of breathing, clavicular, seems to be the easiest to identify. The patient elevates the shoulders on inhalation, using the neck accessory muscles as the primary muscles of inhalation. This upper chest breathing, characterized by noticeable elevation of the clavicles, is unsatisfactory for good voice for two reasons: First, the upper, apical ends of the lungs, when expanded, do not alone provide an adequate respiration; and, second, the strain in using the neck accessory muscles for respiration is often visually apparent, with individual muscles "standing out" (particularly the sternocleidomastoids, as they contract to elevate the upper thorax). Although little research evidence clearly identifies the negative effects on speech of clavicular breathing, no serious singer would waste time developing such a shallow, upper-lung reservoir of air. Clavicular-type breathing requires too much effort for too little breath and contributes to excessive muscle tension.

Diaphragmatic–abdominal breathing may well be the preferred method of respiration, especially if the patient has heavy vocal demands, as in singing or acting without electronic amplification. If the patient is employing diaphragmatic–abdominal breathing, this should be noted on the voice evaluation form. This use of lower thoracic breathing is usually identifiable by the presence of abdominal and lower thoracic expansion on inspiration, and a gradual decrease in abdominal–lower thoracic prominence on expiration. When asked to take in a deep breath, such a patient will demonstrate, on inhaling, relatively active expansion of the lower thorax and little noticeable upper-chest movement.

We can perhaps obtain a more accurate assessment of how patients breathe for speech when we ask them to demonstrate various voices, such as a pulpit voice, a calling-the-kids voice, a talking-to-superiors voice, and so on. Most voice patients exhibit breathing patterns that are somewhere in-between clavicular and diaphragmatic–abdominal breathing, and for these persons we use the somewhat nondescript term *thoracic* on voice evaluation forms. Thoracic breathers exhibit no noticeable upper thoracic or abdominal expansion on inhalation. The general mode of breathing can often be assessed if the clinician observes the patients closely as they speak and demonstrate their typical voice production mode.

Measurement of Pitch.   Observations of voice pitch tell us whether a voice is low or high for the patient's age and sex, but only when we measure pitch can we determine the exact fundamental frequency of a voice. Of the various aspects of voice, frequency as measured in cycles per second now in Hertz (Hz) is one of the most useful and perhaps the most measurable. As part of a voice evaluation, the patient's total frequency range (lowest to highest note) should be determined as a prelude to finding that person's best pitch level (the patient's easiest and most compatible voice pitch) at which to begin therapy probes. Measurements should be made of the patient's habitual pitch (the most frequently occurring or modal pitch level used by the patient). We first discuss some of the instruments available for measuring these aspects of frequency and pitch.

The Visi-Pitch (Figure 5.13) is an excellent clinical instrument for measuring different aspects of frequency, frequency range, and best pitch. We use the term *best pitch* here because *optimal pitch* is not a real entity as has been demonstrated. We are aware, for example, that if there were an actual optimum pitch the singer would only sound best at that pitch and would be severely limited in range and repertoire. The Visi-Pitch offers both a digital display of frequency and an oscilloscopic display. For determination of range, the patient is asked to say the /i/ vowel (e-e-e) at a comfortable pitch and loudness level and then repeat the /i/ at decreasing musical steps, down to the lowest "note" the patient can produce. The patient is then asked to produce successively higher notes until reaching the top of his or her range. Even though the clinician will have a digital writeout of fundamental frequency for each separate vocalization, the productions can be stored on the scope, and frequency values can be determined after the patient has completed the sequence. A cursor feature on the Visi-Pitch allows the clinician to search the stored tracings on the scope to determine the exact frequency of any particular phonation. The lowest and highest frequencies the patient is able to produce represent the patient's range.

As we have said, the concept of optimal pitch can be challenged (and has been in the literature) for a number of reasons, but there is some clinical utility in the notion of a pitch level that is best for the patient during the period of initial voice retraining. One level of pitch usually sounds better in vocal quality, and thus the facilitating approaches of chant talk and pitch shifts take advantage of this observation (see Chapter 6). "Best Pitch" (the pitch level that produces the least

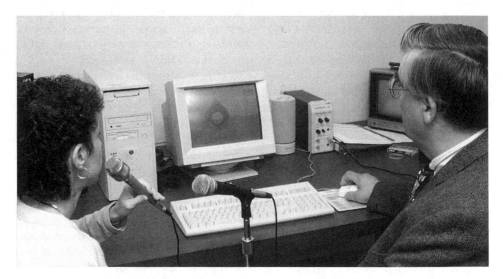

FIGURE 5.13 The Visi-Pitch II *The patient is able to use the visual feedback from the Visi-Pitch screen to modify her pitch and intensity output. Using the split screen (upper/lower) capability, the patient and clinician can compare typical performance with performance under clinical stimulation.*

amount of hoarseness or roughness) can be determined by careful listening to the voice quality at various pitches and by using the jitter and shimmer values computed by the Visi-Pitch. The best pitch is usually the frequency that sounds slightly louder and clearer in quality; relative changes in both intensity and quality can be determined by using jitter and shimmer values. Habitual pitch can be determined by having the patient produce live conversation or oral reading directly into the Visi-Pitch microphone for a time period of eight seconds; frequency can be instantly analyzed and measured. The most often occurring frequency can be easily identified. The Visi-Pitch has been designed as a clinical instrument that will easily provide frequency data both at the time of the evaluation and as ongoing feedback information during voice therapy. Each new version of the Visi-Pitch provides more useful clinical information.

The Phonatory Function Analyzer, mentioned in our earlier discussion of flow rate and volume, provides an excellent measure of pitch during sustained vowels. If a mask is used, the pitch can be measured in connected speech. With a disposable mouthpiece as shown in Figure 5.9, only sustained vowels may be analyzed. Of particular value is the fact that this instrument is capable of five simultaneous measures of voice. The instrument provides a hard copy printout for the patient's chart and also five dials (corresponding to each parameter) that the patient can monitor during voice production.

The new Computerized Speech Lab (CSL) 4300B by Kay Elemetrics provides a useful multidimensional voice program (MDVP) 4305 that has nearly twenty-two different vocal parameters displayed, in addition to the more familiar jitter, shimmer, signal to harmonic ratio, and so forth. While the various parameters are useful and informative for the clinician, they tend to confuse the patient at times and their usefulness as patient feedback is at times compromised. The clinician must draw the patient's attention to the most critical parameters to be viewed, ignoring other parameters.

Another relatively inexpensive clinical instrument for the measurement of pitch is the electric keyboard shown in Figure 5.14. This device is used while the patient is producing a sustained vowel or /m/. Repeated syllables, such as /mimimi/or /bibibi/, and voiced phrases, such as "Miami millionaire" and "Momma made lemon jam" (see nasal glide stimulation in Chapter 6) can be produced by the patient and matched on the keyboard by the clinician. The keyboard can be useful in establishing a new pitch level to begin facilitating techniques such as chant talk, tongue protrusion /i/, or glottal fry (see Chapter 6). The patient's habitual pitch level, pitch range, and best pitch level can be determined with the keyboard. When the musical note is played in step-by-step notes the patients are asked to match the note with their own voice.

It is possible to measure frequency range and make other measures of frequency using a real piano or a pitch pipe. An initial voice recording made at the time of a patient's first clinic visit is a useful tool for analyzing the patient's habitual pitch level. This analysis can be made after the patient has left the clinic. One method we have used is to stop the recorder at random points and attempt to match the voice pitch level with a pitch pipe, an electric keyboard, or a piano. After some experience with a pitch pipe, it is possible to match pitch levels between the pitch pipe frequency and the patient's voice. This is facilitated by remembering key pitch values

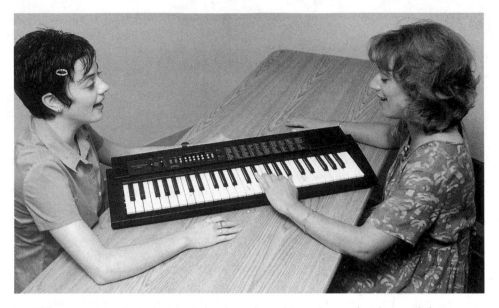

FIGURE 5.14   A typical electronic keyboard used in voice evaluation and therapy.

for average voices. For example, in cycles per second, the typical adult male voice is somewhere near C_3 (128 cps), and therefore is not very different from the C_3 note on a pitch pipe or piano. Using the pitch pipe, we would start at C_3 and then go by gradations (sharps and flats) until we reached "near" the recorded level of the patient's voice. With an adult female, we might select as our beginning pitch A_3 (213 cps) and go up or down to match the patient's voice. A typical starting place for a prepubertal child would be middle C (256 cps). In a two- or three-minute sample from a voice recording, we might select seven or eight voice samples for analysis of pitch level. After we have determined the approximate pitch of the patient's voice samples, we then count the various pitch levels and look for the modal pitch value (the pitch level that occurs most often), and record this as the patient's habitual pitch level. Using the modal pitch gives us a more valid habitual pitch than averaging the obtained sample values and using the mean.

A patient's pitch range can also be determined by using voice models. This may be done by asking the patient first to match a pitch level provided by the clinician. It is usually easier for patients to match their own voice with another person's voice than to a generated pitch level from some instrument such as a piano, a pitch pipe, a loop playback instrument, and so on. For this reason, it is most useful to have on hand some recordings of normal voices (adult male, adult female, several children's voices) producing vowels, prolonging each vowel for about three seconds. These samples can be recorded on small cassette tapes or discs. On playing the sample voice, which should be close to the patients' observed pitch levels, we ask the patients to say "ah" with the sample voice, matching it as closely as possible. This allows us to provide the patients with a model, showing how we want them to sing down to the lowest note they can make, descending by one full note on the musical scale for each production. In our model sample, we prolong each note for about three seconds. Patients' performances should be recorded on tape, whenever possible, and the actual frequency analyses done later in the laboratory. Patients now attempt to sing down to the lowest notes they can produce, then sing up one full note at a time, until reaching the highest notes they can produce, including the falsetto, and then sing down, one note at a time, until reaching their lowest note again. Finally, when the lowest notes are reached, they are asked once again to sing up to the highest note of their ranges. This pitch–range task is usually easiest for patients if they are instructed to sing one note at a time, taking a breath between each three-second production. Many voice patients, and perhaps the population in general, have real difficulty matching their own voices to a pitch model and producing a range of their lowest to their highest pitch productions. It may be impossible for some patients with vocal fold pathology, such as nodules or polyps, to vary the pitch of their voice much. By providing various models and encouragement at the right times, the experienced voice clinician can usually obtain some pitch–range information. Fortunately, for purposes of voice therapy, shifts do not have to be large shifts.

Each individual seems to have a voice pitch level that can be produced with an economy of physical effort and energy. This relatively effortless voice production is a concept we call *best pitch* and is apparently the pitch level at which the thyroarytenoids and other intrinsic muscles of the larynx can produce vocal fold adduction with only minimal muscular effort. It is simply the most efficient pitch for the patient's larynx to produce at this time, given the lesions or habitual phonational set of the patient. The vibrating frequency emitted from the approximated vocal folds is directly related to the natural length and mass of the thyroarytenoids, without much lengthening or shortening. The classic notion of optimum pitch may not be valid but a clinical use of "best" pitch is helpful. Using the Visi-Pitch, we can confirm a pitch level with jitter below .6 percent and shimmer below 2.4 percent. This will sound better in vocal quality and may be accompanied by an increase in loudness without any increase in vocal effort and is the patient's best pitch. When the patient produces such a phonation with clinical stimulation and we ask then "How did that voice feel?" they nearly always say, "It felt good" or "It was no work to make that voice." Such responses by patients are their way of noting the difference between the habitual disordered voice and the newly stimulated voice that is produced in response to clinical stimulation.

Therefore, although the concept of optimum pitch has been questioned (Thurman, 1958), the concept of an "easy, natural" pitch level is useful in voice therapy. Because so many voice patients seem to have problems of vocal hyperfunction, an attempt to have patients produce easy, relatively effortless phonations has obvious diagnostic and therapeutic implications. If a patient can produce a good voice easily, such a voice can become an immediate therapy goal. When best pitch has been determined, the patient should be asked to produce various other vowels and words at that general pitch level. We have used various vowels to determine which produce the best vocal quality at different pitch levels. Our experience with voice disordered patients has revealed that the /i/, /u/, and /o/ vowels almost always produce the best voices, whereas the /a/ and /ae/ always produce the poorest. A qualitative judgment should be made as to how the voice sounds.

To determine the best pitch with which to begin voice therapy, we might ask the patient to yawn and sigh (the relaxed phonation of a sigh is often the best speaking pitch) and also to say "uh huh" (this somewhat automatically produced, affirmative utterance often approximates the best pitch level) (Boone, 1997). These two methods usually yield pitch levels that are close to one another, even if not the same. Indications from the Visi-Pitch further help the determination of optimum pitch. Remember, however, that for clinical purposes we are interested in a particular area of the frequency range (usually a note or two, several notes above the bottom of the total range) that seems to produce the "best" voice with the least amount of effort. This best pitch provides the basis for the chant talk and pitch shift facilitation techniques discussed in Chapter 6.

Variations in Pitch as a Diagnostic Aid.   An inappropriate pitch level may at times contribute to the development of a voice disorder. Some vocal fold pathologies, on the other hand, produce changes in voice pitch, often because of the weighting or increased mass–size of the involved fold(s). Some functionally produced low-pitched voices may be called "the voices of profundity." A young professional person may employ an artificially low-pitched voice to assert authority and knowledge; a preacher may try to "hit the low ones" in his sermon; a young professional woman may think a low-pitched voice is more professional sounding. Conversely, a high-pitched voice is often symptomatic of general tension and difficulties in relaxation. In addition, a postmutational falsetto in a postpubertal male may be the result of a psychological identity problem, or may serve the patient little or not at all and persist out of habit. If a patient's pitch appears incongruous with his or her chronological age (as discussed in Chapter 2) and sex, the clinician should first determine if that patient has the functional ability to speak at a pitch level more compatible with his or her overall organism. If pitch variation is impossible, the condition might be the result of superior laryngeal nerve paralysis, or from certain virilizing drugs that have permanently changed the vocal folds, or of glandular–metabolic changes. These conditions require medical evaluation.

Variations in Loudness.   Some patients are observed to speak too loudly or too softly for particular vocal situations. There is no optimal loudness level for any one individual, as voice loudness will vary according to the situation, the speaker's mood, and the topic. In an evaluation session a clinician can make a judgment about the loudness of the patient's voice. If it appears to be impossible for the patient to speak in a loud enough voice, the dysphonia may be related to vocal fold paralysis, or to increases in the mass of the folds (for example, due to vocal nodules), or to bowed vocal folds worn out from continuous use (myasthenia larynges). Myasthenia larynges is a functional loss of muscle strength without a neurological basis; it is functional—from overuse. It represents a "tired larynx." The vocal folds may bow in this condition.

Soft voices may also be heard in patients who feel relatively inadequate and inferior, and their softness of phonation is consistent with their overall self-image, or the too soft voice may be a symptom of a conductive hearing loss. There are some neurological disorders, such as Parkinson's disease and bulbar palsy, in which the patient characteristically speaks in a voice that may be barely audible. At the other end of the spectrum are patients who speak with voices that may be perceived as uncomfortably loud. Some dysphonic patients, particularly those who speak with hyperfunction, may have inappropriately loud voices as part of their total problem or as a symptom of a sensorineural hearing loss. Another intensity variation that may be observed at the time of voice evaluation is a patient who speaks with little or no fluctuation in loudness (monoloudness), and perhaps with no variation in pitch (monopitch).

Because the loudness of the voice frequently varies according to the setting, the interactions of the speaker–listener, background noise levels, and so forth, it is difficult to measure a representative intensity of someone's speaking voice. One of the best ways we have of measuring loudness is to use a sound–pressure level meter that gives the sound–pressure level of the voice for a particular distance (from speaker's mouth to sound-level microphone). To measure voice intensity, patients are seated so that their mouth is about one meter from the microphone. The intensity level of the voice can be read from the sound-level meter dial in terms of decibels. Remember, however, that this laboratory measure of intensity does not have practical application to the loudness levels the patients may be using in more natural settings.

The Visi-Pitch and Computerized Speech Lab can also provide data for the interaction of frequency and intensity, because the instruments allow the simultaneous plotting of both values. Typically, the speaker, or singer for that matter, uses higher intensity levels for higher frequency levels. With practice it is possible for speakers to hold their pitch level constant and vary the intensity curve without altering frequency. The Visi-Pitch intensity values are relative but direct measurements of sound–pressure level can be made as well.

As mentioned earlier in this chapter, the Phonatory Function Analyzer makes careful intensity measurements in dB SPL as intensity interacts with airflow, frequency, total volume of air, and total phonation time in seconds. This makes the instrument helpful both diagnostically and therapeutically with dysphonic patients. Most measures of voice intensity level should be related to other information specific to airflow and air pressure, frequency, relative opening of the mouth, body position, and so on. If intensity measurements are possible, they are usually supplemented by rating scale judgments of loudness, as discussed earlier in this chapter. In practice the perceptual judgments of loudness may be the most important and useful data on vocal intensity.

Assessment of Vocal Quality.   One early diagnostic sign of a voice problem is the emergence of some kind of vocal quality disorder, such as hoarseness or breathiness. Usually some form of *dysphonia* (the term used through this text for all disorders of voice quality) signals to the patient that he or she has a voice problem. At the time of evaluation, the clinician should listen closely to how the patient speaks and attempt to describe what is heard. The verbal description of dysphonia is extremely difficult, however. Until the state of the art improves, voice clinicians will simply have to grope for terms to describe the voices they hear. Traditionally, three quality conditions, breathiness, harshness, and hoarseness, have been related to difficulties in optimal approximation of the vocal folds on phonation.

In breathiness, we can usually hear an audible escape of air as the approximating edges along the glottis fail to make optimum contact. Breathiness may be related to a patient's functional inability to bring the folds firmly together: the person may have the functional capability of firmer vocal fold approximation, but, for whatever reason, prefers to speak with a breathy voice. Some patients with rheumatoid arthritis take various muscle relaxants that produce excessively breathy voice quality as a side effect. Sometimes breathiness is related to growths on the folds, such as nodules or polyps, that prevent optimum adduction; sometimes it results from cord paralysis, which prevents optimum fold adduction. In a voice signal that is characterized as breathy, the periodicity of vocal tone is reduced and aperiodicity or noise is increased. We frequently observe at the beginning of an utterance marked aperiodicity that decreases as the vocal folds begin to vibrate. The breathy voice is often produced by the vocal folds approximating slowly together after the initiation of the outgoing airstream has already begun.

The spectrograph provides a visual display of what we hear. Figure 2.20 shows that the breathy voice produces noise across the sound spectrum with less definition of a periodic sound wave, as seen in the distinct print of the first three formants in the normal voice spectrogram. Other laboratory measures for quantification of breathiness can be made (with the PFA or Aerophone mentioned earlier), such as measuring airflow–air pressure, spectral noise levels (Sansone and Emanuel, 1970), and determining jitter (variations or perturbations in frequency) and shimmer (variations in cycle to cycle amplitude) as described by Michel and Wendahl (1971). These can be measured by use of the Computerized Speech Lab. The perceptual judgments of the clinician and other listeners continue, however, to play an important role in the observation and diagnosis of breathiness.

A harsh voice is usually heard by listeners as unpleasant. Ainsworth (1980) described the difficulty of defining harshness:

> Verbal descriptions of harshness are difficult to make without using "impressionistic" terms, i.e., *grating, rasping, rough, guttural, raucous.* There often are frequent and "hard" glottal catches, i.e., the initiation of tones with an explosive release of air by the vocal folds, and excessive glottal (vocal) fry which is a low-pitched "popping" sound (p. 7).

Aperiodicity of laryngeal vibration can be seen in the spectrogram for the harsh voice. Often abrupt initiation of voice is characterized by hard glottal attack. Patients sound as if they are working hard to speak. A harsh voice may be described as *strident, metallic,* or *grating;* whatever the description used, the connotation is unpleasant. The Visi-Pitch or any kind of spectrum analyzer like the spectrograph will display harshness with increased aperiodicity across the spectrum, a reduction of fundamental frequency, a scatter of resonance across the spectrum, and abrupt glottal attack as observed in sudden initiation of phonation. In our judgments of harshness we often focus on the metallic aspects of resonance, whereby the voice seems to come out of a pharynx and oral cavity that appear to be in a state of hypercontraction. Instead of hearing softness and some absorption of higher frequency sound waves, we hear a hardness described by Coffin (1981) as a "voice produced by hard, reflective surfaces rather than by soft, absorbing surfaces." It is difficult to verbalize a description of the harsh voices we sometimes hear. Hoarseness is the most common laryngeal quality disturbance, although the term is often used in a meaningless manner to label any kind of laryngeal problem in phonation. Anything that interferes with optimum vocal fold adduction can produce hoarseness. Many patients exhibit it on a purely functional basis: that is, because they approximate the vocal folds too tightly or too loosely together, they produce hoarseness. Typical dysphonic patients display the kind of hoarseness we hear in patients with some form of laryngitis. The hoarse voice heard in patients with bilateral vocal nodules includes a breathy escape of air, and is often accompanied by hard glottal attack as patients attempt to compensate for their phonation difficulties. Hoarseness may be related to mucus on the vocal folds, or sometimes to destruction of all or a part of the folds. The spectral printout of the hoarse voice in Figure 2.20 confirms the combination of breathiness and harshness, as we see increased noise across the spectrum with a heavier concentration of acoustic energy in the first formant at the bottom of the spectrogram.

Many patients with hoarseness begin to compensate for their poor voices by driving the mechanism even harder; they may feel, for example, that they must have abrupt initiation of glottal attack to "get their voices started." The Visi-Pitch is easy to use to determine the abruptness of glottal attack combined with hoarseness. Any kind of air-pressure instrument can likewise verify sudden onset of expiration.

The electroglottograph (EGG) is an excellent device to demonstrate glottal activity and depicts the ratio of long open phase to short closed phase that characterizes the breathy voice. The device also displays aperiodic vocal fold vibration by clearly demonstrating the lack of similarity from wave to wave. The more dissimilar each wave is from the preceding and following waves, the more aperiodicity in the voice. Figure 5.15 shows a glottogram or laryngogram of a prolonged /i/ vowel produced with a very hoarse voice quality. This laryngogram may be contrasted with one of a normal vocal quality and one of a breathy vocal quality during the production of the /i/ vowel.

A clinician's judgment of hoarseness must supplement any instrumental measurements we are able to make. The advantage of some kind of instrument quantification of hoarseness at the time of the initial evaluation is that the measurement data can be compared with data taken subsequently during and at the end of therapy. It has also been our experience that the instruments that provide evaluation data can be used to provide feedback to patients in therapy about particular components of voice. For example, for a patient with hoarseness, it may be advantageous to provide visual feedback on the oscilloscope relative to improvement of periodicity as the voice is heard to be "less hoarse." Like most evaluation data, it should be used not only in the diagnostic–decision process in planning therapy, but also given to patients as continuing feedback and confirmation of their therapy progress (Chapter 6). This can be extremely motivational. This data can be used to make prognostic statements (McFarlane et al., 1998, Weiss and McFarlane, 1998)

Perceptual Judgments of Vocal Quality.   Other variations in vocal fold approximation may produce symptoms of glottal fry, register variations, pitch breaks, and phonation breaks. Most voice evaluation forms have checkoff lists that would include these terms. Glottal fry can be detected using the Visi-Pitch. Instead of a single tracing line representing a single fundamental frequency, the voice is represented by two or more broken lines, indicating that the patient is producing two or three, more or less, simultaneous fundamental frequencies The multiple phonation pulses are, usually of low frequency and are usually observed at the bottom of the patient's frequency range. The phenomenon of fry is usually observed as slight hoarseness that comes into the individual's voice toward the bottom of the

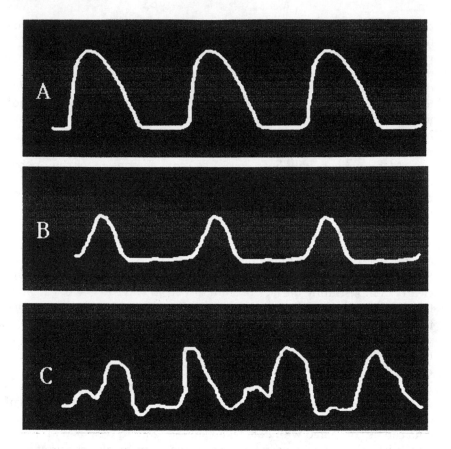

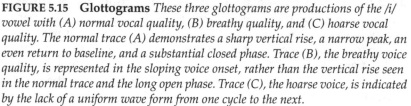

FIGURE 5.15   Glottograms *These three glottograms are productions of the /i/ vowel with (A) normal vocal quality, (B) breathy quality, and (C) hoarse vocal quality. The normal trace (A) demonstrates a sharp vertical rise, a narrow peak, an even return to baseline, and a substantial closed phase. Trace (B), the breathy voice quality, is represented in the sloping voice onset, rather than the vertical rise seen in the normal trace and the long open phase. Trace (C), the hoarse voice, is indicated by the lack of a uniform wave form from one cycle to the next.*

pitch range. It has been described as sounding like an outboard motor boat, a creaking door, popcorn popping, and so on. Moore and von Leden (1958) termed glottal fry *dicrotic dysphonia*. Others have described the vocal folds during the production of fry as thick, with the ventricular bands in close contact with the superior surface of the true vocal folds. It is undoubtedly this thickness of folds that produces the lower fundamental pitch that is characteristic of glottal fry. With some elevation of voice pitch, the fry will often decrease. We consider glottal fry to be a normal vocal register. Register variations, rarely mentioned in United States speech pathology texts, do exist as clinical problems in some voice patients. The concept of vocal register comes from the organ stop, which in German is called *register*. Luchsinger and Arnold (1965) wrote:

In chest voice, the cords vibrate over their entire breadth, whereas the falsetto voice reveals vibration limited to the inner cord margins. When phonating low tones, the cords appear rounded, full, and relaxed, while they are sharp-edged, thin, and taut for falsetto tones. These differences may readily be seen on frontal laryngeal tomograms (p. 97).

Register variation is related to the relative changes in the cross-section of the vocal folds, produced by differential contraction of the vocalis section of the thyroarytenoid muscle. In his classic article, "The Mechanism of the Larynx," Negus (1957) used the terms *thick* and *thin* to correspond to the cross-sectional differences seen in the production of the chest register and the head register. Sometimes we observe voices that seem incompatible with the resonating bodies of the patient. Certain patients may produce variations by attempting to speak at their lower pitches with vocal folds approximated in the manner typical of high-pitched head register. Conversely, sometimes higher pitches are produced with the folds approximated in their fullest broad dimension, the typical pattern of the low-pitched chest register. Register variation (fold approximation incompatible with the desired pitch level) can best be confirmed by frontal X-ray of the approximating glottal surfaces, as seen in frontal tomograms.

When pitch break is observed, it is usually in a voice that is pitched too low. As the patient is phonating, the pitch level suddenly breaks upward to a falsetto level, often one octave above the pitch level the person was using. Pitch breaks may also be observed in a voice pitched too high, and then the break is downward, usually a full octave below the previous pitch level. In an adult patient, voice breaks can be extremely embarrassing. Sometimes pitch breaks are a patient's primary, and perhaps sole, reason for seeking voice therapy. Pitch breaks in children are much more common, but are rarely considered to be clinical problems. Curry (1949) found, in his voice studies of adolescents, that although voice breaks can occur in males in prepuberty, they are much more common at around the age of fourteen, when rapid pubertal changes take place. In eighteen-year-olds, Curry found virtually no pitch breaks. Pitch breaks in children, particularly in males at around the time of puberty, are, in fact, fairly common and usually disappear with continuing physical maturation. In adults, pitch breaks are relatively rare and appear most often to be symptomatic of inappropriate habitual pitch levels—too low a pitch with involuntary pitch breaks upward, or too high a pitch with the breaks occurring downward.

The phonation break or abductor spasm (see Chapter 7) is a temporary loss of voice that may occur for only part of a word, a whole word, a phrase, or a sentence. An individual may be phonating with no observable difficulty when suddenly a loss of voice or phonation break occurs. Patients who experience voice breaks usually exhibit some degree of voice hyperfunction as they speak. They *work too hard* at talking. Typical patients with voice breaks may use their voices a lot, such as teachers. After prolonged speaking, they begin to experience vocal fatigue and try to improve the sound of their voice by raising or lowering the voice pitch or speaking through clenched teeth. The result is increased vocal tension. Finally, while they are phonating, the vocal folds spontaneously abduct and they temporarily lose their voice. By throat-clearing, coughing, swallowing water, or whatever, they restore phonation until the next phonation break. Most voice patients, even if they have occasional phonation breaks, will not exhibit such temporary voice loss during evaluation sessions.

The two different types of phonation breaks or abductor spasms result from different causes. First, as we have described, is the cessation of phonation that results from the sudden abduction of the vocal folds, or from the loss of sufficient glottal resistance, such as when two opposing nodules meet and allow too much air to escape. Too little subglottic pressure remains to drive the cords, and phonation is lost momentarily. A second type of phonation break occurs when there is a phonatory arrest, as in spastic dysphonia, hyperkinetic dysphonia, or ventricular phonation. The vocal folds are simply overadducted, which prevents phonation.

Resonance Testing.   Our focus in this chapter on voice evaluation has been on the evaluation of patients with phonation disorders. That is not to say that patients may not have accompanying resonance disorders; phonation and resonance disorders may go hand in hand. Many patients, however, have voice problems that are primarily of voice resonance. We discuss the problems of voice resonance, their evaluation, management, and therapy in Chapter 9. Many of the neurological disorders discussed in Chapter 4 also have resonance components that may be addressed therapeutically by the methods described in Chapter 9 and Chapter 6, which deal with clinical facilitation techniques.

Two Example Cases Compare Noninstrumental and Instrumental Approaches

These are brief examples from actual cases. The reports are not complete but represent the main facts or observation for each case.

Noninstrumental Approach.   Case #1 is a young adult male with unilateral (right) recurrent vocal fold paralysis. The case history and ENT information would be very similar for both approaches. In the noninstrumental approach the description of the voice would be most critical. It is important to note that the patient has no difficulty swallowing and can produce an adequate cough.

The clinician would note that the voice is weak in loudness, extremely breathy, vocally rough in quality (a dry hoarseness), and of short duration of phonation. It may be noted that the patient states that he cannot be heard and that he constantly runs out of breath and must keep taking extra breathes while talking. These observations can be scaled on a form such as that presented in Figure 5.6. Duration of phonation may be determined by a stopwatch or by counting the seconds by "one thousand one, one thousand two, one thousand three, and so on." In this case, the duration of phonation is found to be three seconds. The pitch of the voice may also be lower or higher than normal, a judgment that should be scaled on the observation of perceptions form (Figure 5.6). In this case the voice was high for a male fundamental pitch. Resonance will be observed and the absence of hypernasality noted.

Clinical stimulation and the response to clinical probes will be noted on the form as well. It may be observed that the extreme breathiness and the low loudness are improved by the head-turning technique and the digital pressure to the larynx technique, both mentioned in Chapter 6. Also a downward pitch shift improves the voice by increasing loudness without extra effort and the breathiness is further reduced. It is noted that phonation time is extended to 6.5 seconds. A tape recording of the evaluation and the response to clinical facilitation techniques will be made. An oral examination will be completed and the results, likely negative, will be noted. The ENT report of vocal fold paralysis will be used because the clinician will likely not have access to endoscopy or stroboscopy.

Instrumental Approach. We use the instrumental–noninstrumental form (Figure 5.6) at this point. Case #1. The instrumental approach with the same young male with unilateral right vocal fold paralysis would be reported in a different manner on the same form. The airflow rate may be reported as 400 ml/sec, rather than as "extremely breathy in quality." The "weakness in loudness" may be reported as 70 dB SPL from the Phonatory Function Analyzer. The fundamental frequency would be reported as 165Hz rather than as "high for a male fundamental." Vocal roughness will be reported as a jitter value of 1.35 percent with a shimmer of 4.36 percent. These values will be noted on the form rather than the perception of "rough, dry hoarseness." Phonation time will be reported as three seconds. Electroglottographic traces will be reported as short closed phases and long open phases of a ratio of 1:4 in time. The irregularity of the wave form from one cycle to the next will be noted. The videostroboscopic results were of a shorter appearing right vocal fold that is fixed in the paramedian position. The right vocal fold adducts and abducts normally. The left vocal fold is lacking tone and flutters during phonation, giving rise to an asymmetrical vocal fold vibration and an open glottal chink during phonation. With application of the lateral digital pressure technique and head turned to the left the glottal gap is markedly reduced and phonation time is increased to 6.5 seconds.

The perceptual report is longer than the instrumental report because instrumentation has allowed us to be parsimonious in the use of words. The instrumental approach has also has allowed us to quantify our findings. This makes comparison of performance at subsequent sessions much easier.

Case #2. Is an adult female (age fifty-six years) with muscle tension dysphonia.

Noninstrumental Approach. This woman demonstrates extreme strain and effort during phonation attempts. She has a vocal quality with marked strained–strangled aspects. Her airflow rate appears low but phonation time is also short, at about five seconds. Voice pitch is low and her rate of speaking is slow. Vocal loudness is generally low but at times is explosive.

Response to clinical stimulation is very positive. With yawn–sigh and tongue protrusion /i/ and upward pitch shifts the voice is much less effortful to produce. The strained–strangled quality is greatly diminished. Phonation time is increased to twelve seconds. The patient reports that this voice is much less effortful to produce and she feels freer during talking than she has in months. Her voice sounded normal in vocal quality and pitch.

Instrumental Approach. Acoustical analysis revealed a jitter score of 1.60 percent and a shimmer value of 3.241 percent. The fundamental frequency was 165 Hz. Duration of phonation was five seconds. The airflow rate was 75 ml/sec. EGG traces were irregular with long closed phases and short or absent open phases. During videostroboscopy the vocal folds were tightly pressed together during phonation with some overlapping of the folds along the glottal margins. Some shortening of the vocal folds was noted as the epiglottis and arytenoids were brought closer together. The false vocal folds were brought into activity overlapping the true vocal folds, making them appear only half their true width. Clinical stimulation using yawn–sigh, tongue protrusion /i/, and upward pitch shifts reduced the excessive glottal valving and extended phonation to twelve seconds. Using the same clinical facilitation techniques during acoustical analysis, the jitter and shimmer were normalized at .62 percent and 2.12 percent, respectively.

Summary

The voice evaluation is the time when the clinician first meets the voice patient, providing opportunity for observation and testing. The evaluation begins when the patient is observed in the waiting room and continues as part of every therapy session, particularly as the clinician continually searches with the patient for new vocal behaviors. The speech–language pathologist must continue to evaluate and observe the patient's respiratory, phonatory, and resonance functions. Whenever possible, these functions should be quantified with instrumentation. Perceptual judgments are also extremely valuable in describing the patient's voice disorder and the manner in which it is produced. The patient's voice data are used for comparison purposes, to quantify vocal changes between the first visit, subsequent therapy sessions, and the final outcome session. Patient performance, both as observed and as measured, is offered to the patient as continuing feedback, helping the patient become aware of voice performance. The evaluation enables the voice clinician to decide on which management steps to take for the patient. If voice therapy is indicated, the evaluation will help the clinician to develop a therapy plan and to predict the patient's outcome prognosis. Two actual voice cases were used to demonstrate the perceptual (noninstrumental) and the instrumental approaches to voice evaluation on a similar evaluation form (Figure 5.6).

CHAPTER

6

Voice Therapy

After the initial voice evaluation is completed, the search for causal and maintaining factors continues. Some voice problems may require only the management of professionals outside of the profession of speech–language pathologists (SLP); for example, a small supralaryngeal cancer may be treated only by the laryngeal surgeon. A problem of vocal paralysis may be managed by both the surgeon and the SLP who will see the patient at different times during the recovery process. Many voice problems are best managed by the SLP, who will provide the needed voice therapy and possibly seek the help of other professionals. For example, the patient with spasmodic dysphonia may be referred by the SLP to an ENT or a neurologist (as discussed in Chapter 4), who will play a primary role in the management of the patient's voice. The SLP may alone provide the voice therapy needed for the patient who has functional aphonia (no voice) or for the child with vocal nodules that have developed as part of a hyperfunctional voice disorder.

What is offered for management and therapy (and by whom) is dictated by the presenting causal and maintaining factors that were identified at the time of the initial diagnostic evaluation (Behrman and Orlikoff, 1997). Even during voice therapy, there must be a continuous search for a possible change in the maintenance factors of the voice problem, which could then dictate a different management or therapy offering.

While many of the management strategies differ among voice patients according to whether their problems are organic, neurogenic, or functional, our voice therapy approaches may not be differentiated according to such causal factors. For example, if the patient is exhibiting a problem in breath control, while the cause of the problem may get primary attention, the techniques for using more efficient breath for voice are selected from a pool of approaches for improving breath control. Perhaps the most commonly observed voice problems are related to vocal hyperfunction for which there are many therapy approaches designed to "take the work" out of speaking. A voice therapy approach for a particular person with vocal hyperfunction would be selected from an array of such approaches, with the selection again related to causal and maintaining factors. A young man who exhibits hard glottal attack might profit from learning to slow down his rate of speech, opening his mouth a bit more, learning more of a *legato* (smooth, easy flow) style of voicing, and practicing vocal chanting. Accordingly, his SLP would select those therapy approaches that help facilitate this easy, smooth style of voicing.

There are some differences in overall management and voice therapy between preschool children, school aged children, and adolescents and adults. The age of the person and the physical size of vocal mechanisms, coupled with cognitive understanding of the goals of therapy, will often dictate what can be done. Let us look separately at some of the issues shaping management and voice therapy for young children and adolescents–adults.

Voice Management and Therapy for Young Children

Track
6 & 10

When the preschool child with a voice disorder is brought to the voice clinic, the problem usually has a physical cause. The functional components of the voice problem at this age are minimal. Consequently, most of the early management emphasis is on evaluation. A sudden hoarseness, perhaps accompanied by laryngeal stridor (noise on inhalation), may cause concern that the child may have a serious laryngeal disease, such as papilloma or laryngeal web. Even at very young ages, the otolaryngologist skilled in endoscopy can use a pediatric endoscope and view the larynx. If papilloma or web and other laryngeal diseases were identified, the primary management of the problem would be medical–surgical. If the hoarseness appears to be related to vocal fold thickening or nodules, which have developed after continuous vocal hyperfunction, some parent counseling may usually be in order. Direct voice therapy with the child may be deferred until the preschooler is cognitively able to understand the importance of curbing particular hyperfunctional behaviors, such as yelling and making continuous "funny" noises. Voice therapy might well be delayed until kindergarten or first grade. The primary voice management role in the preschool child is the identification and possible treatment of laryngeal disease rather than as a preliminary evaluative step for voice therapy.

The most common voice problem in the school-aged child is hoarseness related to vocal hyperfunction. On endoscopy, such children will usually reveal the presence of vocal fold thickening or vocal nodules or polyps. Occasionally, other laryngeal diseases may be identified. This is why management and voice therapy cannot be initiated until the cause of the problem is identified. The organic and neurogenic causal factors discussed in Chapters 3 and 4 will require special medical–surgical management and voice management–therapy consistent with such diagnoses. Again, let us say that the majority of voice problems seen in the school-aged population are related to vocal hyperfunction. The overall thrust of voice therapy for vocal hyperfunction in school-aged children is identifying their voice abuses and voice misuse (see facilitating approach 7, p. 183) and reducing the occurrence of such behaviors.

The clinician can probably do nothing more effective than identify those situations in which the child is vocally abusive, such as yelling at a ballgame, screaming on the playground, crying, imitating noises below or above his or her speaking pitch range, and so on. Many children maintain their vocal pathologies simply by engaging in abusive vocal behavior for only brief periods each day. It is usually not possible to identify these vocal abuses through interview methods or by observing the child in the therapy room; rather, the child must be observed in various play settings, in the classroom, and at home. This need for extensive observation requires that clinicians solicit the help of the children themselves to determine where they might be yelling or screaming. Teachers can provide some helpful clues about the child's vocal behavior both on the playground and in the classroom. Meeting with parents will often reveal further situations of vocal abuse, and the parents may be asked to listen over a period of time for abusive vocal behavior in the child's play or interactions with various family members. At times, we have had good luck using the siblings or peers to help us determine what a child does vocally in certain situations.

Once the abusive situations are isolated, clinicians should obtain baseline measurements of the number of times a vocal abuse is observed in a particular time unit (an hour, a recess period, a day, and so on). Figure 6.1 shows a vocal abuse graph, which plots the number of abuses a child had recorded over a period of two weeks.

Notice that the first plot on the abscissa is the first day's baseline measurement, which tells on the ordinate how many times the child caught himself yelling on that particular day—for this child, eighteen separate yells. The overall contour shows a linear decrement in voice yelling, which is a somewhat typical curve for young children. Having to monitor his offensive behavior seems to motivate the child to reduce it. The child may keep a card in his pocket on which to mark down each occurrence; at the end of the day, he tallies that day's occurrences and plots the total figure on the graph. The review of the plotting graph is a vital part of the therapy, and the child's pride in his graph (which usually shows a decrement in the behavior) helps him continue to curb the vocal abuse. Some children require assistance in making this kind of plot, and sometimes we ask teachers, parents, or friends to also keep tally cards to record the number of events they observed in a particular time period. If children are given proper orientation to the task and clearly know why they must reduce their number of vocal abuses, their tally counts seem to be higher, and perhaps more valid, than the counts of external observers.

Another variation of the tally method requires the child to take his tally card for the date and plot his voice abuse–misuse against that reported by another

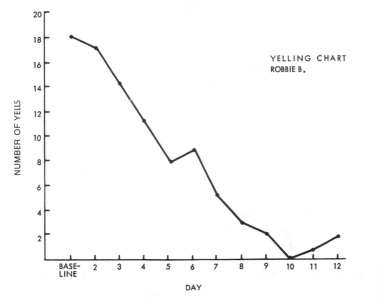

FIGURE 6.1 **A Vocal Abuse Graph**

child or the clinician. For example, in *The Boone Voice Program for Children* (1993) are play materials for a hot-air balloon race in which the clinician "races" the child in plotting changes (in this case abuse–misuse) with hot-air balloons across a sky backdrop. Setting up some kind of reward, such as winning the balloon race, helps the child to become more aware of the desirability of curbing voice abuse–misuse.

An important prelude to the tally method—indeed, to any form of speech therapy, particularly voice therapy—is for the clinician to explain to the child what the problem is, what the child seems to be doing wrong vocally, and what can be done about it. Obviously, a child must first know that there is a voice problem (rarely does a child recognize such a problem independently) before he or she can do anything about it. Such explanations are also especially important because most children with voice problems are not self-referred. Their dysphonias have been discovered by someone else. To the child, there may be no problem.

Voice Therapy for Adolescents and Adults

The abusive vocal behaviors of adults are likely to be more difficult to isolate than those of children. It is the relatively rare adult voice patient whose vocal abuses are bound only to particular situations. Preachers or auctioneers whose voice problems appear only on the job may be excellent examples of vocal misuse; however, dysphonic adolescents or adults generally have hyperfunctional sets toward phonation. They work to talk in most situations. Sometimes, the exaggerated effort experienced by some voice patients toward vocalization is related to a generalized tension that may become more acute in particular situations, such as when they speak to authority figures or when they try to make favorable impressions on their listeners. A more generalized anxiety might best be treated through counseling or psychological therapy. It has been the authors' observation, however, that even patients with a more generalized anxiety can often take the tension out of their voices by employing voice therapy approaches that seem to open up and relax the structures of the airway. Many adult voice patients appear capable of producing a good, optimum voice, providing someone (the clinician) will only help them "find" it.

Therefore, the primary task of voice clinicians is to explore with patients the various therapy techniques that might produce that "good" voice. We advocate the same approach with adults as we do with children: using facilitating techniques as therapy probes. The approach that works is then used as a therapy practice approach. Once the patients are able to produce a model of their own best voice, this model and the techniques used to achieve it become the primary focus of voice therapy.

Voice clinicians also provide patients with needed psychological support, and together they explore various facilitating techniques to be used in particular situations. Hierarchies of stress can often be identified (Boone, 1982; Wolpe, 1987), and behavioral approaches used at these times of stress may minimize symptoms. Patients are taught to isolate those situations in which they experience poor voice and to substitute at those times more optimum forms of behavior—that is, easier voice.

Voice disorders in adolescents and adults often have a negative impact on their lives because they may interfere with life interactions and employment. Some patients become desperate over their vocal problems, and so seek professional help. The family physician is often the first professional who identifies a voice problem as a disorder that needs the expert help of an otolaryngologist or speech–language pathologist. The physician subsequently refers the patient for a voice evaluation that, more often than not, involves the evaluation–diagnostic procedures described in Chapter 5. Voice therapy is often the recommended step after the diagnostic evaluation.

Voice Therapy Facilitating Techniques

In this text, we call our therapy approaches *facilitating approaches.* That is, the selected therapy technique facilitates a "target" or a more optimal vocal response by the patient. The techniques may be used with patients with various kinds of voice disorders: organic, neurogenic, or functional. Part of voice therapy is searching with patients to find the facilitating approach that seems to help them produce the desired vocal response. Many patients with the same voice disorder, such as functional dysphonia, may require different therapy approaches for the same problem. It is important to remember that no *one* specific therapy approach is facilitative for all patients with the same voice problem.

The accomplished voice clinician will have many voice therapy techniques to use for particular voice problems with certain patients. In addition to the current list of 25 approaches in this edition of *The Voice and Voice Therapy,* there are many other therapy approaches described in the literature: Andrews (1995); Aronson (1990); Boone (1997); Case (1996); Colton and Casper (1996); Greene and Mathieson (1991); Kotby (1995); Morrison and Rammage (1994); Stemple, Gerdeman, and Glaze (1994).

The facilitating approaches in Table 6.1 are listed alphabetically. After each approach a notation (X) is made to indicate the voice parameters that the particular approach has the potential to influence. For example, approach 1, auditory feedback position, in most cases has little influence on the pitch or loudness of the voice; its biggest influence is usually on vocal quality. Consequently, for the three columns in Table 6.1—pitch, loudness, quality—only the quality column is marked with an X. Other techniques, such as 25, Yawn–Sigh, influence all three parameters of pitch, loudness, and quality. Some experienced voice clinicians combine various facilitating approaches in their search with the patient to find the target voice. Each of the twenty-five facilitating approaches in Table 6.1 is discussed from the following four perspectives: (1) Kinds of problems for which the approach is useful; (2) procedural aspects of the approach; (3) typical case history showing utilization of the approach; and (4) evaluation of the approach.

1. Auditory Feedback

A. Kinds of Problems for Which the Approach Is Useful.   Many voice patients profit from using some kind of auditory feedback in and out of voice therapy. Those patients who displayed a window of voice improvement during the evaluation session (such as when masking was used as a diagnostic probe resulting in an immediate improvement in voice) will often benefit from the use of auditory feedback during therapy sessions. Regardless of the causal factor of the disorder (organic,

TABLE 6.1   Twenty-Five Facilitating Approaches in Voice Therapy

Facilitating Approach	Parameter of Voice Affected		
	Pitch	Loudness	Quality
1. Auditory feedback	X	X	X
2. Change of loudness	X	X	X
3. Chant talk		X	X
4. Chewing			X
5. Counseling (explanation of problem)	X	X	X
6. Digital manipulation	X		X
7. Elimination of abuses		X	X
8. Establishing a new pitch	X		X
9. Focus	X	X	X
10. Glottal attack changes		X	X
11. Glottal fry		X	X
12. Head positioning	X		X
13. Hierarchy analysis	X	X	X
14. Inhalation phonation	X	X	
15. Laryngeal massage	X		X
16. Masking	X	X	X
17. Nasal/glide stimulation			X
18. Open-mouth approach		X	X
19. Pitch inflections	X		
20. Relaxation	X	X	X
21. Respiration training		X	X
22. Tongue protrusion /i/	X		X
23. Visual feedback	X	X	X
24. Warble	X		X
25. Yawn–sigh	X	X	X

neurogenic, or functional), the patient's voice may improve with such feedback. There are different kinds of auditory feedback that may enhance patient response, such as using real-time amplification and letting patients hear themselves on headphones as they are speaking. Voice improvement is best secured by listening real-time on amplification equipment that has a speech–voice range focus, such as the commercially available instruments as the Hearit or the Facilitator. Some motor speech patients might profit from the use of an auditory metronome that can pace either an increased or decreased rate of response modeling for the patient; for example, a metronome set at about 60 words per minute can result in a marked slowing down of the Parkinson patient's speech rate, which may increase both voice quality–volume and articulation intelligibility. Most voice patients profit from auditory modeling, hearing either their own voice on auditory playback or an external model (perhaps a speaking pitch note or the clinician's voice). Auditory modeling, to be effective, must be immediate. The clinician may stop recording on a cassette, rewind, and play for the patient a recording of the model and the patient response. The auditory playback is easier on loop-playback recorders, such as the tape-loop Phonic Mirror or the solid-state loop auditory feedback mode found on the Facilitator.

B. Procedural Aspects of the Approach. Let us separate the application approaches for three forms of auditory feedback: real-time amplification, metronome pacing, and loop playback.

1. Real-time amplification of one's speech and voice enables one to hear oneself clearer than would be possible without such self-amplification and auditory focus. Real-time amplification requires the clinician to use an amplifier, microphone, and headset with the patient. The clinician uses a cassette recorder, a boom box, or an amplifying instrument that provides real-time feedback as the patient speaks.

> **a.** The patient is asked to listen on the headphones closely to what he or she will be saying. Usually another facilitating approach is used, such as chanting or focus, that the patient will use while speaking. The patient then listens closely to the sound of the voice or speech while he or she is using the approach.
> **b.** The patient is asked to evaluate the appropriateness of his or her response. If adjustments are made, they are listened to with real-time amplification again.

2. The clicks or beats of a metronome may provide good auditory pacing for those patients who need to slow down or increase their rate of speech.

> **a.** The rate of clicks per minute is set on the instrument. All wind-up or electronic metronomes have a setting switch. On the Facilitator, the click pacing ranges from 50 to 150 clicks per minute.
> **b.** The best pacing practice is achieved by the patient matching the clicks by shortening or prolonging the vowel duration of the practice material. Changing vowel duration is a preferred way to change rate over altering pause duration between words or phrases.

3. Loop playback allows the patient to hear immediately what was just said. The Phonic Mirror and Language Master were designed for immediate replay feedback.

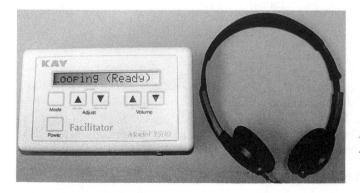

FIGURE 6.2 KAY FACILITATOR, Model 3500 *The Facilitator is an auditory feedback device with five modes of feedback: real-time amplification, loop feedback, delayed auditory feedback (DAF), masking (speech range), and metronomic pacing.*

The authors have constructed cassette loops (Boone, 1982) that enable the patient to hear an immediate playback. The more recent Facilitator (1998) has a solid-state loop system that allows the patient who wears a headset an immediate playback (from 1–6 secs) of what was just said. These procedures are used for the Facilitator:

a. The patient wears a headset and lapel mike. The mode switch on the Facilitator is turned to "LOOPING (READY)." To record a model and/or patient response, the UP (↑) arrow is pressed and released.

b. When playback is wanted, the DOWN (↓) arrow is pressed and released. This stops the recording and provides an immediate playback. Tapping the down arrow again will provide a repeat playback; a new playback of the same utterance will occur with each successive tap of the down arrow.

c. The patient is asked to evaluate the immediate playback. The clinician, who may wear another headset with microphone, provides some feedback specific to the appropriateness of the patient's response. The patient may be asked to repeat the utterance and steps (3a) and (3b) are repeated.

C. Typical Case History Showing Utilization of the Approach.   J. W., a forty-nine-year-old social worker, had a two-year history of functional dysphonia. At the time of the initial interview it was found that elevating her pitch slightly at the end of a phrase or sentence seemed to eliminate all hoarseness. Loop playback was very effective in helping her realize that raising pitch slightly in an upward inflection cleared the hoarseness out of her voice. Working with her SLP using loop playback, she practiced repeating sentences in two different ways: one, with the usual downward inflection (which caused hoarseness), and two, saying them with upward inflection. Using immediate loop feedback in a few practice sessions appeared to be a primary approach in developing better functional voice out of the clinic, especially in her work as a social worker.

D. Evaluation of the Approach.   Voice improvement is often enhanced by listening closely to one's voice. The use of auditory feedback is often an important step in therapy for articulation, language, fluency, and voice disorders. Real-time amplification, loop playback, and using external metronomic pacing can be effective auditory aids in voice therapy. A holistic approach to correcting a voice disorder, such as listening to one's voice, is often preferred over fractionating various voice components (breathing, pitch, loudness, etc.) with separate practice for each component.

2. Change of Loudness

A. Kinds of Problems for Which the Approach Is Useful.   Some patients have voices that have inappropriate loudness, too loud or too soft. Many of the vocal pathologies experienced by children are related to such excesses of loudness as screaming and yelling. Weak, soft voices may develop as a consequence of the prolonged hyperfunctional use of the vocal mechanism that results in the eventual breakdown of glottal approximation surfaces—for example, a patient with vocal nodules who loses much airflow around the nodules and is unable to produce an intense enough vocal fold vibration to achieve a sufficiently loud voice. Some speaking environments require a loud voice, and untrained speakers or singers may push for loudness at the level of the larynx rather than adjust their respiration. Inappropriate loudness of voice is most often not the primary causative factor of a voice problem, but rather a secondary, if annoying, symptom. Reducing or increasing the loudness of the voice lends itself well to direct symptom modification through exercise and practice, and often, if other facilitating techniques are being used, does not even require the use of loudness techniques per se.

B. Procedural Aspects of the Approach

1. For a decrease in loudness:

   a. See that the patient has a thorough audiometric examination to determine adequacy of hearing before any attempt is made to reduce voice loudness. Once it has been established that the patient has normal hearing, the following steps may be taken.

   b. For young children, ages three through ten, the change of loudness steps in *The Boone Voice Program for Children* (1993) are useful. Ask the child to develop awareness of five different voices:

      i. Voice 1 is presented as a whisper.
      ii. Voice 2 is presented as the voice to use when not wanting to awaken a sleeping person, a quiet voice.
      iii. Voice 3 is the normal voice to use to talk to family and friends.
      iv. Voice 4 is the voice to use to talk to someone across the room.
      v. Voice 5 is the yelling voice to call someone outside.

   c. With patients over ten years old, discuss with the patient the observation that he or she has an inappropriately loud voice. The patient may be unaware of the loud voice and should listen to tape-recorded samples of his or her speech. The best demonstration tape for loudness variations would include both the patient's voice and the clinician's, to provide contrasting levels of loudness. Then ask the patient, "Do you think your voice is louder than mine?"

   d. Focus on making the patient aware of the problem. Once the patient becomes aware that his or her voice is too loud, ask, "What does a loud voice in another person tell you about that person?" Loud voices are typically interpreted to mean that the speaker feels "overly confident," or "sure of himself," or that the speaker is putting on a confident front when he or she is really scared, or that he or she is mad at the world, impressed with his or her own voice, trying to intimidate listeners, and so on. Some discussion of these negative interpretations is usually sufficient to motivate the average patient to learn to speak at normal loudness levels.

   e. Practice using a quiet voice (voice 2 in section b). The practice for the quiet voice can be facilitated by using instruments that give feedback specific to intensity, such as the Vocal Loudness Indicator and the Visi-Pitch. The Vocal Loudness Indicator, for example, has a series of lights that are illuminated by increases in voice intensity. Keeping the instrument at a fixed distance, the patient can quickly learn to keep his or her voice at a lower intensity level to prevent the light (all or a few) from coming on.

2. For an increase in loudness:

   a. Determine first that the inappropriate softness of the voice is not related to hearing loss, general physical weakness, or a severe personality problem; for these cases, a symptomatic approach is not indicated. The steps that follow are for voice patients who are physically and emotionally capable of speaking in a louder voice.

   b. Discuss with the patient the soft voice. A tape-recorded playback of the patient's and clinician's voices in conversation will usually illustrate for the patient the inadequacy of the loudness. After the patient indicates some awareness of his or her soft voice, ask, "What does a soft, weak voice tell us about a person?" Inadequately loud voices are typically interpreted to mean that the speaker is afraid to speak louder, is timid and shy, is unduly considerate of others, is scared of people, has no self-confidence, and so on. Some discussion of these negative interpretations is usually helpful.

   c. By exploring pitch level and fundamental frequency, try to achieve a pitch level at which the patient is able with some ease to produce a louder voice. If the patient habitually speaks near the bottom of his or her pitch range, a slight elevation of pitch level will usually be accompanied by a slight increase in loudness. The Visi-Pitch has been useful in helping patients associate changes in pitch with relative changes in intensity. Certain frequencies produce greater intensities. When the patient finds the "best" pitch level, he or she should practice sustaining an /a/ at that level for five seconds, concentrating on good voice quality. He or she should then take a deep breath and repeat the same pitch at a maximum loudness level. After some practice at this "home base" pitch level, ask the patient to sing /a/, up the scale for one octave, at one vocal production per breath; then have him or her go back down the scale, one note per breath, until he or she reaches the starting pitch.

   d. Explore with the patient his or her best pitch—that is, the one that produces the best loudness and quality. Auditory feedback devices (such as loop tape recorders) should be employed, so that the patient can hear what he or she is doing. Some counseling may be needed about the practice pitch used because the patient may be resistant to using a new voice pitch level. Note that the practice pitch level may well be only a temporary one, and not necessarily the pitch level the patient will use permanently. It is important that the work be pursued both in and out of therapy. A change in loudness cannot be achieved simply by talking about it. It requires practice.

   e. Sometimes respiration training (which we discuss later in the chapter) is necessary for a patient with a loudness problem. Remember, however, that even though loudness is directly related to the rate of airflow through the approximated vocal folds, little evidence indicates that any particular way of breathing is the best for optimum phonation. Any respiration exercise that produces increased subglottal air pressure may be helpful in increasing voice loudness.

   f. For those patients who seem unable to increase voice loudness, we might employ the Lombard effect (Newby, 1972). The Lombard effect is observed when patients reflexively voice at louder levels when reading or speaking against increasing competing noise. For example, as the patient reads aloud, the clinician introduces about 75 dB of speech–range masking from the Facilitator (see facilitating approach 16 for application procedures).

   3. Occasional patients or people wanting to improve their voices demonstrate little or no loudness variation. Fluctuation in loudness can be helped by:

   a. Make a tape recording of the patient's voice. Ask the patient how he or she likes the voice on playback. People who become aware of the monotony of their voices, and who are concerned about it, can usually develop loudness variation (and pitch inflection) with practice.
   b. Use a loop-playback system. Record speech or oral reading and then listen back immediately. Ask the patient about the relative appropriateness of loudness or loudness variation.
   c. Most voice and diction books include practice materials for developing loudness variation in the voice.

C. Typical Case History Showing Utilization of the Approach.   C. T., a thirty-one-year-old teacher, complained for more than a year of symptoms of vocal fatigue—that is, pain in the throat, loss of voice after teaching, and so on. Laryngoscopy revealed a normal larynx, and the voice evaluation found that the man spoke at "a monotonous pitch and low loudness level, with pronounced mandibular restriction, at times barely opening his mouth." Early efforts at therapy included the chewing approach, with special emphasis given to varying pitch level and increasing voice loudness. The patient was highly motivated to improve the efficiency of his phonation; he requested voice therapy three times a week and supplemented the therapy with long practice periods at home. After nine weeks of therapy, pretherapy and posttherapy recordings were compared, and the patient agreed with the clinician that he sounded "like a new man." Speaking in a louder voice for this patient seemed to have an immediate effect on his overall self-image, resulting in an almost immediate increase in his total communicative effectiveness. Not only did the patient achieve a better-sounding speaking voice, but he reported no further symptoms of vocal fatigue.

D. Evaluation of the Approach.   Inappropriate loudness of voice penalizes the patient. Happily, many of the facilitating techniques described in this chapter have some influence on voice loudness, and inadequate loudness is also highly modifiable. In fact, more often than not the use of various other facilitating techniques will have an indirect effect on voice loudness, obviating the need for loudness techniques per se.

3. Chant Talk

A. Kinds of Problems for Which the Approach Is Useful.   Voice problems related to hyperfunction are often helped by the chant approach. The chant in music is characterized by reciting many syllables on one continuous tone, creating

in effect a "singing monotone." We hear chanting in some churches and syna-
gogues, performed by clergy and select groups. The words run continuously
together without stress or a change in prosody for the individual word segments.
In singing, the *legato* is very similar to the chant we use in voice therapy. A
common dictionary definition of legato is "smooth and connected with no break
between tones." The chant in therapy is characterized by an elevation of pitch,
prolongation of vowels, lack of syllable stress, and an obvious softening of glottal
attack. Once a patient can produce the chant in its extreme form (such as in a Gre-
gorian chant), it can usually be modified to resemble conversational phonation.
We have used chanting with other facilitating approaches, such as chewing, open
mouth, and yawn–sigh.

B. Procedural Aspects of the Approach

1. The chant–talk approach is explained to the patient as a method that reduces
the effort in talking. It is important to point out to the patient that the method will
only be used temporarily as a practice method and will not become a permanent
and different way of talking. Demonstrate chant talk by playing a recording of a
religious chant. Then imitate the recording by producing the same voicing style
while reading any material aloud.

2. Urge the patient to imitate the same chant voicing pattern. Most patients are
able to do this with some degree of initial success. For those who cannot chant in
initial trials, present a chant recording again and then follow it with the patient's
own chant production. Some lighthearted kidding is useful to tell the patient that
the chant is a different way of talking and will only be used briefly as a voice training device. If the patient cannot chant after several attempts, use another facilitating approach. For those patients who can chant, go on to step 3.

3. The patient should now read aloud, alternating the regular voice and the
chant voice. Twenty seconds has been found to be a good time for each reading
condition. Ask the patient to read aloud first in the normal voice, then in a chant,
then back to normal voice, then in a chant, and so on.

4. Record the patient's oral reading. On playback, contrast the different sound
of the normal voice with the chanted voice. Discuss the pitch differences, the phonatory prolongations, and the soft glottal attack.

5. Once patients are able to produce chant talk with relative ease, they should
try to reduce the chant quality, approximating normal voice production. Slight
prolongation and soft glottal attack should be retained as the patient reads aloud
in a voice with only slight chant quality remaining.

C. Typical Case History Showing Utilization of the Approach.   C. C. was a

twenty-eight-year-old woman who sold telephone directory advertising. She began
to experience increased dysphonia and "dryness of throat," particularly toward the
end of a busy day of calling on customers. On endoscopic examination, she was
found to have bilateral vocal nodules with unnecessary supraglottal participation
during phonation. She spoke at an inappropriately low pitch, with mandibular
restriction and noticeable hard glottal attack. Twice a week she received voice ther-

apy designed to "take the work out of phonation." The chewing approach, coupled with the chant–talk approach, dramatically changed her overall voicing style. She was able early in therapy to incorporate the soft glottal attack of the chant into her everyday speaking voice. Other approaches, such as open mouth and yawn–sigh, were added with various self-practice materials she could use. The patient reported that she practiced throughout the day in her car, driving between appointments. In about twelve weeks, videoendoscopy revealed that the nodules had disappeared and that her supraglottal larynx stayed open during normal voicing. There was no evidence of hard glottal attack at the time of her clinic discharge.

D. Evaluation of the Approach.   The chant–talk approach is easy for most patients to use. Initially, it is important to let the patient know that chanting is only a temporary behavior, designed to take the work out of phonation. We have found that the method works well with children, who seem to enjoy the "different" way of talking. For those patients who need to reduce hard glottal attack, the chanting approach seems to produce dramatic results for softening voicing onsets.

4. Chewing

A. Kinds of Problems for Which the Approach Is Useful.   The authors have restored chewing as a facilitating approach in this edition. We see too many people with vocal hyperfunction who appear to speak through clenched teeth with very little mandibular or labial movement. Such patients profit from using the chewing approach. We often kiddingly ask such patients, "Have you ever been a ventriloquist?" We then reply to their usual answer of "no," "You certainly could be because you barely move your mouth when you speak." Many hyperfunctional voice patients, after being asked the ventriloquist question, develop immediate insight as to their relative lack of mouth opening. Chewing is helpful for the patient who speaks with great tension and hard glottal attack. During simultaneous voicing and chewing, we often hear less strain in the voice, easier glottal attack, and an improvement in voice quality.

B. Procedural Aspects of the Approach

1. We first do what is necessary to help the patient become aware of the need for greater mouth opening while speaking. Following the ventriloquist question, we may view talking on a real-time video monitor or by looking in a mirror. Immediate video playback after talking is a good method for instructing the patient specific to the relative amount of mouth opening he or she is using.

2. The clinician and patient look in a mirror as the clinician demonstrates exaggerated chewing. Care is given to have both good vertical and horizontal movements of the mouth. We pretend that we are chewing a stack of three crackers at one time with an open mouth. Ask the patient to imitate exaggerated chewing as has been demonstrated. Point out to the patient the amount of mouth opening by saying something like, "You see we let our jaw drop down with our lips open wide. If we were actually chewing crackers, the crumbs would all drop out of our open mouth." Spend as much time as needed to develop good open-mouth chewing.

3. We now add light voice to the chewing. Here we have to be careful to avoid the same kind of monotonous sound, like "yam-yam-yam," that can come from chewing in the same pattern while voicing. To mix the sounds (and the mouth movements) up a bit, we may have the patient say in a chantlike way such nonsense words as "ah-la-met-erah" or "wan-da-pan-da." Stay with such nonsense words until the patient masters the simultaneous chewing–speaking. It should be noted here that most children like to do chewing and take easily to the approach. Some adults may resist doing it, or be unable to do it; if so, the approach should be abandoned and other approaches used, such as the open-mouth approach.

4. Once simultaneous chewing–speaking is established, ask the patient to count and chew. It will take several practice attempts before the patient can do it. Listen and watch the first attempts on video playback. Tell the patient at this point that the chewing is "a means to the end of producing a more relaxed voice." The patient should be counseled that the exaggerated chewing is only used temporarily, and that we will soon cut down the movements to resemble more "the mouth movements of normal speakers."

5. Now use words and phrases for practice chewing. When the patient can do this, we would then practice sentences. Avoid going too fast. Go back to earlier levels if the chewing seems to be "fading."

6. After several weeks of practice in chewing, the patient should be taught how to diminish the exaggerated chewing to resemble more normal mouth movements. Practicing oral reading with chewing is a good final step. Videotaping the practice session will allow the patient to study his or her success on video playback.

7. Ultimately, the patient just "thinks" the chewing method. By this time, the patient has developed an awareness of what oral openness and jaw movement feel like and has experienced the vocal relaxation that accompanies the feeling.

C. Typical Case History Showing Utilization of the Approach.   S. J., a forty-four-year-old realtor, began to experience extreme vocal fatigue toward the end of her working day. At the voice evaluation, she reported, "Sometimes I lose my voice altogether at the end of the day, or after I talk a lot, it hurts right here" (as she pointed to the general hyoid area). As she volunteered her history, little mouth opening was observed with her voice sounding at an inappropriate high pitch with the end of sentences characterized by "squeezed phonation." On endoscopy, her vocal folds showed "posterior redness, suggestive of reflux with no middle or anterior pathology noted." A diagnosis of "muscular tension dysphonia" was made with a special notation made relative to "speaking through clenched teeth." Early in voice therapy, the patient worked on developing better respiration skills for voicing and developing more natural oral movements (less mandibular restriction). While there was some initial resistance by the patient to using the chewing approach, after she began to experience increased oral relaxation as she practiced the chewing, she incorporated greater oral movements into her everyday speaking pattern. The patient experienced a very good voice result from both reduction of her reflux by a medical regimen and eliminating her dysphonia and vocal fatigue from voice therapy (with early emphasis given to using the chewing approach).

D. Evaluation of the Approach.   The chewing approach is not a panacea for all voice problems, but its positive effectiveness in reducing muscular tension dysphonia or vocal hyperfunction is observed soon after it is applied. It appears that when oral structures are involved in the automatic function of chewing, according to Brodnitz and Froeschels (1954) who first introduced the technique, these oral structures (facial muscles, mandible, tongue) appear capable of "more synergic, relaxed movement." It appears that relaxing the overall vocal tract while chewing also relaxes the phonatory function of the larynx and pharynx. By employing a commonly used action, such as chewing, the patient is able to achieve relaxation of the vocal tract from a holistic or *gestalt* point of view, without attempting to relax particular muscles. For the voice patient who appears to be talking between clenched teeth, the chewing approach is a good way to develop more open, natural oral movements. This approach may be contraindicated for the patient with TMJ (temporomandibular joint) syndrome.

Track 7

5. Counseling (Explanation of Problem)

A. Kinds of Problems for Which the Approach Is Useful.   One cannot easily separate the person from his or her voice. Some voice problems may be among the visible symptoms of someone with serious personality problems, or sometimes the voice problem may be the cause of psychological maladaptive reactions. Counseling the voice patient, including direct explanations of the voice problem, may be more effective with the patient than applying various symptomatic voice therapy techniques.

Putting the voice problem in its proper perspective can often free the patient from overwhelming concern. Patients with hyperfunctional voice disorders, in particular, profit from hearing the clinician describe the voice problem in words they can understand. Clinical experience has taught these authors that if they can help individuals know why they have the voice problem, sometimes nothing more is needed to change a phonation style or to curb vocal abuse–misuse. In the case of those dysphonias that are wholly related to functional causes (such as hyperfunction), it is important that clinicians not confront patients with the implication that they "could talk all right if they wanted to." Instead of saying, "You are not using your voice as well as you could," a clinician might say, "Your vocal folds are coming together too tightly." The latter statement absolves the patient of the guilt he or she might experience if the clinician indicated that the patient was doing things "wrong." The patient will be much more receptive to a statement that puts the blame on the vocal folds. For patients with structural changes of the vocal folds, such as nodules or polyps, it may be necessary to explain that the organic pathology may well be the result of prolonged misuse, and that by eliminating the misuse, the patient will eventually experience a reduction of vocal fold pathology.

B. Procedural Aspects of the Approach.   Counseling the patient is highly individualized. One of the most common counseling approaches in voice therapy is helping the patient to put his or her voice problem in its proper perspective. For some patients, the voice problem is the cause of all of their ills, such as poor job performance, social inadequacy, or general unhappiness. The clinician must have some sensitivity to the depth of the patient's overall attitude and self-image. If the clinician senses psychological or social problems well beyond his or her counseling–psychological training to deal with such problems, referral should be made to professional counselors, psychologists, or psychiatrists. More often than not in voice therapy, a direct explanation of the patient's problem proves to be most effective.

In voice problems related to vocal hyperfunction, it is important to identify for the patient those behaviors that maintain the dysphonia. No exact procedure for this can be laid down; each case has its own rules. For problems related to abuse and misuse of the voice, identify the inappropriate behavior and demonstrate to the patient some ways in which it can be eliminated. In the vocal abuse reduction section of our voice program for children (Boone, 1993), we put much focus on having the child cognitively approach the problem of vocal abuse. By using comic pictures with an accompanying story text, we help the child understand the consequences of continued abuse and emphasize what can be expected (a better voice) if he or she reduces or eliminates such abuses.

For truly organic problems, such as unilateral adductor paralysis, the same explanations must be made, but in terms of inadequate and adequate glottal closure. Most voice patients want to understand what their problems are and what they can do about them. Make use of medical and diagnostic information, but explain things to the patient in language the patient can understand. Such imagery as "your vocal cords are coming together too tightly," or "you seem to place your voice back too far in your throat," may lack scientific validity but may help the patient understand the problem. Make explanations brief and to the point, but take care not to put the patient psychologically on the defensive during the first visit. If, after the evaluation, it appears that some psychological or psychiatric consultation is necessary, further diagnostic-therapy sessions may have to be held before the patient can agree to find out more about his or her feelings.

C. Typical Case History Showing Utilization of the Approach.   C. V., a sixty-two-year-old widow, came to the clinic with a voice problem that first resembled spasmodic dysphonia. As she volunteered her history, her voice sounded tight, strangled; it sounded as if she were crying. She differed from the typical patient with spasmodic dysphonia in the diagnostic session and early therapy periods by demonstrating normal voice repetition skills, and she could count or read aloud with normal phonation. Spontaneous narratives, however, about her former work as a department store buyer or details about her personal life were portrayed vocally with great struggle, sometimes accompanied by actual tearing. Early in voice therapy, her SLP was sensitive to the continuous observation that her voice symptoms were part of an overall picture of loneliness and general unhappiness about life. The woman was referred to a counseling psychologist, who, together with the SLP, has helped the patient make a happier life adjustment and consequently experience a better-sounding voice for most situations.

D. Evaluation of the Approach.   With a little guidance by the clinician in helping the patient understand his or her voice problem, what causes it, and what can be done about it, the typical voice patient can often make progress in overcoming the voice problem. Both children and adults profit from an explanation of their voice problem and from understanding how particular behaviors, like yelling or clearing one's throat excessively, keep their voices in trouble. Sometimes an explanation of the problem is the primary treatment with no other facilitating approaches required. For those patients who need much practice with various approaches, they seem to make better progress when they understand the rationale behind what they are practicing. Voice clinicians must remain sensitive to the psychological needs of voice patients and recognize that some of their patients have personal needs greater than improving their voices per se. Such patients should be referred appropriately to other counseling or psychological professionals.

Track 7

6. Digital Manipulation

A. Kinds of Problems for Which the Approach Is Useful.   Finger pressure on the thyroid cartilage can be applied by the clinician in different ways for different problems. For males, who for functional reasons are using higher F_0 values than they should, light pressure anteriorly on the thyroid cartilage appears to nudge the thyroid cartilage back slightly, shortening the overall length of the vocal folds. This shortening thickens the folds, resulting in a lower F_0. This anterior pressure approach is particularly effective for postadolescent males whose pitch levels seem to remain at prepubescent levels. Another form of digital manipulation is placing the fingers lightly on the thyroid cartilage and monitoring the vertical positioning of the larynx. During the swallow or in a fear–tension state or when singing notes toward the upper end of one's singing range, the overall larynx appears to rise; lowering of the larynx is achieved during the yawn–sigh (Boone and McFarlane, 1993) or singing at the lower end of one's range or during a very relaxed state. The digital monitoring of laryngeal height is a good technique for anyone who appears to have excessive laryngeal vertical movement or who is concerned about laryngeal posturing at high or low levels. Analysis of voice therapy effectiveness for patients with unilateral vocal fold paralysis (McFarlane et al., 1991, 1998) is another form of digital manipulation found to be effective. McFarlane and others found that finger pressure on the lateral thyroid cartilage wall can often produce better vocal fold approximation, resulting in stronger phonation.

B. Procedural Aspects of the Approach.   The three digital procedures used in voice therapy are quite distinct from one another, both in the procedural steps used and the kind of voice problems for which they are helpful. We list the steps separately for each of the three procedures:

1. Digital pressure for lowering pitch.

    a. With the exception of some men with falsetto voices, patients will respond to digital pressure by producing a lower voice pitch. Ask the patient to prolong a vowel (/a/ or /i/). As the vowel is prolonged, apply slight finger pressure on the thyroid cartilage. The pitch level will drop immediately.

    b. Ask the patient to maintain the lower pitch after the fingers are removed. If the patient can do this, he or she should continue practicing the lower pitch. If the high pitch quickly reverts back, repeat the digital pressure.

    c. If the method is used to let the patient hear and feel a lower pitch, the patient should practice producing the lower pitch with and without digital pressure on the thyroid cartilage.

2. Monitoring the vertical movements of the larynx.

   a. For a patient with excessive pitch variability and tension related to much vertical movement of the larynx, demonstrate how to place the fingers on the thyroid cartilage and monitor laryngeal vertical movement while phonating.

   b. Ask the patient to produce a pitch level several full musical notes off the bottom of his or her lowest note. Keeping the fingers on the thyroid cartilage, ask the patient to lower pitch one note at a time to the lowest note in his or her pitch range. Usually, the larynx will lower its position in the neck at the low end of the pitch range. Then ask the patient to sing one note at a time up to the top of the singing range, exclusive of falsetto. Toward the top of the scale, the patient should feel (through the fingertips) a slight elevation of the larynx. Review both the lowering and rising of the larynx at the extremes of the pitch range.

   c. Once the patient has experienced vertical movement in the preceding steps, point out that in production of a speaking voice that is relatively free of strain, no vertical movement of the larynx should be felt during digital monitoring. Oral reading and speaking should be developed with little or no vertical laryngeal movements. Practice in oral reading with encouraged pitch variability can then be monitored by slight digital pressure of the thyroid cartilage with the patient's confirming (hopefully) no vertical movement.

3. Unilateral digital pressure for patients with unilateral vocal fold paralysis.

Track 7

   a. While there appears to be a slight phonation improvement by pressing on the thyroid lamina on the side of the paralysis, this is not always found. We begin, however, by having the patient posture the head straight–forward (looking slightly down rather than upward). The patient is asked to phonate and extend a vowel. While the patient phonates, the clinician exerts medium finger pressure on the lateral thyroid wall on the side of the vocal fold paralysis. If a louder, firmer voice is produced with this pressure, continue various phonation tasks, coupled with finger pressure on the thyroid cartilage on the side of the involvement.

   b. If louder voice was not achieved in step (a) above, the patient continues to look forward while the clinician applies pressure to the opposite side of the thyroid cartilage (pressing the side opposite the vocal fold paralysis). Attempt various phonation tasks while exerting this lateral finger pressure.

   c. If lateral pressure to either thyroid lamina while the patient looks ahead has not produced an improvement in voice, provide lamina pressure with the head turned to one side. If the head is turned to the left, first apply pressure to the left lamina; if unsuccessful, keep the head turned left with pressure then given to the right lamina. If this produces better voice, continue phonation tasks with the head turned to the left and finger pressure on the side that seems to produce the best voice.

   d. The last posture is for the head turned to the right with each side pressed in an attempt to find the better, more functional voice.

   e. It should be noted again that it has been our experience that one cannot predict which head posture (straight ahead or turned laterally) and/or which side receives finger pressure will produce a better-sounding voice, whether or not the left or right vocal fold is paralyzed. More often than not, however, digital manipulation following steps a–d will often provide for the patient a better, more functional voice.

C. Typical Case History Showing Utilization of the Approach.   J. F. was a seventeen-year-old male who had been raised exclusively by his mother until her sudden death about a year before. Since that time he had lived with a maternal uncle who was concerned about the boy's effeminate mannerisms and high-pitched voice. Laryngeal examination revealed a normal adult male larynx. The boy was found to have a habitual pitch level of around 200 Hz, well within the adult female range, but below the level of falsetto. The most effective facilitating technique for producing a normal voice pitch was to apply digital pressure on the external thyroid cartilage. The young man was able to prolong the lower pitch levels with good success, but any attempt at conversation would be characterized by an immediate return to the higher pitch. After three therapy sessions, he was able to read aloud using the lower pitch but was unable to use the lower voice in conversation except with his male clinician. Subsequent psychiatric evaluation and therapy were initiated for "identity confusion and schizoidal tendencies." Voice therapy was discontinued after two weeks, when it was clearly demonstrated that the patient could produce a good baritone voice (125 Hz) whenever he wanted. Unfortunately, follow-up telephone conversations several months after therapy revealed that he was using his high-pitched, pretherapy voice exclusively.

D. Evaluation of the Approach.   The effectiveness of any one of the three digital manipulation approaches can be determined immediately. Either the anterior digital pressure to the thyroid cartilage will lower voice pitch or it will not. If the speaking pitch is lowered with digital pressure, it affords an excellent "window" for the patient (such as a young man with puberphonia) to experience producing a lower-pitched voice. Tracking the vertical movements with light finger pressure can often help the patient appreciate the amount of unnecessary laryngeal movement he or she may be experiencing. Finally, in the search for a more functional voice after unilateral vocal fold paralysis, digital pressure on the thyroid lamina with or without head turning may uncover a functional voice. Developing such an uncovered voice in the patient with unilateral vocal fold paralysis may obviate the need for various surgical procedures in the quest of restoring a functional voice (McFarlane and others, 1991).

7. Elimination of Abuses

A. Kinds of Problems for Which the Approach Is Useful.   There are many ways that one can abuse or misuse the voice. *Vocal abuse* comprises various behaviors and events that have some kind of deleterious effect on the larynx and the voice, such as:

1. Yelling and screaming
2. Speaking against a background of loud noise
3. Coughing and excessive throat-clearing

4. Smoking
5. Excessive talking or singing
6. Excessive talking or singing while having an allergy or upper respiratory infection
7. Excessive crying or laughing
8. Weight lifting

Vocal misuse means improper use of voice, such as:

1. Speaking with hard glottal attack
2. Singing excessively at the lower or upper end of one's range
3. Increasing vocal loudness by squeezing out the voice at the level of the larynx
4. Speaking at excessive intensity levels
5. Cheerleading (Case, 1996)
6. Speaking over time at an inappropriate pitch level
7. Speaking or singing (such as a prolonged show rehearsal) for excessively long periods of time

We could, obviously, add other abuses and misuses to such a list. Identification and reduction of vocal abuse–misuse are primary goals in voice therapy for hyperfunctional disorders such as functional dysphonia with or without such physical changes as vocal nodules, polyps, or contact ulcers. Therapy cannot be successful until contributory vocal abuse–misuse can be drastically reduced. Optimum usage of the voice, such as the vocal hygiene program outlined in Chapter 7, also requires identifying possible abusive voice situations and making deliberate efforts to minimize their occurrence.

B. Procedural Aspects of the Approach

1. Time must be given early in voice therapy to identifying possible vocal abuse. Once a particular vocal abuse is identified, the patient and clinician should develop a baseline of occurrence. This will often require that the clinician hear and observe the patient in and out of the clinic environment, such as on the playground, at the pulpit, or in a nightclub. The number of times the particular event occurred must be tallied.

2. Children with vocal abuse must become aware of the impact of such abuses on their voices. With children we use the "Vocal Abuse Reduction Program" (Boone, 1993), which recommends: an explanation of how additive lesions occur, using the story *A Voice Lost and Found*; a review of the child's abuses; and a systematic reduction of the child's abuses, using the voice tally card, the voice counting chart, and the hot-air balloon race (p. 7). The focus of the reducing abuse program is to make the child cognitively aware of the relationship of vocal abuse–misuse to increasing symptoms of voice. The story in the program is pictorially illustrated with various vocal behaviors related to changes of "the little bumps on the vocal cords."

3. Discuss identified vocal abuses with the patient, emphasizing the need to reduce their daily frequency. Assign to the patient the task of counting the number of times each day he or she engages in a particular abuse. Perhaps a peer or sibling could be brought in, told about the situation, and asked to join in on the daily count. Depending on the age of the patient, a parent or teacher, spouse, or business associate might be asked to keep track of the number of abuses that occur in their presence. At the end of the day, the abuses should be tallied for that day.

4. Ask the patient to plot his or her daily vocal abuses on a graph. Along the vertical axis, the ordinate, the patient should plot the number of times the particular abuse occurred, and, along the base of the graph, the abscissa, the individual days, beginning with the baseline count of the first day. Instruct the patient to bring these graphs to voice therapy sessions. Keeping a graph usually increases the patient's awareness of what he or she has been doing and results in a gradual decrement of the abusive behavior. The typical vocal abuse has a sloping decremental curve, indicating its gradual disappearance. Greet any decrement in the plots of the people observing the patient, but particularly in those compiled by the patient, with obvious approval.

C. Typical Case History Showing Utilization of the Approach. Joyce was a twenty-seven-year-old secretary who complained of a voice that was often hoarse and that tired easily every day. Subsequent indirect laryngoscopy confirmed a slight bilateral thickening at the anterior–middle third junction. A detailed history and observation of the patient found that she constantly cleared her throat. The throat-clearing had become a habit. She rarely felt that she was able "to bring up any mucus" but just cleared her throat in an attempt to make her voice clearer. A high-speed motion picture depicting throat-clearing was shown to the patient. She was counseled to try to reduce its occurrence. The patient subsequently began to tally her throat-clearing and coughing as they occurred, plotting them on a graph at the end of the day. Within two weeks, she was able to change her throat-clearing habit. Her vocal quality improved immediately and she never needed formal, long-term voice therapy.

D. Evaluation of the Approach. Identifying vocal abuses and attempting to eliminate them by plotting their daily frequency on a graph are effective in helping young children with voice problems. Adolescents are equally guilty of vocal abuses and profit from keeping track of what they are doing. Typical adult abuses, such as throat-clearing, are often eliminated after a week or two of graph plotting by motivated patients. The effectiveness of this approach, in fact, is highly related to the skill of the clinician in motivating the patient to eliminate the abusive behavior. The value of the plotting is more in developing awareness of the frequency of the problem than in the actual count per se. Reduction of vocal abuse has become a primary part of most voice therapy programs for children (Andrews, 1995; Boone, 1993; Stemple, Gerdeman, and Glaze, 1994) and for adults (Boone, 1997; Case, 1996; Morrison and Rammage, 1994).

8. Establishing a New Pitch

Track 3 & 4

A. Kinds of Problems for Which the Approach Is Useful. Although it is well established that there is no absolute optimum pitch on which a particular person should speak, some people with voice problems may profit from speaking at a different pitch level. A change of pitch will often have positive effects on voice, such as improving vocal quality and loudness. Speaking at the very bottom of one's pitch range requires too much force and effort. Similarly, speaking habitually toward the top of one's range can be vocally fatiguing. Because a number of instruments available today can portray fundamental frequency in real time (while one is phonating), awareness and feedback of one's ongoing pitch level play prominent roles in establishing new pitches through therapy.

B. Procedural Aspects of the Approach

1. If pitch needs to be raised or lowered, describe where the patient is and where the target pitch is. The methods for determining habitual and optimum pitches described in Chapter 5 can be applied here. Make a tape recording of the patient producing various pitches, including feedback about the old pitch and the projected target pitch. The playback should always be followed by some discussion comparing the sound and the feeling of the two pitches.

2. Most voice patients can imitate their own pitch models, once they have been produced by the appropriate facilitating technique. Occasionally patients cannot initiate a pitch to match a model, as Filter and Urioste (1981) found in testing college women with normal voices. A useful model can be produced by having the patient extend an /i/ at the target pitch level for about five seconds and recording the phonation on a loop recorder. The patient will immediately hear the target production. The loop tape playback will provide the patient with a continuous playback of his or her own voice model of the target pitch. There are many advantages to using the patients' own voices as their voice models, in that they already have voicing experience producing the sounds they are now trying to match. Remain with the loop model /i/ for considerable practice before introducing a new stimulus.

3. Several excellent instruments available today can provide real-time display of fundamental frequency, both with a digital write-out and on a display screen on a monitor: PM 100 Pitch Analyzer, Phonatory Function Analyzer, Visi-Pitch, and B & K Real-Time Frequency Analyzer (see reference section at end of book). Usually, these instruments permit the clinician to display patient voice values specific to frequency and intensity. The PM 100 and Visi-Pitch both offer split-screen capabilities, whereby a voice model can be put on an upper screen and the patient's production displayed on a lower screen, permitting comparisons between model and trial productions. Any instrument that can display fundamental frequency information can provide valuable feedback to a patient attempting to establish a new voice pitch.

4. Using any four of the instruments described in step 3 above, the patient can receive exact feedback relative to the frequency he or she is using. Any deviation below or above the target F_0 can be given in immediate feedback. Of great benefit for the patient is developing the immediate awareness when he or she is producing the target F_0.

5. Establishing a new pitch is facilitated by working first on single words, preferably words that begin with vowels. Each word is repeated in a pitch monotone (using the target pitch). Occasionally a patient has more difficulty using the new pitch with certain words. Any such "trouble" words should be avoided as practice material because what is needed at this stage of therapy is practice in rapidly phonating a series of individual words at the new pitch level.

6. Once the patient does well at the single-word level, introduce phrases and short sentences. It is usually more productive at this stage to avoid practice in actual conversation because the patient is better able to use the new phonation in such neutral situations as reading single words, phrases, and sentences. When success is achieved at the sentence level, assign the patient reading passages from various voice and diction books. Success in using the new pitch level can be verified by using the instruments described earlier, in step 3.

7. After reading well in a monotone, the patient may try using the new pitch in some real-life conversational situations. In the beginning he or she may have more success talking to strangers, such as store clerks; patients often find it difficult to use the new pitch level with friends and family because their previous "sets" may prevent them from utilizing their new vocal behavior. Whatever conversational situation works best for the individual should be the one initially used.

8. It is helpful in therapy to tape-record the patient's voice as he or she searches to establish a new and different pitch level. When the patient is able to produce a good voice at the proper pitch level, his or her own "best" voice can then become the therapy model.

C. Typical Case History Showing Utilization of the Approach.   John, a ten-year-old boy, was referred by his public-school speech clinician for a laryngeal examination because of a six-month history of hoarseness. The findings included a normal larynx and a "low-pitched dysphonic voice." John could readily demonstrate a higher phonation, which was characterized by an immediate clearing of quality. In the discussion that followed the tape-recorded playback of his "good" and "bad" voice, John stated that he thought he had been trying to speak like his older brother. The clinician pointed out to him that his better voice was more like that of other boys his age, and that the low-pitched voice he had been using was difficult for others to listen to. In subsequent voice therapy with his public-school clinician, John focused on elevating his voice pitch to a more natural level. His success was rapid, and therapy was terminated after six weeks.

D. Evaluation of the Approach.   The pitch of the voice changes constantly, according to the speaker's situation. In some patients, however, the pitch level appears to be too high or too low for the overall capability of the laryngeal mechanism. In other people, an aberrant pitch level is just one manifestation of the total personality. Patients with additive masses to the folds (nodules, papilloma, polyps, and so on) may have lower pitch levels than normal because the thicker vocal folds vibrate more slowly, emitting a lower fundamental frequency. As the lesion is reduced or eliminated, the frequency of the voice becomes higher, perhaps approaching normal limits. For patients with additive laryngeal lesions due to vocal hyperfunction, it is often best to work slowly toward increasing pitch level to approximate levels of the patient's age and sex peers. Some patients use aberrant pitch levels because of personality factors. Counseling such patients and helping them want to change pitch levels might well have to precede actual symptomatic therapy to alter pitch. Typically, however, voice patients who may need to change pitch levels can do so rather quickly, after experiencing marked improvement in overall voice quality because of pitch change.

9. Focus

A. Kinds of Problems for Which the Approach Is Useful. Good focus of the voice is characterized by the voice coming "from the middle of the mouth, just above the surface of the tongue" (Boone, 1997, p. 71). Problems in "horizontal" voice focus occur when the tongue is too far forward or too far backward within the mouth. The "thin" or baby-sounding voice is produced by carrying the tongue high and forward. The back-focused voice, sounding like the country bumpkin voice or the voice of the television character Alf, is produced by carrying the tongue elevated in the back of the mouth.

The most common focus problem we see in patients with voice disorders is the voice sounding as if it were deep in the throat. Many patients focus on their throats as the anatomical site of their problem. Such patients profit from this approach because it shifts their mental imagery from the throat to the upper vocal tract.

Perkins (1983) has written that "voice that feels focused high in the head" is a more efficient voice, and it can survive extensive vocalization. The clinician helps the patient focus on the area of his or her face under the cheeks and across the bridge of the nose. Most patients with chronic dysphonia experience both difficulty finding their voices and continued expectancy of vocal failure. They clear their throats continually, they make phonation rehearsals, and they worry about the poor vocal quality they are likely to have the next time they attempt to speak. For these patients successful voice clinicians often employ two techniques, respiration training and placing the voice in the facial mask, for two reasons: (1) to improve respiratory control and resonance; (2) to transfer the patient's mental focus away from the larynx and place it with the activator (respiration) and the resonator (supraglottal vocal tract).

B. Procedural Aspects of the Approach

1. An explanation of focus is facilitated by having the patient review Figure 6.3 with the clinician. Determination is first made as to what kind of remedial focus is needed: Is the voice too far forward, too back, or sounding deep in the throat? Although cited in the Figure 6.3 line drawing, a nasal focus is not presented as a focus problem.

2. For anterior focus, the clinician points to the left side (labeled Front) of the horizontal line A in Figure 6.3, saying to the client, "It appears that your voice sounds too far forward in your mouth. This seems to be caused by carrying your tongue high and forward in your mouth. This makes the voice sound babyish or thin." If possible, the clinician should imitate a thin, front sounding voice, commenting afterward, "I made the thin voice with my tongue carried forward."

   a. Front-of-the-mouth focus can often be corrected by producing back-of-the-mouth sounds in rapid succession. We ask the patient to repeat "kuh-kuh-

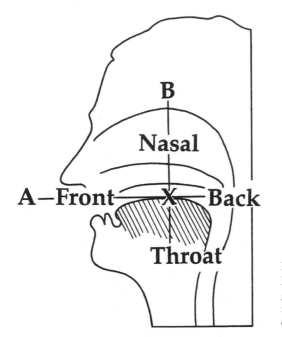

FIGURE 6.3   Voice focus sites.
X = normal. Used with permission by Singular Publishing Group Inc., San Diego, California, from D. R. Boone's *Is Your Voice Telling on You?* 1997.

kuh-kuh" in a rapid series, stressing the back consonant /k/ and other low back vowel sounds like "kah," "guh," and "gah."

   b. For other exercises designed for correcting anterior focus, the clinician might use the exercises from Boone's *Is Your Voice Telling on You?* (1997, pp. 79–80).

   c. Compare the old thin voice with the back voice, using some kind of loop or recorded feedback.

  3. For posterior-focused voice, the clinician points to the right end of the A line in Figure 6.3 marked Back. We say to the patient, "Your voice sounds back in your mouth, which seems to come from your tongue placed too far back. We can bring your tongue forward by practicing some front-of-the-mouth sounds."

   a. We seem to get posterior-to-anterior shift of focus quicker when only whisper is used on the first practice words. The patient is instructed to repeat front-of-the-mouth words like *peep*, *pipe*. Each word is said rapidly four or five times, like "peep-peep-peep-peep-peep."

   b. TH (voiceless) words like *this* or *that* are whispered in rapid succession, four or five times.

   c. /s/ words like *see* and *sat* are whispered in a rapid series.

   d. The whispered series for each word is then repeated with light voice. Posterior focus exercises may be found on pp. 80–81 in *Is Your Voice Telling on You?*

  4. Poor vertical focus, with the voice sounding as though it is focused down deep in the throat, produces poor vocal quality. Of the three focus problems (front–back–throat), the throat focus voice is the most common problem seen in the voice clinic. Getting the voice "out of the throat" is a problem of mental imagery.

Although the clinician and the patient can hear the low-throat voice focus, it is not possible to find an exact anatomic site where the low voice is produced. Rather, we use the imagery of "placing the voice in the facial mask" or in the middle of the face, as shown in the drawings of Figure 6.4. Or we tell the patient, referring back to Figure 6.3, "Your voice should sound like it's coming from the X, where the two lines cross, or from the surface of your tongue."

a. Time should be given in developing the imagery of taking the voice "out" of the throat and "placing" it in the front of the face, or the facial mask. Many clinicians and voice scientists profess skepticism over the construct of focus; however, functionally a change of focus can produce an immediate and dramatic change in the sound of the voice. While physiologically we cannot demonstrate focus, its immediate sound effects produce measurable changes in voice (less perturbation, formant shifts, quality differences).

b. Give as much time as possible to step a above. A good way to begin higher focus is with increased nasalization. Have the patient say "one-a-one-a-one" with exaggerated nasality. Place the fingers along the bridge and sides of the nose to feel the sound vibrations in the nose. Use other monosyllabic nasal words like *mom, me, many,* and exaggerate their nasality.

c. If the patient confirms feeling the vibrations of the nasal consonants and the nasalized vowels, practice reading short nasal sentences with exaggerated nasal resonance, such as "many men want some money." Practice reading /m-n-ng/ phrases and sentences. Contrast the feeling of the higher-focused nasal voice with the lower throat voice. The two voices should sound and feel differently.

d. If the nasal consonants have facilitated a higher focus from the throat focus, introduce some high front vowels and words like *baby, beach, take,* emphasizing the resonance in the facial mask.

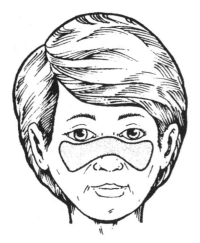 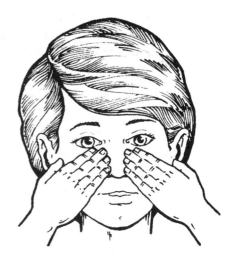

FIGURE 6.4 *The imagery of "placing" the voice in the middle of the face is helped by using these two pictures.* (The Boone Voice Program for Children, *2nd ed. Austin, TX: Pro-Ed, 1993).*

e. This is a good time to listen critically to the higher-focused resonance. Use the loop playback of the Facilitator, or listen to the voice and look at the tracings on the Visi-Pitch. Contrast the old lower focus with the higher mouth focus, contrasting the sound and the "feel" of the two voices. Oral reading and conversation in the voice clinic should emphasize the feeling of higher focus and the "set" the patient assumes to achieve it.

C. Typical Case History Showing Utilization of the Approach. Lilly was a forty-nine-year-old financial planner who decided that her voice was "too small for the kind of work I do." A subsequent voice evaluation found her to have a habitual voice pitch around 260 Hz (near middle C) with a thin, front-of-the-mouth resonance. An endoscopic examination found her to have a normal larynx. When she listened to her voice on cassette playback, she commented, "That's the kind of baby voice I always seem to have." Our subsequent voice therapy empha-sized developing a more posterior focus to her voice. In a few therapy sessions, she developed a voice that sounded like it came from "further back," with a noticeable improvement in overall voice resonance. She was also able to lower her voice pitch two full notes to 195 Hz (near an A3). After eight therapy sessions, she consistently showed a more mature voice with normal resonance. On a two-year follow-up interview, she continued to demonstrate a normal voice.

D. Evaluation of the Approach. For the patient with a thin, front voice or a back, "Alf" voice, or a low in the throat voice, changing one's voice focus appears to be an easily attained goal. Contrasting the sound of the voice from front, back, or low with a voice that sounds like it is coming from the middle of the mouth or higher in the facial mask is a vital step in using focus in therapy. If the patient can change the sound focus of his or her voice after clinician instruction and modeling, the impact on improving voice is almost immediate. Successful use of focus can be coupled with other therapy approaches, such as auditory feedback, establishing a new pitch, nasal/glide stimulation, and the open-mouth approach. Occasional voice patients will be unable to hear the difference between a deep-focused voice and a higher-placed facial mask voice; for such patients, the focus approach cannot be used.

10. Glottal Attack Changes

A. Kinds of Problems for Which the Approach Is Useful. The phenomenon of glottal attack is related to the onset of voicing. While most patients speak with normal glottal attack, problems in glottal attack are heard either in an abrupt "hard" attack or in the opposite breathy, "easy" onset of voice. An abrupt, bombas-tic, glottal attack is heard in voicing that begins with sudden onset. Severe abrupt glottal attack was listed as a laryngeal misuse in facilitating approach 7, Elimina-tion of Abuses. Speaking with abrupt vocal onset is taxing on the vocal folds, as reported by Pershall and Boone (1986), who found on endoscopy of a normal sub-ject that continuous staccato phonation (abrupt-onset phonation) caused slight edema and redness on the anterior–middle third site of the glottal margin. Hard glottal attack, an example of vocal hyperfunction, is often heard in patients with posterior lesions, such as contact ulcers or contact granuloma.

An excessively easy, breathy glottal attack may be heard in patients with uni-lateral vocal fold paralysis or in occasional patients with an aging voice (as dis-cussed in Chapter 7). Greene and Mathieson (1991) have used the label *phonasthenia* for the tired voice, with or without vocal fold bowing, that will often have soft, breathy phonation onsets.

B. Procedural Aspects of the Approach.   The two changes in glottal attack (reducing hard attack or developing hard attack) use two distinctively different ther-apy approaches. For reducing hard glottal attack we would use these procedures:

1. Hard glottal attack is a fairly common phenomenon among actors, politicians, and untrained singers. Play recordings of the voices of such people, and of the patient, for the patient, and then demonstrate the contrasting soft, easy glottal attack. The length of the demonstration should depend on the patient's insight.
2. Demonstrate a child's vocal attack by letting the patient contrast a recording of his or her own voice with the normal voice of a peer. Then practice using words beginning with /h/, taken from various lists. Select monosyllabic words, beginning with the aspirate /h/ for soft attack practice. When the /h/ words are produced correctly, introduce other words beginning with unvoiced consonants for similar practice. Then use words beginning with vowels.
3. Use the whisper–phonation technique. Choose a few monosyllabic words, each beginning with a vowel. The patient's task is to whisper very lightly the initial vowel, prolonging it by gradually increasing the loudness of the whis-per until phonation is introduced and, finally, the whole word is said. The whisper blends into a soft phonation.
4. The yawn–sigh approach is particularly effective in eliminating hard glottal attack.
5. By definition the chant approach eliminates hard glottal attack by its initiat-ing legato into the speaking voice. It can often be successfully combined with the yawn–sigh or the chewing approach.
6. Simultaneous chewing and chanting make abrupt onset of phonation impossible.
7. Once the patient is able to produce easy-onset phonation by chanting, chew-ing, or yawning sighing, a good therapy procedure is to have the patient contrast the easy-onset phonation with abrupt-onset phonation. The lack of effort of easy onset and the obvious effort of abrupt onset make a convincing contrast between the two modes of voice onset.
8. Various instruments are useful in providing the patient feedback about the severity of his or her glottal attack or suddenness of initiation of phonation. The display from a spectrograph or the Visi-Pitch can show the relative onset time of phonations; a vertical tracing at the beginning of the word indicates hard, abrupt vocal attack as opposed to a sloping onset tracing that displays a more gradual onset. Using various facilitating approaches, the clinician and the patient can visually confirm the relative suddenness of onset by the slope of the onset curve.

For the weak voice, where increasing hard glottal attack might be of some benefit, we follow these procedures:

1. Demonstrate hard glottal attack for the patient. A graphic way to do this is to purse the lips for the sudden release of a labial plosive, blow the cheeks slightly out, and then suddenly produce words like *pop, peep, pick, bob, beet, beak,* and so on. Have the patient imitate the production, visually tracking the plosive release by watching in the mirror or on video playback.
2. Repeat the production of monosyllabic plosive words, saying one word per breath. Place the tracings on an oscillograph or on the Visi-Pitch screen. Observe the abrupt vertical lines, depicting sudden onset. Contrast the sudden production with the gradual onset of words beginning with /h/, as seen in the sloping onset curve of /h/ onset words.
3. The old "pushing" approach (Froeschels, Kastein, and Weiss, 1955) could be used briefly to demonstrate sudden onset. One method of the "pushing" approach was to raise the arms to about shoulder height, and then extend the arms suddenly down, saying a plosive-onset word timed with the sudden arm extension. Another method was to bring the fists up to the chest, suddenly releasing them downward as a plosive-onset word is said. Effort should be made to say the word suddenly, timed with the arm movements.

C. Typical Case History Showing Utilization of the Approach. Louis was a thirty-five-year-old assistant professor of hydrology who came to the voice clinic with the sole complaint of "pain in the throat and hoarseness" after lecturing for more than an hour. A subsequent voice evaluation and visitation to his classes found that Louis was lecturing with a "different voice" from the one he used conversationally. His lecture voice appeared to be at the bottom of his vocal pitch range, and he spoke with excessive glottal attack. He felt (perhaps correctly) that his low-pitched voice and his abrupt way of saying things made him sound a bit more authoritative and "in charge of my subject matter." Although some work in voice therapy involved raising his voice pitch two full steps, focus was on eliminating hard glottal attack. Within a few weeks of starting voice therapy, he reported no discomfort after lecturing, and the dysphonia after prolonged lecturing began to disappear.

D. Evaluation of the Approach. Optimizing glottal attack is often easily accomplished in voice therapy. More commonly, efforts are usually successful in reducing hard glottal attack, resulting in less effort expended for voicing–speaking. Hard glottal attack is often part of a more generalized vocal hyperfunction, resulting in muscle tension dysphonia and often a tense sounding voice, unpleasant to the ears of one's listeners. Likewise, the excessively breathy glottal attack can often be sharpened with voice therapy, resulting in a voice that often sounds louder, contributing to increasing one's overall speech intelligibility.

11. Glottal Fry

A. Kinds of Problems for Which the Approach Is Useful. True glottal fry is produced in a relaxed manner with very little airflow and very little subglottic air pressure (Zemlin, 1998). Glottal fry, considered a normal voice register, is valuable for patients with vocal nodules as well as for patients with other hyperfunctional problems such as polyps, cord thickening, functional dysphonia, and even spasmodic dysphonia and ventricular phonation. Although glottal fry can be an extremely powerful facilitating technique to improve voice in the dysphonic patient and is a useful diagnostic vocal probe, it has a second use, as well: It can be an index of vocal fold relaxation. In order to produce a glottal fry of 65 to 75 Hz, which is desirable, the vocal folds must be relaxed. A patient may not always be able to achieve this fry in the first session, but the accomplishment of a "good fry" of about 70 or 75 Hz is an index that the larynx has been relaxed. The glottal fry can be produced on either inhalation or exhalation. After producing glottal fry phonation for five to ten seconds and then being asked to say a phrase such as "easy does it," a patient with nodules often experiences normal or near-normal vocal quality for the first time in months.

B. Procedural Aspects of the Approach

1. A common pencil eraser or very dry hard raisin can represent a vocal nodule. When placed between the pages of a hardback book, the eraser keeps the pages apart with a gap on either side of the eraser; likewise, nodules produce a gap between the vocal cords, as was shown in Figure 3.3. If the eraser is placed between two marshmallows instead of between the pages of a book, the marshmallows "wrap around" the mass of the eraser. In glottal fry, the compliant vocal cords can "wrap around" the nodules and improve approximation. A clinician can see this with stroboscopic videoendoscopy and demonstrate it to the patient.

2. Ask the patient to let out half of his or her breath and then say /i/ softly, holding it until it dies away slowly. Encourage the patient to stretch the /i/ as long as possible.

3. Once the patient has a well-sustained /i/ in the glottal fry mode, have him or her open the mouth medium wide and protrude the tongue. Then have the patient make the tone "larger" by "opening the throat." The desired tone is a deep, resonant, slow series of individual pops, which we describe as sounding "like dragging a stick along a picket fence."

4. Have the patient attempt to produce the same tone on inhalation as on exhalation. Some people are better able to produce the glottal fry on inhalation. Also have the patient alternately reverse the tone—first on exhalation, then on inhalation. Next, have the patient say words such as *on* and *off* and *in* and *out* in the glottal fry mode. Suggest that the patient slightly prolong these words and say them on both inhalation ("on," "in") and exhalation ("off," "out"), alternately back and forth between ingressive and egressive airflow. Tape-record the glottal fry so the patient has a model or target.

5. When the patient is able to produce these words well and can produce the sustained /i/ or /a/ in glottal fry, ask him or her to say "easy does it," "squeeze the peach," or "see the eagle" in a normal voice. These are almost always produced with greatly improved or normal vocal quality. The patient will generally be able to say only a few words with the improved quality and will then need to go back to the glottal fry mode. Tape-record these phrases and contrast them with the patient's typical voice. Also ask the patient to judge the two.

6. When the correct glottal fry is learned, instruct the patient to practice for a few minutes several (ten or more) times each day. To assist the patient in practice, suggest that he or she tie practice to the environment—for example, by producing the fry each time he or she sees a bus or a red car, or during the last two minutes of each hour. The patient must be producing the fry appropriately before you allow practice.

C. Typical Case History Showing Utilization of the Approach.   Mark, a ten-year-old boy, and Brian, an eleven-year-old boy, were referred for voice evaluation by an otolaryngologist who had diagnosed bilateral vocal nodules. Both boys had low-pitched, hoarse voices with frequent phonation breaks during connected speech. They had had these voices for nearly one year. After teaching glottal fry as just described, we had "contests" to see who could fry the longest and at the slowest rate. We had the boys say words in the fry mode back and forth to each other. We saw each boy twice a week, once together and once individually, for forty-five-minute sessions. In three months, their voices were normal, and the nodules were completely gone. We should note that with one boy, we reduced vocal abuses during his soccer activity, as well.

D. Evaluation of the Approach.   The approach appears to work because very little subglottic pressure and very little airflow are required to produce the glottal fry. Therefore, there is little stress on the folds. The compliant folds seem to reduce the amount of friction as they meet during phonation. This allows the nodules to be reduced or reabsorbed even though the patient continues to talk. The new talking is produced with far less vocal fold tension.

Track
7 & 9

12. Head Positioning

A. Kinds of Problems for Which the Approach Is Useful.   Basic to good vocal performance (acting, lecturing, singing) is good posture and head positioning. Also, changing head position may facilitate a better voice in patients with various kinds of voice problems. Patients with unilateral vocal fold paralysis will sometimes demonstrate a stronger voice by lateralizing head position, with or without digital pressure on the lateral lamina of the thyroid cartilage (see facilitating approach 6, Digital Manipulation). Finding optimum head positioning has been found to be helpful in chewing and swallowing with patients with various neurological disorders. The symptoms of dysarthria involving both speech and voice may be minimized in a particular patient by a specific head position. We find that a patient with symptoms of vocal hyperfunction can often experience a better, more relaxed voice by placing the head in a different position. Several distinct head positions can be tried in therapy in an attempt to find one that facilitates better voice:

1. Normal straight ahead
2. Neck extended forward with head tilted down, face looking up
3. Neck flexed downward with head tilted down, face looking down
4. Neck flexed unilaterally with head tilted to either the left or right, with tilted face looking forward
5. Head upright and rotated toward left or right, face looking in that direction

Any one head position may change pharyngeal–oral resonating structures in such a way that a change in vocal quality (either better or worse) may occur.

B. Procedural Aspects of the Approach

1. Introduce the approach by demonstrating various head positions, either by photograph, video, or live demonstration. A simple explanation of the technique should accompany the demonstration: "Sometimes changing the positions of our heads can improve the sound of our voices. The head can be tilted either down or back, or to the left or right. Sometimes we can improve the sound of our voices simply by turning our heads to one side or the other. No one head position seems to help everyone. Let us try a few and listen to any changes in voice we hear."

2. The best voicing task to use to search for head position influence is the prolongation of vowels, such as /i/, /ɪ/, /ɛ/, /æ/, /o/, or /u/. Once a helpful position is discovered, any kind of voice practice material can be used.

3. Many gradations in positioning are possible between the normal head position and one of the extreme head positions described previously. For example, when flexing the neck and bringing the head down in a gradual movement, perhaps at the beginning of the movement, a voice change can be noted. As soon as change can be noted, if it is to occur, the head should be kept at that position without going to the full range of the movement.

4. Neurologically impaired patients may experience some oral–pharyngeal asymmetry from their disease—that is, one side of the neck or oral cavity may function better than the other side. A particular lateral movement of the head may make a sudden and noticeable improvement in voice in such patients. If so, then ask the patient to practice voice material with the head in the lateral position.

5. Patients with vocal hyperfunction—that is, patients who use too much effort to talk—often profit most from neck flexion with the chin tucked down toward the chest. Such downward carriage of the head seems to promote greater vocal tract relaxation. If an easy, target voice is achieved with neck flexion, this head-down position should be held during voice practice attempts.

C. Typical Case History Showing Utilization of the Approach.
Mary was a fifty-five-year-old housewife who had had vocal difficulties for the past five years. A subsequent voice evaluation found that she had a moderately severe functional dysphonia accompanied by neck tension with severe mandibular restriction, hard glottal attack, and an inappropriately high voice pitch. Voice therapy was scheduled twice weekly with therapy focus on increasing her mouth opening, developing an easy glottal attack with "a legato phonatory style." The chewing and open-mouth approaches were unsuccessful until changing head position was added to the therapy. Mary was instructed to "tuck in her chin," flexing the anterior neck muscles with her face looking downward. Keeping her chin down, she was able to reduce neck tensions; she experienced immediate improvement in vocal quality. In subsequent therapy sessions, she developed an awareness that much of her past vocal strain was related to her tendency to hyperextend her neck; by using the opposite head position with anterior neck flexion, she was able to produce voice with relatively little strain. This change of head position, coupled with other therapy techniques designed to promote greater oral openness and ease of vocal production, helped Mary reestablish a normal voice.

D. Evaluation of the Approach.   Changing to another head position by flexing or extending the neck can have an immediate positive effect on voice quality. Such an approach is usually used in combination with other voice therapy approaches, such as using the open-mouth approach or digital manipulation. Whereas patients with severe functional tensions often profit from anterior neck flexion, such as Mary above, voice problems caused by some neurogenic diseases are often minimized by using some of the other head positions described earlier, in section A. Lateralization of the head by looking to one side or the other can often produce a stronger voice in patients with unilateral vocal fold paralysis. Changing head positions to facilitate better voice requires much trial and error. If a particular head position works, it should be used; if not, other head positions should be tried.

13. Hierarchy Analysis

A. Kinds of Problems for Which the Approach Is Useful.   In hierarchy analysis, the patient lists various situations in his or her life that ordinarily produce some anxiety and arranges those situations in a sequential order from the least to the most anxiety-provoking. Individual patients may instead prepare a hierarchy of situations, ranging from those in which they find their voices best to those in which they find them worst. This technique is borrowed from Wolpe's (1987) method of reciprocal inhibition, which teaches the patient relaxed responses to anxiety-evoking situations. After identifying a hierarchy of anxiety-evoking situations, the patient begins by employing the relaxed responses in the least anxious of them and, in therapy, works his or her way up the hierarchy, thereby eventually deconditioning his or her previously established anxious responses. The identification of hierarchical situations (less anxiety–more anxiety; worst voice–best voice) is a useful therapeutic device for most patients with hyperfunctional voice problems, which by definition imply excessive overreacting. Patients with functional dysphonia, or with dysphonias accompanied by nodules, polyps, and vocal fold thickening, frequently report that their degrees of dysphonia vary with the situation. Such patients may profit from hierarchy analysis.

B. Procedural Aspects of the Approach

1. Begin by developing in the patient a general awareness of the hierarchical behavior to be studied. If, for example, the patient is to be asked to identify those situations in which he or she feels most uncomfortable, discuss with the patient the symptoms of being uncomfortable. Or if the patient is going to develop a hierarchy of situations in which he or she experiences variation of voice, discuss and give examples of what is a good voice or a bad voice. Explain that the patient must develop a relative ordering of situations, sequencing them from "good" to "bad." Some patients are initially resistant to this sort of ordering, perhaps because they never realized that there are relative gradations to their feelings of anxiety or relative changes in their quality of voice. They may not be aware that the degree of their anxiety or hoarseness is not constant.

2. Although the majority of voice patients are soon able to arrange situations into a hierarchy, a few require practice sequencing some neutral stimuli. On one occasion, a woman was taught the idea of sequential order by arranging five shades of red tiles from left to right, in the order of the lightest pink to the darkest red. Having done this, she was then able to sequence her voice situations, proceeding gradually from those in which her voice was normal to those in which it was extremely dysphonic.

3. As a home assignment, have the patient develop several hierarchies with regard to his or her voice. One hierarchy might center on how the patient's voice holds up with the family, another on how it is related to the work situation, and a third on what happens to it in varying situations with friends. After these hierarchies have been developed by the patient at home, review them in therapy.

4. In therapy, use the "good" end of the hierarchical sequence first. That is, begin by asking the patient to recapture, if possible, the good situation. The goal of therapy is to duplicate the feeling of well-being or the good voice that the patient experienced in the situation rated as best. Efforts should be made in therapy to recall the good factors surrounding the more optimum phonation. If the patient is successful in re-creating the optimum situation, his or her phonation will sound relaxed and appropriate. The re-created optimum situation thus serves as an excellent facilitator for producing good voice. After some success in re-creating the first situation on the hierarchy, capturing completely his or her optimum response (whether this is relaxation or phonation or both), the patient will then be able to move on to the second situation. Again the goal is to maintain optimum response. The rate of movement up the hierarchy will depend entirely on how successfully the patient can re-create the situations and maintain optimum response. By using the relaxed response in increasingly more tense situations, the patient is conditioning himself or herself to a more favorable, optimum behavior.

5. Although some patients can re-create situations outside the clinic with relative ease, some cannot. As soon as possible, have the patient practice the optimum response outside the clinic under good conditions, so that he or she will eventually be able to use it in the real world in more adverse situations. The patient must not lose sight of the goal of maintaining the good response in varying situations outside the clinic.

6. Not all patients can go all the way up the hierarchy, maintaining good voice at each level. Such patients should be counseled that most people experience anxiety or poorer voice in some situations, such at the highest level of the hierarchy. Some practice might be given at one step lower in the hierarchy where good performance is still maintained.

C. Typical Case History Showing Utilization of the Approach.   Jamie was a twenty-eight-year-old transsexual who was in counseling for gender transference from male to female. As part of her overall gender-change program it was recommended that she "receive speech–voice therapy to develop a more feminine speaking style." In voice therapy, Jamie reported that her out-of-clinic voicing was continually changing, "very dependent on what kind of situation I find myself in." Jamie was employed full-time as a secretary–receptionist in an area agency for aging. Her speech–language pathologist worked with her to develop this nine-step hierarchy in which she found she had the best female voice all the way down to the level where it seemed hardest to convey her femininity:

Best Voice

1. I always have my best new voice with my mother.

2. The director of our agency. She is always a great listener to everyone.

3. I answer the phone at work with a very good voice.

4. The doctor at the clinic doesn't listen as well as he should. He wants me to try harder to be a woman.

5. Some salespeople are hard to talk to and especially car mechanics.

6. I think some people at the church are bigots.

7. I still date my old boyfriend who doesn't understand me anymore.

8. Meeting new men tends to make me nervous and my speech breaks down.

9. Talking with my dad is hardest. He won't accept me and still calls me Jim.

Worst Voice

D. *Evaluation of the Approach.* Most voice patients report great variability in voice quality, depending on how much they have been using the voice, the time of day, and the psychodynamics of the speaking situations. Hierarchy analysis is often helpful for dealing with vocal inconsistencies experienced while talking with different people in various situations. By analyzing the hierarchical situations in which voice deteriorates or improves, the patient develops an awareness of those situational cues that are causing voice changes. Perhaps for the first time, the patient realizes that voice quality is not a constant, and that vocal quality fluctuations are somewhat dependent on how relaxed one feels, how comfortable one is with his or her listeners. Therapy then focuses on using the best voice found low on the hierarchy. The patient attempts to use that optimum voice in those situations in which he or she has previously experienced difficulty. Hierarchy analysis is consistently useful in voice therapy.

14. Inhalation Phonation

A. *Kinds of Problems for Which the Approach Is Useful.* Patients who have functional aphonia and functional dysphonia often profit from inhalation phonation. It introduces the high-pitched inhalation voice, which, according to Lehmann (1965), is always produced by true vocal fold vibration. This can be a helpful technique for the patient who perseverates using ventricular phonation and often demonstrates difficulty "getting out of it." Likewise, it can be helpful for the patient with functional dysphonia who has developed some maladaptive voice that seems to resist change. On videoendoscopy, when the voice patient is asked to produce an inhalation voice, we see the true folds in a stretched position (lengthened in their respiratory length) suddenly adducted and set in vibration. It is the relative thinness of the folds on inspiration that seems to produce the high-pitched voice. The ease with which most patients can produce the technique (inhaling with voice and exhaling with a near-matched voice) makes the approach readily useful in establishing or reestablishing true vocal fold vibration.

B. Procedural Aspects of the Approach

1. This particular approach, which is similar to masking, is perhaps better demonstrated than explained. Demonstrate inhalation phonation by phonating a high-pitched sound while elevating the shoulders. It is important to time the initiations of the inhalation with shoulder elevation. Elevate the shoulder so you can mark for the patient the contrast between inhalation (shoulders raised) and exhalation (shoulders lowered).

2. After demonstrating several separate inhalations with simultaneous shoulder elevation and phonation, say, "Now, I'll match the high-pitched inhalation voice with an expiration voice." Inhale, raising the shoulders and simultaneously humming in a high pitch, then dropping the shoulders on exhalation and producing the same voice. Repeat the inhalation–exhalation matched phonations several times.

3. Ask the patient to make an inhalation phonation. He or she should repeat the inhalation phonation several times. Now again repeat the inhalation–exhalation matched phonation, taking care to make the associated shoulder movements. Then tell the patient, "Now drop your shoulders on expiration, making the same high-pitched voice as you do it." With a little practice, most patients are able to do it.

4. After the patient has produced the matching hum, say, "Now, let us extend the expiration like this." Demonstrate a continuation of the high pitch, sweeping down from your falsetto register to your regular chest register on one long, continuous expiration. Repeat this several times. Then say to the patient, "Once I've brought my vocal cords together at the high pitch, I then sweep down, keeping them together, to the pitch level of my regular speaking voice."

5. If the patient is unable to produce this shift from high to low, repeat the first four steps. If the patient can make the shift down to the regular speaking register, say, "Now you're getting your vocal cords together for a good-sounding voice." Take care at this point not to rush the patient into using the "new" voice functionally. Rather, have the patient practice some similar hum phonations. After some practice just phonating the hum, give the patient a word list containing simple monosyllabic words for "true" voice practice.

6. Once the patient is able to produce inspiration–expiration without difficulty, he or she should be instructed to no longer use the pronounced shoulder movements. Elevating and dropping the shoulders are only necessary to mark the difference between inspiration and expiration.

7. Stay at the single-word practice level until normal voicing is established. We often spend several therapy periods practicing the new phonation as a motor practice drill without attempting to make the voice conversationally functional. You might say, "Now we're getting the vocal folds together the way we want them." This places the previous aphonia or ventricular phonation "blame" on the mechanism rather than on the patient. Counseling with the patient at this time is important. The motor practice gives the patient time to adjust to the more optimum way of phonating.

C. Typical Case History Showing Utilization of the Approach.   Derek, a five-year-old boy, was found to have small bilateral vocal nodules. His speech clinician placed him on complete voice rest, which unfortunately was enforced for five continuous months. At the end of five months, the nodules had disappeared, and Derek was instructed by both the physician and the speech pathologist to resume normal phonation. Despite all his efforts, Derek could only whisper. He became completely aphonic but whispered easily to all people with much animation and relative comfort. This functional aphonia remained for two months, after which he was instructed, "Go back and talk the normal way." Derek gestured that he wanted to use his voice but could not "find it." Therapy efforts for restoring phonation were begun about seven months after Derek's phonations had ceased. Inhalation phonation was initiated, and at the first therapy session Derek was able to produce a high-pitched inhalation sound and to follow his clinician well by matching the inhalation with an expiration sound. He was able to use an expiration phonation, appropriate in both quality and pitch, by the end of the first therapy session. He was scheduled for two other appointments within a twenty-four-hour period, during which he practiced producing his regained normal voice. He was counseled that his "voice is working now and you'll never have to lose it again." The boy has had normal phonation since his voice was restored using the inhalation phonation technique. Counseling to curb yelling and other vocal abuses appeared to be successful, as Derek has experienced no return of the bilateral vocal nodules.

D. Evaluation of the Approach.   Some patients who experience either aphonia, dysphonia, or ventricular phonation for any length of time lose their ability to initiate normal true fold phonation. The longer the aphonia or dysphonia persists, the harder it might be to use normal voice. Inhalation phonation is a simple way to produce true cord approximation and voicing. The high-pitched voice on inhalation probably results from the folds being longer in their inhalation posture, and even though they may adduct on command, they remain in their longer configuration. This elongated posture thins them, resulting in the higher-pitched phonation. The important part of the approach, however, is matching the inhalation voicing with exhalation voicing. Once the patient can produce the exhalation voice without the inhalation prompt, the inhalation practice is no longer needed.

15. Laryngeal Massage

A. Kinds of Problems for Which the Approach Is Useful.   This particular approach follows the procedures, modified slightly, for manual circumlaryngeal therapy, as presented by Aronson (1990), which offer gentle manipulation and massage of the larynx. The approach is recommended for use with patients with functional voice disorders in which structural or neurogenic causal factors cannot be identified. While the most commonly used professional term for such voice disorders is *functional dysphonia,* a few authors have recommended that these functional disorders be classified as *psychogenic dysphonia* (Aronson, 1990) or *muscle tension dysphonia* (Morrison and Rammage, 1994). As introduced earlier in this text, we use the term *functional dysphonia* generically to include hoarseness without identified structural or organic cause, ventricular dysphonia, puberphonia, falsetto, and voicing with discomfort (pain, scratchy throat, etc.). Stress, psychological conflict, and overall systemic tension often appear to worsen the symptoms of functional dysphonia. Manual circumlaryngeal therapy offers gentle laryngeal manipulation and massage, resulting in lower laryngeal carriage and greater intrinsic–extrinsic laryngeal muscle relaxation.

There are two studies in the literature (Roy, Bless, Heisey, and Ford, 1997; Roy and Leeper, 1993) that both report successful use of manual circumlaryngeal therapy as a primary therapy for patients (N = 17 and 25, respectively, in the two above studies) with functional dysphonia. Of startling clinical significance is that positive reduction of voice symptoms was achieved for each patient in only one therapy session using this laryngeal manipulation–massage therapy. Although the present authors can report good results with this technique, we have also achieved lower laryngeal posturing with greater muscle relaxation using the yawn–sigh technique (Boone and McFarlane, 1993). Therefore, in our clinical practice, we employ the yawn–sigh first with the patient with a high larynx and laryngeal tension. If the patient is not successful employing the yawn–sigh, our next approach is the use of manual circumlaryngeal therapy as described by Aronson (1990).

B. Procedural Aspects of the Approach

1. Our first step is to screen for a high larynx and probable excessive laryngeal–neck muscle tension. If not present, other facilitating approaches are used. If present, we continue.

2. The yawn–sigh is first attempted (see facilitating approach 25). If a lower larynx and greater muscle relaxation are achieved by using the yawn–sigh, we do not apply laryngeal manipulation and massage.

3. We follow Aronson's procedures for reducing "musculoskeletal tension associated with vocal hyperfunction":

   a. Encircle the hyoid bone with the thumb and middle finger. Work back posteriorly until the major horns are felt.
   b. Apply light pressure with the fingers in a circular motion over the tips of the hyoid bone.
   c. Repeat this procedure with the fingers from the thyroid notch, working posteriorly.
   d. Find the posterior borders of the thyroid cartilage (medial to the sternocleidomastoid muscles) and repeat the procedure.
   e. With the fingers over the superior borders of the thyroid cartilage, begin to work the larynx gently downward and laterally at times.
   f. Ask the patient to prolong vowels during these procedures, noting changes in quality or pitch. Clearer voice quality and lower pitch indicate relief of tension. Because of possible fatigue, rest periods should be provided.
   g. Improvement in voice is immediately reinforced. Practice should be given in producing voice in vowels, words, phrases, and sentences.

h. Discuss with the patient how voice tension has been reduced. Repeat the procedures. Can the patient maneuver his or her own larynx to a lower position?

4. We find out whether the patient can experience the same lowering of the larynx with muscle relaxation by producing the yawn–sigh. We discuss how both techniques can be used when excessive laryngeal tension is experienced.

C. Typical Case History Showing Utilization of the Approach. Carl was a twenty-three-year-old graduate student in speech and hearing sciences who complained to his clinical supervisor that in certain situations he experienced "such tightness in my throat, I can hardly get my voice out." A subsequent voice evaluation found him to have unnecessarily high carriage of his larynx accompanied by some evidence of functional dysphonia. He was asked to read Aronson's description of therapy for "musculoskeletal tension (vocal hyperfunction)" (1990, p. 339). Subsequently, the supervisor conducted a full one-hour manual circumlaryngeal therapy session with Carl that had an immediate result of lowering his laryngeal posture and relaxing his voice, resulting in "a voice that was always there with greater intensity and less perturbation." Carl was followed over an eighteen-month period (while in graduate school) and was able to maintain a normal voice following the one session of laryngeal manipulation and massage.

D. Evaluation of the Approach. One only has to see a demonstration of this manipulation–massage technique to be impressed with its sudden effectiveness in reducing muscular tension and producing a more relaxed, lower-pitched, resonant voice. We have been impressed with the results of laryngeal massage. Aronson has described his approach as "maneuvering the patient's laryngeal and hyoid anatomy," which fits the term *massage,* described as "the act of rubbing, kneading, or stroking the superficial parts of the body with the hand" (Blakiston, 1985, p. 913). The studies by Roy and Leeper (1993) and Roy, Bless, Heisey, and Ford (1997) suggest short-term benefits from using laryngeal massage or manual circumlaryngeal therapy with functional dysphonic patients.

Track 13

16. Masking

A. Kinds of Problems for Which the Approach Is Useful. Patients with functional aphonia are often able to produce normal phonation under conditions of auditory masking. Using masking with patients who have functional dysphonia will often reveal a "window" of improved phonation. It appears that many such patients produce faulty voices because of poor real-time auditory monitoring. The use of masking in both diagnostic testing and therapy will often reveal changed phonation states that can then be recorded and used as voice models in subsequent therapy. The masking facilitating approach uses a voicing–reflex test, used by audiologists as the Lombard test (Newby, 1972). In fact, the Lombard test was first introduced as a method of finding voice in patients with functional aphonia. When asked to phonate in a loud-noise background, patients with functional aphonia sometimes used light voice. In the voice-reflex situation, the patient wears earphones and is asked to read a passage aloud. As the patient is reading, a masking noise is fed into the earphones. The louder the masking, the louder is the patient's voice. At loud masking levels the patient cannot monitor well either the loudness or the clearness of his or her voice. Some patients with functional dysphonias actually experience clearer voices when they cannot monitor their productions because of loud masking. Some care should be given to the amount of masking intensity that is used, particularly when using white or pink noise masking (ASHA, 1991). The use of speech–range masking, such as that provided by the Facilitator (1998), permits effective masking at relatively low intensity levels.

B. Procedural Aspects of the Approach

1. The masking approach is best used without any prior explanation. The increased voicing experienced under masking conditions is produced on a reflexive, nonvolitional basis.

2. Masking should be presented with the patient wearing headphones and not presented free-field. The patient is seated by a masking source, such as the white noise of an audiometer or the speech–range masking of the Facilitator. The patient is asked to read aloud and to keep reading no matter what kind of interruption he or she may hear. We typically have the patient read (or very young children are asked to count) about ten seconds, introduce masking for five seconds, go back to reading without masking, then reintroduce masking. We record the patient's oral reading, and on playback we can hear the changes in voice that are introduced when masking occurs.

3. An audiocassette recording should be made as the patient reads aloud. An aphonic patient's whisper may change to voice under conditions of masking. It is important to have recorded the emergence of voice, which the patient can use in step 5. The dysphonic patient (functional, ventricular, or puberphonic) should also be recorded while using the masking approach. Marked differences in voice quality between the absence and presence of masking conditions will probably be evident.

4. Five- or ten-second exposures to masking are introduced to the patient bilaterally. The intensity levels should be in excess of 70 dB SPL, which is sufficiently loud to mask out the patient's own voicing attempts. Whenever an aphonic patient hears the loud masking, he or she may attempt some feeble vocalization. Under masking a dysphonic patient will produce a louder voice and often a voice with more normal vocal quality, as well.

5. Do not use the masking method beyond the trial stage with those few voice patients who do not demonstrate the voice-reflex effect. If it works well, and produces voice improvement, the method may be used as part of every therapy period. You might then experiment by having the patient listen to tapes of himself or herself, to see whether the patient can match volitionally his or her voice under masking conditions. Recordings can then be made contrasting the voice without masking (attempting to re-create the same voice as heard under masking) and the voice with masking. Try to have the voices sound alike.

6. A patient may profit from reading aloud under masking conditions, and then having the masking abruptly ended to see if he or she can maintain the better voice. Many other variations using the masking noise can be initiated by inventive clinicians.

C. Typical Case History Showing Utilization of the Approach.   Lillian was a nine-year-old girl who had a history of vocal nodules that had been previously treated successfully with voice therapy. Several months after therapy had been terminated as successful (no nodules, normal voice), Lillian developed a severe influenza that left her with no voice. She was completely aphonic and could communicate only by whispering and using good facial expressions and gestures. The aphonia continued for one month (over the December holiday break) before she returned to the voice clinic. The masking approach was used with Lillian after attempts at modeling and request for voice failed. Lillian was asked to read aloud under conditions of 70 dB masking. Her reading attempts were recorded on a twenty-second loop tape. As soon as masking was introduced, light phonation was heard and recorded on the loop cassette. The masking and oral reading were stopped, and Lillian was asked to hear her good voice on the tape. The child clapped her hands in joy that she now had a returned voice. Further masking followed by ear training was used as her voice became stronger. After two follow-up therapy sessions, Lillian was discharged with a normal voice. The pushing approach—producing the word *patch* with sudden extension of arms—was then demonstrated for Lillian to use "if you ever lose your voice again." Hopefully, her "believing" in pushing as a protection against future voice loss will function as a placebo effect and prevent any recurrence of aphonia. Lillian has had no voice problem in the two years since the one month of aphonia.

D. Evaluation of the Approach.   The masking approach is most helpful with aphonic patients. It is also helpful for patients with some form of functional dysphonia or young men with puberphonia. If the masking noise is loud enough, in excess of 70 dB SPL, patients cannot hear their voices to monitor phonation. If required to continue speaking by reading aloud under conditions of masking, patients will often produce relatively normal voices. Clinicians should use some care in confronting the patients on audiotape playback with their "good" voices. Improved voices under conditions of masking should be used as the patients' models for their own imitation phonations. Clinicians should use the masking approach with some degree of eclecticism—that is, if the approach works, use it; if it does not, quickly abandon it.

17. Nasal/Glide Stimulation

Track
6 & 12

A. Kinds of Problems for Which the Approach Is Useful.   Clinicians frequently note that in voice therapy certain stimulus sounds seem to facilitate an easier-produced, often better-sounding voice. This is particularly true working with children and adults with problems of vocal hyperfunction. Watterson, McFarlane, and Diamond (1993) have found in studying fifteen adult voice patients with vocal hyperfunction and fifteen matched control subjects that nasal and glide consonants facilitated better voicing patterns and were judged by the hyperfunctional subjects as "easier" to produce. The concept of differences in vocal effort has been also investigated by Bickley and Stevens (1987) and Baken and Orlikoff (1988), generally finding that supraglottal resonance-articulatory postures have a direct relationship to laryngeal physiology and function. Using words that contain many nasal and glide consonants, usually coupled with other therapy techniques, often helps the patient produce desired "target" vocalizations. Using nasal/glide consonants as therapy stimuli is particularly useful for patients with functional dysphonia, spasmodic dysphonia, and dysphonias related to fold thickening, nodules, and polyps.

B. Procedural Aspects of the Approach

1. Most therapy techniques require the patient to say something. For example, in the open-mouth approach or in practicing focus, the patient is given a few stimulus words to say. Words that contain nasal or glide consonants will often produce the best-sounding voice or the voice that appears made with the least amount of effort (as compared with words containing other consonants).

2. The clinician can find a number of monosyllabic and polysyllabic words containing nasal consonants for the patient to practice saying as the response when using various facilitating approaches. Here are a few examples: *man, moon, many, morning, many men, moon man, manual lawnmower, Miami millionaire, morning singing.*

3. A variation of the technique is to use nasal monosyllabic words and introduce an /a/ between each word. Ask the patient to say three words in a row with the neutral /a/ between each word. For example, "man a man a man" or "wing a wing a wing."

4. We use the same procedure for words containing glide consonants. It has been found, however, that nasal consonants combine very well with the /l/ and /r/ phonemes, and many of our glide words contain nasal consonants: *loll, lil, rare, rah, lilly, arrow, marrow, married, married women, one lonely memory, Laura ran around, remember many lawmen.*

5. Using monosyllabic /l/ and /r/ words with an /a/ between them seems to produce good voice, such as "lee a lee a lee" or "rah a rah a rah."

C. Typical Case History Showing Utilization of the Approach.

Louise was a sixty-six-year-old housewife who was forced to divorce her husband of some forty-two years. She experienced a number of somatic symptoms following the divorce, including a severe functional dysphonia. Endoscopic–stroboscopic examination revealed a high carriage of the larynx with moderate vocal fold compression. The yawn–sigh approach was found to be effective in lowering her larynx and encouraging a more optimal vocal fold approximation. Under the sigh condition, she was asked to say various words. It was found that words with many nasal and glide consonants facilitated the easiest-produced and best-sounding voice. Intensive self-practice and twice-weekly voice therapy for nine weeks, supplemented by concurrent psychological counseling, resulted in a good functional return of normal voice.

D. Evaluation of the Approach.

Clinicians are always looking for voicing tasks that facilitate good voice production. Recent research has validated that certain sounds, particularly nasal and glide consonants, facilitate voice production. Among patients with vocal hyperfunction, nasal/glide consonant words are perceived by patients as producing voice with less effort (Watterson, McFarlane, & Diamond, 1993). Word stimuli containing many nasal/glide consonants appear to facilitate in voice therapy a voice that sounds better and is produced (according to patient self-evaluation) with less effort.

18. Open-Mouth Approach

A. Kinds of Problems for Which the Approach Is Useful.   Encouraging the patient to develop more oral openness often reduces generalized vocal hyperfunction. Opening the mouth more while speaking and learning to listen with a slightly open mouth allow the patient to use his or her vocal mechanisms more optimally. The open-mouth approach promotes more natural size–mass adjustments and more optimum approximation of the vocal folds, and this helps correct problems of loudness, pitch, and quality. Opening the mouth more is also recommended to increase oral resonance and to improve overall voice quality. The voice also sounds louder. Developing greater openness should be part of any voice therapy program wherein the patient is attempting to use the vocal mechanisms with less effort and strain.

B. Procedural Aspects of the Approach

1. Have the patient view himself or herself in a mirror (or on a videotape playback, if possible) to observe the presence and absence of open-mouth behavior. Identify any lip tightness, mandibular restriction, or excessive neck muscle movement for the patient.

2. Children seem to understand quickly the benefits of opening the mouth more to produce better-sounding voices. In our voice program for children (Boone, 1993), we use a brief story that illustrates two boys, one who talks with his mouth closed and one who speaks with his mouth open. We then introduce a hand puppet and ask the child if he or she has ever been a ventriloquist. The ventriloquist is described as someone who does not open the mouth, in contrast to the puppet, who makes exaggerated, wide-mouth openings.

3. The ventriloquist–puppet analogy also works well with adults. Let the patient observe the marked contrast between talking with a closed mouth and talking with an open one. Ask the patient to watch himself or herself speak the two different ways in a mirror. Instruct the patient that what he or she is attempting will at first feel foreign and inappropriate. The initial stages of letting the jaw relax are frequently anything but relaxed.

4. To establish further this oral openness, ask the patient to drop the head toward the chest and let the lips part and the jaw drop open. Once the patient can do this, have him or her practice some relaxed /a/ sounds. When the head is tilted down and the jaw is slightly open, a more relaxed phonation can often be achieved.

5. In order for patients to develop a feeling of openness when listening, and as a preset to speaking, they must first develop a conscious awareness of how often they find themselves with tight, closed mouths. One way to develop this awareness is to have patients mark down, on cards they carry with them, each time they become aware that their mouths are closed unnecessarily. The marking task itself is often enough to increase a patient's awareness, and over a period of a week the number of mouth closings will decrease notably. Another way of developing an awareness of greater orality is to have patients place in their living environments (on a dressing table, desk, or car dashboard) a little sign that says "OPEN" or perhaps has a double arrow or any other code that might serve as a reminder.

6. Greater oral openness requires a lot of self-practice to overcome the habit of talking through a restricted mandible. Steps 3 and 4 facilitate greater mouth opening and are good practice tasks. After some practice in using greater mouth opening, the patient should confirm what it looks like by viewing videotape playback in practice sessions. Practice materials for improving greater mouth opening may be found in practice kits for children (Blonigen, 1994; Boone, 1993) and in voice books such as Andrews (1995), Boone (1997), Brown (1996,) Case (1996), Colton and Casper (1996), and Stemple, Gerdeman, and Glaze (1994).

C. Typical Case History Showing Utilization of the Approach. J. J., a seventeen-year-old high school girl, was examined by a laryngologist about one year after an automobile accident in which she had suffered some injuries to the head and neck. Laryngoscopic examination found all visible laryngeal structures normal in appearance and function, despite the fact that since the accident the girl's voice had been only barely audible. The speech pathologist was impressed "with her relatively closed mouth while speaking, which seemed to result in extremely poor voice resonance." Voice therapy combined both the chewing and the open-mouth facilitating approaches. It was discovered in therapy that for three months after the automobile accident the girl had worn an orthopedic collar that seemed to inhibit her head and jaw movements. It appeared that much of her closed-mouth, mandibularly restricted speech was related to the constraints imposed upon her by the orthopedic collar. When using the open-mouth approach with her head tilted down toward her chest, she was immediately able to produce a louder, more resonant voice. The open-mouth approach was initiated before beginning chewing exercises, and both achieved excellent results. Therapy was terminated after six weeks, with much voice improvement in both loudness and quality.

D. Evaluation of the Approach. The voice, both normal and dysphonic, improves in quality with greater mouth opening. On opening the mouth a bit more, the voice usually improves immediately. Besides opening the mouth more while speaking, the approach also encourages slight mouth opening while listening. A gentle opening of less than one finger wide between the central incisors keeps the teeth apart and generally fosters a relaxed oral posture. The open-mouth approach has been particularly effective with performers who often open their mouths well during performance (acting, singing) but may forget the importance of opening their mouths during conversation.

19. Pitch Inflections

A. Kinds of Problems for Which the Approach Is Useful. The prosodic and stress patterns of the normal speaking voice are characterized by changes in pitch, loudness, and duration. In some individuals, the lack of pitch variation is notice-able because the resulting voice is monotonous and boring to listeners. Speaking on the same pitch level with little variation, which for the average speaker is impossible to maintain, requires the inhibition of natural inflection. It is usually observed in overcontrolled people who display very little overt affect. Fairbanks (1960), who describes pitch variation as a vital part of normal phonation, defines inflection and shift: "An *inflection* is a modulation of pitch during phonation. A *shift* is a change of pitch from the end of one phonation to the beginning of the next" (p. 132). Voice therapy for patients with monotonic pitch seeks not only to establish more optimum pitch levels but also to increase the amount of pitch vari-ability. Any voice patient with a dull, monotonous pitch level will profit from attempting to increase pitch inflections. Many patients with functional dysphonia related to vocal hyperfunction appear to speak with little pitch fluctuation, often part of a pattern of oral and mandibular tightness with the lips and mandible in a fixed, nonmoving pattern.

B. Procedural Aspects of the Approach

1. The patient must first become aware of his or her vocal monotony in play-back of a recorded utterance on a cassette or on loop playback on an instrument like the Facilitator. Play samples of lack of pitch variability and follow with sam-ples of good pitch variability, as provided by the clinician. Follow the listening with evaluative comments.

2. Begin working on downward and upward inflectional shifts of the same word, exaggerating in the beginning the extent of pitch change. Helpful sources for increasing pitch variation may be found in Boone (1997), Brown (1996), McKin-ney (1994), Morrison and Rammage (1994), Stemple and Holcomb (1988), among many others.

3. Using the same practice materials, have the patient practice introducing inflectional shifts within specific words.

4. Pitch inflections can be graphically displayed on many instruments such as the Visi-Pitch or PM 100 Pitch Analyzer. Set target inflections for the patient, to see if the patient can make his or her pitch level reach the same excursions or move-ment as the target model on the scope.

5. Record and play back for the patient various oral reading and conversational samples, critically analyzing the productions for degree of pitch variability.

C. Typical Case History Showing Utilization of the Approach.   Dr. T., a fifty-one-year-old economics professor, received severe course evaluations from his students, who complained of his "monotonous" voice. On a subsequent voice eval-uation, during both conversation and oral reading, he used "the same fundamental frequency with only minimal excursion of frequency." His voice was indeed monot-onous, not only in pitch but in loudness, as well. He also used the same duration characteristics for most vowels. Dr. T. was highly motivated to improve his speaking voice and manner of speaking. Subsequent therapy focus was on increasing pitch inflections and improving loudness variations. He was provided with audiocassette

tapes, which he practiced daily, matching the target model productions with his own voicing attempts. After six weeks of voice therapy and intensive self-practice, Dr. T. demonstrated improvement in both his conversational and lecture voices. Unfortunately, his lack of overall animation and boring affect still resulted in poor course evaluations. However, his conversational voice with increasing pitch inflections appeared to make a much more favorable impression on those around him.

D. Evaluation of the Approach.   Voice quality in functional dysphonias is often improved when overall effort in speaking is reduced. Speaking for an extended period of time in a monotone is tiring (to both the speaker and the listener). People who wish to improve the quality of their speaking voices can often profit from increasing pitch variability as they speak. Using auditory feedback, listening to one's voice on playback, appears to be a good way of improving pitch variability in one's voice.

20. Relaxation

A. Kinds of Problems for Which the Approach Is Useful.   It is not possible for most students, working adults, and retirees to have a world that is free of tension. As Eliot (1994) has written in describing the need for relaxation and a reduction in life's stresses, "When you can't change the world, you can learn to change your response to it" (p. 87). Because encountering stress is part of the human condition, what becomes important is how we react to stresses. Our patients with hyperfunctional voices often develop vocal symptoms as part of their stress reaction. Among the particular voice symptoms Boone (1997) related to stress are diplophonia, dry throat and mouth, harshness, elevated pitch, functional dysphonia, and shortness of breath. Accordingly, a frequent goal in voice therapy is to take the "work" out of phonation by using such voice therapy techniques as the open-mouth and yawn–sigh approaches along with symptomatic relaxation.

Symptomatic relaxation methods might well relax components of the vocal tract but may not lead to overall relaxation from stress reduction (Feldman, 1992). It is usually useless to imply to voice patients that if they "would just relax," their voice symptoms would lessen and their voices improve. If our patients could relax, they would. The clinician must recognize that a certain amount of psychic tension and muscle tonus is normal and healthy; however, some individuals overreact to their environmental stresses and live with "a fast idle," expending far more energy and effort than a situation requires. When such psychic effort is causative or coupled with voice symptoms, some encouragement for increasing the patient's relaxation abilities is in order. By relaxation, therefore, we mean a realistic responsiveness to the environment with a minimum of needless energy expanded.

B. Procedural Aspects of the Approach

1. For children, we develop an understanding of principles of relaxation, following some of the recommendations and materials offered by Wilson's *Voice Problems of Children* (1987) or Andrews's *Voice Therapy for Children* (1991). For adults, it is helpful to have voice patients read the chapters on stress management and methods for reducing stage fright in Boone's *Is Your Voice Telling on You?* (1997) or read about posture and release in Brown's *Discover Your Voice* (1996).

2. Introduce to the patient the concept of differential relaxation as outlined by Feldman (1992). The classical method of differential relaxation might be explained to the patient and applied. Under differential relaxation, the patient concentrates on a particular site of the body, deliberately relaxing and tensing certain muscles, discriminating between muscle contraction and relaxation. The typical procedure here is to have the patient begin distally, away from the body, with the fingers or the toes. Once the patient feels the tightness of contraction and the heaviness of relaxation at the beginning site, he or she moves "up" the limb (on to the feet or hands, and thence to the legs or arms), repeating at each site the tightness-heaviness discrimination. Once the torso is reached, the voice patient should include the chest, neck, "voice box," throat, and on through the mouth and parts of the face. With some patients, we start the distal analysis with the head, beginning with the scalp and then going to the forehead, eyes, facial muscles, lips, jaw, tongue, palate, throat, larynx, neck, and so on. Some practice in this progressive relaxation technique can produce remarkably relaxed states in very tense patients.

3. Various biofeedback devices can help the patient develop a feeling of relaxation. Such feedback as galvanic skin response, pulse rate, blood pressure, and muscle responsiveness through electromyographic tracings all seem to correlate well with patients' feelings of anxiety and tension. By performing a particular relaxed behavior, such as yawning, a patient can confirm his or her particular arousal state by the biofeedback data. Using such biofeedback devices, the patient can soon learn what it "feels" like to be relaxed or free of tension.

4. Wolpe (1987) combines relaxation with hierarchy analysis. The patient responds to particular tension-producing cues with a relaxed response, such as feeling a heaviness or warmth at a particular body site, and maintains a relaxed response in the tension situation. The patient may instead develop a situational hierarchy specific to tension and voice by attempting to use a relaxed voice at increasingly tense levels of the hierarchy, as outlined in the adult voice program by Boone (1982).

5. Head rotation might be introduced as a technique for relaxing components of the vocal tract. The approach is used in this way: The patient sits in a backless chair, dropping the head forward to the chest; the patient then "flops" his or her head across to the right shoulder, then lifts it, then again flops it (the neck is here extended) along the back and across to the left shoulder; he or she then returns to the anterior head-down-on-chest position and repeats the cycle, rolling the head in a circular fashion. A few patients will not find head rotation relaxing, but most will feel the heaviness of the movement and experience definite relaxation in the neck. Once a patient in this latter group reports neck relaxation, he or she should be asked to phonate an "ah" as the head is rolled. The relaxed phonation might be recorded and then analyzed in terms of how it sounds in comparison to the patient's other phonations.

6. Open-throat relaxation can also be used. Have the patient lower the head slightly toward the chest and make an easy, open, prolonged yawn, concentrating on what the yawn feels like in the throat. The yawn should yield conscious sensations of an open throat during the prolonged inhalation. If the patient reports that he or she can feel this open-throat sensation, ask him or her to prolong an "ah," capturing and maintaining the same feeling experienced during the yawn. Any relaxed phonations produced under these conditions should be recorded and used as target voice models for the patient. Encourage the patient to comment on and think about the relaxed throat sensations experienced during the yawn.

7. Wilson's *Voice Problems of Children* (1987) includes an excellent presentation on various relaxation procedures for use with children, developed by Wilson and other authors, which seem to have equal applicability to adults. Most of the procedures described can immediately increase relaxation and reduce tension associated with speaking.

8. Ask the patient to think of a setting he or she has experienced, or perhaps imagined, as the ultimate in relaxation. Different patients use different kinds of imagery here. For example, one patient thought of lying in a hammock, but another person reacted to lying in a hammock with a set of anxious responses. Settings typically considered relaxing are lying on a rug at night in front of a blazing fire, floating on a lake, fishing while lying in a rowboat, lying down in bed, and so on. The setting the patient thinks of should be studied and analyzed; eventually, the patient should try to capture the relaxed feelings he or she imagines might result from, or may actually have been experienced in, such a setting. With some practice—and some tolerance for initial failure in recapturing the relaxed mood— the average patient can find a setting or two that he or she can re-create in his or her imagination to use in future tense situations.

C. Typical Case History Showing Utilization of the Approach. M. Y., a thirty-four-year-old missile engineer, developed transient periods of severe dysphonia when talking to certain people. At other times, particularly in his professional work, he experienced normal voice. Mirror laryngoscopy revealed a normal larynx. During the voice interview, the speech pathologist was impressed by the man's general nervousness and apparently poor self-concept. In exploring the area of interpersonal relationships, the patient confided that in the past year he had seen two psychiatrists periodically but had experienced no relief from his tension. Further exploration of the settings in which his voice was most dysphonic revealed that his biggest problem was talking to store clerks, garage mechanics, and persons who did physical labor; some of his more relaxed experiences included giving speeches and giving work instructions to his colleagues. Subsequent voice therapy included progressive relaxation. Once relaxed behavior was achieved, the patient developed a hierarchy of situations, beginning with those in which he felt most relaxed (giving instructions to colleagues) and proceeding to those in which he experienced the most tension (talking with car mechanics). After some practice, the patient was able to recognize various cues that signaled increasing tension. Once such a cue occurred, he employed a relaxation response, which more often than not enabled him to maintain normal phonation in situations that had previously induced dysphonia. As this consciously induced response continued to be successful, the patient reported greater confidence in approaching the previously tense situations, knowing he would experience little or no voice difficulty. Voice therapy was terminated after eleven weeks, when the patient reported only occasional difficulty phonating in isolated situations and increased self-confidence in all situations.

D. Evaluation of the Approach. The popularity of many relaxation and stress-reduction programs today is probably due in part to their offering people with excessive tensions some relief from their agonies. Symptomatic voice therapy focuses on faulty voices and sometimes the tensions associated with (if not the cause of) the vocal problems. A growing number of voice clinicians feel that direct symptom modification, such as teaching relaxed responses to replace previously tense responses, breaks up the circular kind of response that often keeps maladaptive vocal behaviors "alive." In effect, we talk the same way today that we talked yesterday until we learn a better way to respond. Using the voice in a more relaxed manner with less competitive tension is a "better way to respond."

21. Respiration Training

A. Kinds of Problems for Which the Approach Is Useful. Singing teachers and vocal coaches often put more emphasis on respiration training with singers and actors than speech–language pathologists do with patients with voice disorders. While training in breath support is vital for the extremes of vocal performance produced by singers and actors, the typical patient with a functional voice disorder may need only some instruction for developing expiratory control (such as avoiding "squeezing" out final words of an utterance because of lack of adequate breath). Hoit (1995), in an excellent article summarizing studies of diaphragmatic–abdominal muscle physiology, makes a strong point for recognizing the difference in muscle function specific to whether the student/patient's body is supine or vertical. It would appear that increasing abdominal muscle participation while the patient is either sitting or standing would have some relevance to the voice patient with vocal hyperfunction. Management of respiratory limitations related to neurogenic voice disorders and pulmonary disease is discussed in Chapters 4 and 7 of this text. The following procedures are useful with functional voice disorders when there is a demonstrated need to improve respiratory function for voice.

B. Procedural Aspects of the Approach

1. Provide the patient with a simple demonstration on how expiratory air can set up vibration (i.e., place your lips gently together and blow through them, setting up a visual–audible demonstration). If the clinician has difficulty doing this, moistening the lips will often facilitate the vibration and its audible sound. Continue with the explanation by discussing with the patient how our outgoing air passes between the vocal folds, setting them into vibration, which we hear as voice.

2. Demonstrate a slightly exaggerated breath, as used in sighing. The sigh begins with a slightly larger-than-usual inhalation (like a yawn) followed by a prolonged open-mouth exhalation, usually with light, breathy voice. Describe the type of breath used to produce the sigh as the "breath of well-being," the kind of easy breath one might take when comfortable or happy—the sigh of contentment. One of the authors (DB) tells his patients "the kind of noise you make when you first see the Grand Canyon!"

3. Demonstrate the quick inhalation and prolonged exhalation needed for a normal speaking task. Take a normal breath and count slowly from one to five on one exhalation. See if the patient can do this; if he or she can, extend the count by one number at a time, at the rate of approximately one number per half-second. This activity can be continued until the patient is able to use the "best" phonation achieved during the number counts. Any sacrifice of voice quality should be avoided, and the number count should never extend beyond the point at which good quality can be maintained.

4. Various duration tasks, such as prolonging vowels, provide excellent practice in expiratory control. Prolonging an /s/, /z/, /a/, /ɑ/, /æ/, or /i/ for as long as possible provides an expiratory measure that can be used for comparison. Take a baseline measurement in the beginning, such as number of seconds a particular phonation can be maintained, and see whether this can be extended with practice. Avoid asking the patient to "take in a big breath"; rather, ask him or her to take in a normal breath of well-being, initiating a lightly phonated sigh on exhalation. See if the patient can extend this for five seconds. If so, progressively increase the extension to eight, twelve, fifteen, and finally twenty seconds. The voice patient who can hold on to an extended phonation of a vowel for twenty seconds has certainly exhibited good breath control for purposes of voice. Such a patient would not have to work on breath control per se, but he or she might want to combine work on exhalation control with such approaches as hierarchy analysis (to see if he or she can maintain such good breath control under varying moments of stress).

5. Select from various voice and articulation books reading materials designed to help develop breath control. Give special attention to the patient's beginning phonation as soon after inhalation as possible, so as not to waste a lot of the outgoing airstream before phonating. Encourage the patient to practice quick inhalations between phrases and sentences, taking care not to take "a big breath."

6. With young children who need breathing work, begin with nonverbal exhalations. One way to work on breathing exhalation with little children is to use a pinwheel, which lends itself naturally to the game "How long can you keep the pinwheel spinning?" With practice, a child will be able to extend the length of his or her exhalations (the length of time the pinwheel spins). Another method of enhancing exhalation control is to place a piece of tissue paper against a wall, begin blowing on it to keep it in place when the fingers are removed, and keep blowing on it to see how long it can be kept in place. Both the pinwheel and tissue-paper exercises lend themselves to timing measurements. These measurements should be made and plotted graphically for the child; when a certain target length of time is reached, the activity can be stopped.

7. When working with a singer, actor, or lecturer who needs some formal respiration training, you might take the following steps:

  a. Avoid having the patient lie supine on his or her back for the purpose of observing abdominal protusion on inhalation and abdominal retraction on expiration. As Hoit (1995) summarized, the supine chest wall–abdominal muscle movements while supine are not the same as they are with the patient sitting or standing in a vertical position. The only time we recommend watching supine abdominal movements is when the patient appears very tense; the tense patient may profit from watching the passive movements of the abdomen as the diaphragm's displacement moving toward the feet works to protrude the abdominal wall.

b. Formal work on respiration requires good patient posture. Have the patient stand against a wall, with the buttocks and shoulders making some wall contact. Have the patient "stand tall," with the chin slightly tucked in as if the top of the head were suspended by a rope attached to the ceiling.

c. Have patients place one hand on the central abdomen and one hand laterally low on the rib cage (ninth through twelfth ribs). Instruct them to feel the abdomen and rib cage getting larger on inhalation. On exhalation, feel the abdomen tightening and the rib cage getting smaller. This exercise should be repeated as often as required to give the patient the awareness that on inhalation the chest gets bigger and on exhalation it gets smaller.

d. The patient is encouraged to feel the abdomen tightening on expiration. Some practice should be given to following inhalation (accomplished primarily through chest wall expansion) by gradual tightening (contraction) of the abdominal muscles. As soon as the patient demonstrates some ability to contract abdominal muscles on expiration, add phonation activities. The voice patient who has been speaking from the level of the throat, without adequate breath support, will "feel" the difference that a bigger breath makes when phonation is desired. The voice patient who needed respiration training in the first place must have respiration and phonation combined into practice activities as soon as possible.

e. Ask the patient to prolong vowel sounds coupled with continuant-type consonants with and without abdominal muscle support. Provide immediate auditory feedback, such as by using a loop recorder, so that the patient can contrast the voice differences produced with and without abdominal support.

f. Develop with the patient the concept of increasing one's air volume by increasing chest expansion. Explain that with greater air volume available for expiration–phonation, it will be possible to say or sing more words per breath without squeezing or strain at the end of a phrase or sentence. It has been demonstrated (Plassman and Lansing, 1990) that subjects with perceptual cues (such as feeling chest wall expansion) can soon develop strategies to reproduce desired and greater lung volumes.

8. For serious problems in respiration, which are often related to such illnesses as emphysema or bronchial asthma, the clinician should enlist the help of other specialists to help the patient improve efficiency. Physical therapists, respiratory therapists, and pulmonary medical specialists may have the expertise required to assist the patient. The voice clinician can often offer the patient ways of phrasing and using expiratory control to better match what the patient is trying to say and thus can supplement the respiration therapy of these other specialists. For example, we have coordinated a breathing-for-speech program for quadriplegic patients, in which the speech pathologist and the physical therapist work closely with the patient to improve both general respiration and expiratory control for speech phrasing and better voice.

C. Typical Case History Showing Utilization of the Approach.   Libby was a forty-five-year-old special-education teacher who complained of vocal fatigue as a regular part of her teaching day. She felt that when she was not working, her voice was not a problem. Observation of Libby during her voice evaluation revealed that conversationally she often began to speak without an adequate inspiration. After five or six consecutive spoken words, her voice would become dysphonic and strained. Her voice problems seemed to occur when her air volumes were low and she was experiencing inadequate transglottal airflow. Subsequent voice therapy, designed to reduce the amount of work she was putting into vocalization, gave some priority to increasing her inspiratory volumes, reducing the number of words she attempted to speak on one breath, and teaching her to take "catch-up" breaths when she needed them. Loop recordings were used in therapy to monitor her breath support; she would read a ten-word sentence aloud and then immediately listen to a loop playback of the utterance, judging it for respiratory adequacy and lack of strain. After five weeks of twice-weekly voice therapy working on better respiratory control, Libby developed an easy phonatory style and a voice that served her well in her various life situations, including her teaching.

D. Evaluation of the Approach.   A number of voice patients may profit from some kind of respiration training. At the time of the initial voice evaluation, such patients may have done poorly on air-volume and pressure tests or exhibited poor expiratory control. Vocal attempts by such patients are often strained and involve too much effort; symptoms of vocal hyperfunction are common. A slight increase of inspiratory volume may produce an immediate effect of reducing vocal strain and improving overall vocal quality.

Track 3

22. Tongue Protrusion /i/

A. Kinds of Problems for Which the Approach Is Useful.   Many hyperfunctional voice problems are improved by the tongue-protrusion approach. This approach is especially helpful for patients with ventricular phonation (dysphonia plicae ventricularis) or "tightness" in the voice, such as when the laryngeal aditus (laryngeal collar) is held in a somewhat closed position. When the tongue is held in a posterior position or the pharyngeal constrictor muscles are contracted to constrict the pharynx, the voice will sound strained or "tight." A patient with such symptoms is asked to produce /i/ with the tongue extended outside of the mouth (but not far enough to cause discomfort). This works to offset the squeezing of the pharynx. The tongue must not protrude so far outside of the mouth that it causes muscle strain in the area under the chin. The /i/ is produced in a high pitch either at the upper end of the patient's normal pitch range or at the lower end of the falsetto register. This approach can be used simultaneously with the glottal fry or the yawn–sigh.

B. Procedural Aspects of the Approach

1. Demonstrate to the patient what is expected by opening the mouth and protruding the tongue while producing a high-pitched, sustained /i/. Stress that the jaw is to "drop open" comfortably and that the tongue is to be extended comfortably. Many patients are reluctant, at first, to stick out the tongue in the presence of a stranger, so demonstrate and reassure them that this is just what you want. You may touch the patient's chin with the index finger to encourage a little wider jaw opening and say, "Roll the tongue out a little farther."

2. Patient should go up and down in pitch while sustaining the /i/ vowel, with the mouth open and the tongue out. Listen for improved vocal quality. When this is achieved, ask the patient to sustain the tone (McFarlane, Nelson, and Watterson, 1998).

3. Have the patient chant /mimimimi/ at this level with the tongue still out of the mouth. Then instruct the patient to slowly "slip" the tongue back into the mouth while continuing to produce the /mimimimi/.

4. At this point, the pitch is usually still high. Demonstrate a sustained /i/ that is lowered by three steps from the pitch that the patient was producing. This often produces a good quality on the first step or the first two steps, but a return to the poor voice may occur on the third step. Repeat the procedure, but only go down two steps. Sustain the second step. Repeat until the tone is established. You may need to return to the original open mouth and tongue protrusion if the target tone is lost.

5. When the new tone is established, gradually add words to the sustained /i/ —e.g., *be, pea, me, see the peach,* and *easy does it.*

C. Typical Case History Showing Utilization of the Approach. Tammy, a fifteen-year-old girl, was referred with ventricular phonation of more than eighteen months' duration. Her voice, which was consistently hoarse, rough, and low in pitch, was effortful to produce and made her sound like an older male speaker. Tammy had undergone a prolonged bout of flu prior to the onset of the ventricular voice, and she frequently coughed and cleared her throat violently. Strong glottal valving could be heard at times during connected speech. After seven sessions of individual voice therapy using the tongue-protrusion approach just described, Tammy's voice was normal in all situations at home, in school, and at work for the first time in more than eighteen months.

D. Evaluation of the Approach. This approach appears to work because the tongue, when protruded, pulls its root out of the pharynx and opens the laryngeal aditus. Also, the high pitch is made with a light, breathy approximation of only the true vocal cords. The production of voice with the tongue outside of the mouth is sufficiently novel so as not to trigger the typical pattern of phonation that may have become habituated.

23. Visual Feedback

A. Kinds of Problems for Which the Approach Is Useful. With the advent of computer-assisted instrumentation, there is great reliance on the monitor screen as a feedback device. For example, the patient can have a target F_0 line fixed on the screen, and the therapy task is to attempt to match the line with his or her same F_0 production. If the lines converge, this is visual reinforcement of a "correct" production. When we presented using various forms of auditory feedback as a facilitating approach, we recognized that the auditory system may well depend on auditory feedback as a primary mode for modifying speech–language–voice behaviors. However, most voice patients also profit from receiving visual feedback relative to respiratory physiology, acoustic parameters of voice, and various digital feedback values (air volumes–pressure–flow or F_o or percentage of nasal resonance, and so forth). For example, patients working on nasalence problems will often profit from using the Nasometer (Kay, 1994), which provides real-time visual feedback relative to the acoustic balance between oral and nasal resonance; the data generated by the Nasometer can provide visual feedback specific to the success of increasing or decreasing one's nasal resonance. Visual feedback can provide the patient with data specific to his or her voice measurements, as compared with the data found on the same vocal behaviors in the normal population. Visual feedback is valuable in voice therapy with any kind of patient who is working to improve or optimize vocalization.

Any of the evaluation instruments we use in our diagnostic voice evaluations that have visual dials, screens, or write-outs can be used for visual feedback. We compare visually the patient's performance under different conditions, such as visual magnetometer tracings on a screen that depict relative abdominal–chest wall movements under voice intensity conditions (i.e., such as the soft voice versus the loud voice). Making photocopies of visual data provides good feedback for the patient or for the parents of a child with a voice problem who may see the child's voice progress as depicted in visual write-outs (pitch changes, perturbation changes, etc.). Providing visual feedback for the patient can play a prominent role in voice therapy.

B. Procedural Aspects of the Approach

1. Visual feedback instruments should be introduced to the patient. In respiration, any of the measuring devices for air volume and pressure–flow described in Chapter 5 may be useful, particularly in comparing early performance with performance after therapy. Real-time measurements of respiration, such as how long one can prolong /s/, can be useful. Magnetometer tracings can be studied as the patient is performing, providing real-time feedback relative to abdominal–chest wall movements. Flexible videoendoscopy can provide the patient with visual confirmation of adequacy of velopharyngeal closure, pharyngeal and supraglottal participation during voicing, and/or detailed visualization of vocal fold movements. Stopping and restarting video playback provides visual feedback of actual oropharyngeal physiology.

2. The term *feedback* implies ongoing monitoring of some kind, giving back performance information to the patient as he or she is performing. Biofeedback (monitoring galvanic skin response, blood pressure, stress, etc.) is generally fed back to the patient visually, providing changing numeric values or changes in the number or color of lights or line tracings. Some forms of biofeedback include tactual or proprioceptive monitoring, both of which have little relevance to voice feedback, as both the pharynx and larynx are not particularly endowed with tactual or proprioceptive receptors. Acoustic monitoring and monitoring laryngeal physiology, when converted to visual images, can provide useful feedback, particularly when used jointly with another facilitating approach. For example, look at Visi-Pitch tracings and perturbation numeric values when visually tracking voice production under deliberate changes in loudness (facilitating approach 2). Ask patients to match the visual feedback they may be seeing with the loop auditory feedback of what they have just said.

3. Many computer-assisted clinical software programs have vital visual feedback available for patients of all ages. For example, the *Dr. Speech* (Tiger Electronics, 1997) software programs have real-time portrayals (digital, line tracings, cartoons) for such voice parameters as pitch or loudness. Among many other computer-assisted programs is the visual feedback available in the *Computerized Speech Lab* (CSL) (Kay, 1997) software programs that permit looking at twenty-two parameters of a single vocalization, then comparing the data with built-in threshold results.

4. The speech–language pathologist will find an endless number of software programs that can provide visual feedback on some aspect of voice performance. Attempt, however, to use only those programs that provide some ongoing auditory feedback coupled with the visual feedback.

C. Typical Case History Showing Utilization of the Approach. Bill was a twenty-one-year-old college student with vocal nodules and a severe dysphonia. At the time of his voice evaluation, it was found that he spoke at the very bottom of his pitch range. When he elevated pitch two or three notes, his voice became remarkably clearer. Using the Visi-Pitch we were able to set pitch boundaries within which we wanted him to practice. If he dropped his voice too low, he could see his tracing go below our target lines. Jitter and shimmer values dropped considerably near B2 on a piano keyboard, which we used as a target pitch. Bill profited from his clinical practice on the Visi-Pitch, which provided him with immediate visual feedback relative to both his pitch usage and the perturbation values that shifted with the pitch of his voice. Auditory feedback, particularly loop playback, was also effective for Bill in practicing an easy glottal attack with a slightly higher voice pitch. At the end of eight weeks of twice-weekly voice therapy, endoscopic examination found Bill to have "a normal larynx, free of vocal nodules."

D. Evaluation of the Approach. As instrumentation is developed that can portray various aspects (respiration–phonation–resonance) of voice, it can play an important role in providing visual feedback to patients. Once a target behavior has been isolated for a patient, such instrumentation can provide ongoing feedback on the appropriateness of patient production. Feedback presents various visual portrayals (values of frequency, jitter, shimmer, and so forth) of what the patient is hearing. Various facilitating efforts in therapy often produce changes in the sound of voice that are confirmed by different feedback devices. Once an optimal voicing pattern has been established, the use of feedback devices is no longer necessary.

24. Warble

A. Kinds of Problems for Which the Approach Is Useful. When patients have habituated a dysphonia over a long period of time, it is sometimes difficult to break up or interrupt the habitual (almost automatic) mode of phonation producing the hoarse, rough, or breathy voice. In an attempt to break the strongly established pattern, we have used the warble tone phonation. If one has a "muscle set" strongly associated with the onset of phonation, this can be offset by changing the phonatory adjustments of the larynx. This is what happens in the warble approach. Patients constantly change pitch and loudness (to a lesser degree) until they are instructed to extend the tone at a particular level of pitch and loudness. With warble, the pitch is constantly shifted up and down until the phonatory or prephonatory set is disrupted and new vocal tone can be produced free from excessive laryngeal muscle tension and free of the undesirable vocal quality. An instrument that displays the pitch for the patient as well as displays the vocal roughness can greatly aid the patient in his or her use of this technique. The instrument's trace of the frequency and jitter (pitch perturbation) will display the warble tone visually. The "scatter" (produced by jitter in the voice) or departure of the trace from a tight single line trace can easily be seen by the patient as a target for pitch and quality. The Visi-Pitch display works well to display the success of this technique for the patient. Any patient who has a hoarse, rough, strained, or breathy voice may be a candidate for this approach regardless whether the voice is secondary to functional adjustments or related to nodules or other cord pathology such as cord thickening and polyps.

B. Procedural Aspects of the Approach

1. Ask the patient to listen to the clinician produce a tone that is varied up and down in pitch. At the same time, the loudness will usually vary, increasing as pitch is raised and decreasing in loudness with pitch lowering. The patient is instructed to watch the trace on the scope and imitate the clinician.

2. Use some kind of computer screen or oscillographic display screen that will portray the up-and-down continuous tracings of the warble. The patient produces the tone with an /i/ vowel for a comfortable duration at a mid-loudness level, constantly shifting the tone up and down. The clinician watches the trace on the screen and listens to the tone. When the tone sounds best, the trace will be less scattered or more of a solid line. When the best sound tone and most compact trace are achieved, the tone is extended at that level. It is important that the tone not be interrupted or broken but extended at a desired pitch and loudness level.

3. When the patient has successfully produced a warble tone two or three times and has seen these on the screen display, the next task is to make the warble portion shorter and the steady-state vowel portion longer in duration. For example, if the warble is two seconds, extend the steady-state portion for five or six seconds. This is repeated several times.

4. Next the extended portion is produced without the warble. At this point, usually, the inappropriate muscle set is interrupted. If the patient loses the new mode of phonation initiation, the clinician returns to step 1 above. The new phonatory set or mode of phonation is then transferred into vowel-initiated words and all voiced short phrases such as *even now, easy days,* and so on.

C. Typical Case History Showing Utilization of the Approach.   Margaret, a thirty-nine-year-old female with a four-year history of a rough, very hoarse voice (perturbation, jitter level of 2.0) was referred by an ENT physician following recurring bouts of throat infection. There were no instances of clearer voice at any time in her speech. Both the ENT exam and the videostroboscopy demonstrated normal laryngeal structure; however, the stroboscopy study revealed a very lax adjustment of the cords. The mucosal wave was extremely exaggerated. Other facilitating techniques failed to produce an improvement in the voice. Using the warble technique

at a very high pitch broke up her phonatory set, which had persisted for four years. The improved quality of voice production was first extended at 400 Hz and in the same session worked down to 220 Hz. This voice was transferred to the phrase level at 220 Hz with a perturbation level of .4 (which is within the normal range) in the same initial treatment session. In subsequent therapy sessions, the voice was stabilized in conversation and appeared normal in every measure.

D. Evaluation of the Approach.   The effect of this approach appears to be that the warble fluctuations of pitch and loudness are sufficiently novel to interrupt the inappropriate laryngeal muscle set adopted by the dysphonic patient and used subsequently whenever the patient phonates. It also allows the clinician to use a glide of pitch and loudness adjustments, sliding into a new, more appropriate mode of phonation without the patient being aware of the "slide" into normal or near-normal voice.

25. Yawn–Sigh

Track 10

A. Kinds of Problems for Which the Approach Is Useful.   The yawn–sigh is one of the most effective therapy techniques for minimizing the tension effects of vocal hyperfunction. Characteristically, in vocal hyperfunction, we see the larynx rise, the tongue lifted high and forward, the vocal folds tightly compressed, and the pharynx constricted (Boone and McFarlane, 1993). The yawn–sigh provides a dramatic contrast: The larynx drops to a low position, the tongue is more forward, there is a slight opening between the vocal folds, and the pharynx is usually dilated, as seen in Figure 6.5. The yawn–sigh is frequently combined with other therapy approaches for such problems as functional dysphonia, spasmodic dysphonia, and dysphonias related to thickening, vocal fold nodules, and polyps. When it appears that the patient might profit from a lower, more relaxed carriage of the larynx, that patient is a candidate to receive either laryngeal massage (following Aronson's (1990) steps for "maneuvering the patient's laryngeal and hyoid anatomy," p. 34) as outlined in facilitating approach 15 or attempt to use the yawn–sigh approach. It has been these authors' experience (Boone and McFarlane, 1993) that if the patient can readily do the yawn–sigh, we do not have a need to use the Aronson maneuvering approach.

B. Procedural Aspects of the Approach

1. With children, explain this approach using the pictures and narrative from *The Voice Program for Children* (Boone, 1993). Showing a child the appropriate pictures, we read:

> This girl usually has a tight mouth. She uses too much effort when she speaks. Her voice does not sound good. (Demonstrate) This girl is opening her mouth wide and yawning. She is very relaxed. When she sighs at the end of the yawn, it will be her best voice (p. 141).

2. With teenagers and adults, explain generally the physiology of a yawn—that is, that a yawn represents a prolonged inspiration with maximum widening of the supraglottal airways (characterized by a wide, stretching, opening of the mouth). You may show the photograph in Figure 6.5 and contrast it with other CT scans of the pharynx taken while subjects were doing other vocal tasks, as displayed by Pershall and Boone (1986). Then demonstrate a yawn and talk about what the yawn feels like.

3. After the patient yawns, following your example, ask the patient to yawn again and then to exhale gently with a light phonation. In doing this, many patients are able to feel an easy phonation, often for the first time.

4. Once the yawn–phonation is easily achieved, instruct the patient to say words beginning with /h/ or with open-mouthed vowels, one word per yawn in the beginning, eventually four or five words on one exhalation.

5. With teenage and adult clients, there are yawn–sigh exercises available, with explanations that the patient can read, in *Is Your Voice Telling on You?* (Boone, 1997, pp. 121–126).

6. Demonstrate for the patient the sigh phase of the exercise—that is, the prolonged, easy, open-mouthed exhalation after the yawn. Then, omitting the yawn entirely, demonstrate a quick, normal, open-mouthed inhalation followed by the prolonged open-mouthed sigh.

7. As soon as the patient can produce a relaxed sigh, have him or her say the word *hah* after beginning the sigh. Follow this with a series of words beginning

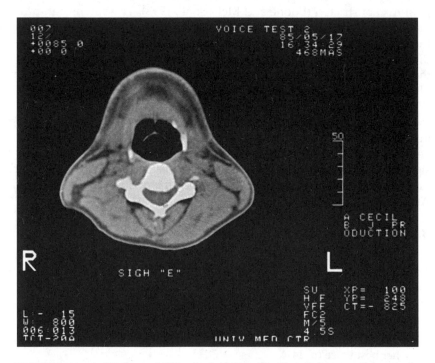

FIGURE 6.5   A CT Scan *A CT scan depicting the dilated pharynx of a normal subject producing a prolonged /i/ vowel on an expiratory sigh. This CT scan was taken near the apex of the arytenocids, showing the horizontal cross-section of the neck and mandible. Vertebral bone is shown in white; the open airway (with a slice of epiglottis across it) is represented in black (absence of tissue).*

with the glottal /h/. Additional words for practice after the sigh should begin with middle and low vowels. Take care to blend in, toward the middle of the sigh, an easy, relaxed, relatively soft phonation. This blending of the phonation into the sigh is often difficult for the patient initially, but it is the most vital part of the approach for the elimination of hard glottal contacts.

8. Once the yawn–sigh approach is well developed, have the patient think of the relaxed oral feeling it provides. Eventually, he or she will be able to maintain a relaxed phonation simply by imagining the approach.

C. Typical Case History Showing Utilization of the Approach.   Jerry, a forty-seven-year-old manufacturer's representative, had a two-year history of vocal fatigue. He often lost his voice toward the end of the workday. After a two-week period of increasing dysphonia and slight pain on the left side of the neck, a consulting laryngologist found that Jerry had "slight redness and edema on both vocal processes." The subsequent voice evaluation also found that he spoke with pronounced hard glottal attack in an attempt to "force out his voice over his dysphonia." Using the yawn–sigh approach, Jerry was able to demonstrate a clear phonation with relatively good resonance. His yawn–sigh phonations were recorded on loop and fed back to him as the voice model he should imitate. Because Jerry reported some stress in certain work situations, the hierarchy analysis approach was used to isolate those situations in which he felt relaxed and those in which he experienced tension. Thereafter, whenever he was aware of tense situational cues, he employed the yawn–sigh method to maintain relaxed phonation. Combining yawn–sigh with hierarchy analysis proved to be an excellent symptomatic approach for this patient because his voice cleared markedly, and no recurrence of the periodic aphonia was evident. Twice-weekly therapy was terminated after twelve weeks, and the patient demonstrated a normal voice and a normal laryngeal mechanism.

D. Evaluation of the Approach.   The yawn–sigh is a powerful voice therapy technique for patients with vocal hyperfunction. During the yawn–sigh, the pharynx is dilated and relaxed. When the patient is asked to sigh an /i/ or an /a/, the voice comes out with little effort and sounds relaxed. For some patients with continued vocal hyperfunction, the voice produced on the sigh will feel relaxed, in dramatic contrast to the patient's normally tense voice.

Summary

Twenty-five facilitating approaches for use in voice therapy have been presented. Four approaches in the last edition of this book have been replaced with four new ones. Our selection is based on which approaches we use the most often. These therapy approaches are only a few among those that the typical clinician may use with voice patients. Voice therapy for most voice problems requires continuous assessment of what the patient is able to do vocally. The selection of which approach to use is highly individualized for the particular patient, and there is no one approach that is helpful for the same voice problem with every patient. Management and therapy for patients with special problems are presented in the next chapter, Chapter 7.

7 Management and Therapy for Special Problems

In previous chapters (3, 4, 5, and 6) we have looked at various voice disorders resulting from a number of causal factors (structural diseases and problems, neurogenic factors, and vocal hyperfunction). In this chapter, we will look at various management strategies and voice therapy approaches to be used with special problems, many of which have been mentioned in previous discussions of disorders, and we will develop management–therapy steps for each problem in more detail. The problem of laryngeal cancer and its management–therapy will be covered in Chapter 8, and voice resonance and its management–therapy will be presented in Chapter 9.

We have organized management–voice therapy for special problems into four major headings (with problems listed alphabetically under each heading) in Table 7.1. The presentation of the order of headings is random.

Management–Voice Therapy for Particular Populations

We will look separately at management–voice therapy for voice patients from various population groups, as listed in Table 7.1.

Voice in Older People (Aging)

It is difficult to present any kind of meaningful summary about the aging voice for several reasons: (1) there is a vast difference between the voices of younger aged persons (sixty-five to eighty years) and older aged persons (over eighty years); (2) the voices of "fit aged" do not differ significantly from those of younger subjects; and (3) voice changes in the aged are more likely to be influenced by disease rather than by physiologic aging (Woo, Casper, Colton, and Brewer, 1992). Those authors question the diagnosis of "presbylaryngis," the old larynx, stating that "presbylaryngis is not a common disorder and should be a diagnosis of exclusion made only after careful medical and speech evaluation" (p. 139).

The elderly are indeed a heterogeneous group and represent the fastest growing segment of the U.S. population, with the over-eighty-five group showing the largest percentage increase of any population segment (Barry and Eathorne, 1994). In studying 151 voice patients over sixty-five, Woo and his colleagues (1992) found that the voice problems of 64 patients had a neurogenic base, 24 had benign

TABLE 7.1   **Management–Voice Therapy for Special Voice Problems**

For Particular Populations	For Respiratory-Based Voice Problems
Older People (Aging)	Asthma
People with AIDS	Emphysema
Children & Adults with Hearing Loss	Faulty Breath Control
Professional Voice Users	Airway Obstructions
Transsexuals	

For Faulty Voice Usage	For Vocal Fold Lesions
Abductor Spasms (Phonation Breaks)	Cysts
Diplophonia	Granuloma
Functional Aphonia	Nodules–Polyps
Functional Dysphonia	Papilloma
Pitch Breaks	Reflux
Puberphonia	Sulcus Vocalis
Ventricular Phonation	

laryngeal lesions, 22 had glottic or supraglottic cancer, 12 had inflammatory problems, and only 11 were classified as functional problems or related to advanced age. Considering these data, one might well conclude that management and therapy should be more focused on various disease processes rather than on aging per se.

It does appear, however, that there are some generalized characteristics of the voices of aged people that lead to their identification as older subjects. Many studies have demonstrated a significant relationship to listener judgment and the aged subject's actual age. We can guess people's ages by the way they sound (Linville, 1987; Shipp, Qi, Huntley, and Hollien, 1992). Several factors have been identified that seem to lend themselves to age identification. The fundamental frequency (Fo) seems to lower with each successive decade of life through age fifty. The female voice continues to lower in Fo throughout the life span; the male Fo begins to rise slightly in the sixties and in each decade after that. There is greater Fo variability among both aged female and male speakers. Elevated perturbation measures (jitter and shimmer) have been found in some studies. A slower speaking rate related to renewing breath more often (probably related to a 40 to 50 percent decrease in vital capacity by age seventy) is another speaking characteristic of the aged person. There have been mixed reports (Hoit and Hixon, 1992; Morris and Brown, 1994) about the voice loudness levels of older people compared with those of younger people; it would appear that voice loudness is not a significant variable in the perception of age in conversational speech.

It would appear that voice is *not* among the distinguishing factors displayed between younger and older people. Rather, the increased voice changes we hear in the older population are related more to disease factors than to a deteriorating vocal physiology. Our management and voice therapy choices are, therefore, more related to minimizing vocal symptoms as part of disease. It would appear from an overall voice management point of view that efforts to improve the overall physical fitness of the aged patient will often have a positive influence on voice. Counseling the patient specific to good vocal hygiene is helpful. Direct work on improving respiratory efficiency can help the older person develop better expiratory control, perhaps saying more words per breath. Direct work on increasing the speed of one's speech can have a "rejuvenating" effect on the sound of the older patient's voice. Among other facilitating approaches found useful in improving the voice of a motivated older person are auditory feedback, focus, glottal fry, masking, respiration training, and visual feedback.

Voice in People with AIDS

The speech–language pathologist in a medical setting, community clinic, or in private practice will occasionally encounter a patient with a voice problem related to HIV (human immunodeficiency virus) leading to infectious AIDS (acquired immunodeficiency syndrome). While in the early stages of AIDS the patient may be symptom-free, in the later stages of the disease, communication may be affected by problems of articulation, voice, language, hearing, and cognition. Looking at management and therapy for voice disorders, we will limit our discussion to problems of voice.

The most common voice problem experienced by an AIDS patient is loss of voice loudness. This soft-intensity voice is often accompanied by a slight dysphonia. This lack of vocal competence can be caused by one or many of these AIDS-related problems: general systemic fatigue and oral, pharyngeal, and/or laryngeal lesions, such as Kaposi's sarcoma, or fungal infection and herpetic infection (Flower, 1991; Kingdom and Lee, 1996). The patient's lack of successful immune response to a host of infectious agents receives the focus of the physician. A sympathetic voice clinician can help the patient with his or her voice weakness by working on improving functional respiratory support of voice, such as by cutting down the number of words said on one breath. The dysphonia, often observed to be slight hoarseness, may be helped by changing voice focus more forward in the facial mask (Boone, 1997) accompanied by a slight elevation of voice pitch. The patient may be most helped by the clinician providing a voice amplifier–speaker, often available through vendors of assistive devices, with specific instruction to the patient on how to use the instrument.

The speech–language pathologist working with the AIDS patient should realize that the risk of infection when working closely with AIDS patients is extremely low. Flower and Sooy (1987) make a strong case that because "HIV is a fragile virus," rudimentary measures of cleanliness and sterilization can give full protection to the clinician and other people in contact with the patient. They cite a study by Gerberding (1988) in which 240 professionals with frequent and intense contact with AIDS patients were studied; the study concluded: "Of the 240 individuals studied, more than one third have sustained needlesticks or other accidents involving contaminated fluids. Researchers found no antibodies to the AIDS virus in any workers who were not coincidentally also members of one of the high-risk groups" (Flower and Sooy, 1987, p. 29).

Care should be taken by the clinician to wear gloves and to take other universal precautions when fitting the AIDS patient with an assistive device like a voice amplifier or hearing aid. Obviously, oral and endoscopic examinations should be preceded by extensive hand-washing, wearing gloves, and washing hands thoroughly after the procedure; the clinician may wish to wear a face mask during the procedure. Equipment, such as a returned voice amplifier or the endoscope, should be sterilized after use. Flower (1991) recommends that "all devices should be wiped with a 1:10 dilution of household bleach" after usage. Personnel with an upper respiratory infection working with the patient should minimize the possibility of infecting the patient by wearing a face mask.

An adequate voice for the AIDS patient is part of overall functional communication for these patients. As we continue to have more success in managing HIV infections with less severity of symptoms with a longer life span, the rehabilitative role of the speech–language pathologist with the AIDS patients will take on more long-range importance.

Voice in Children and Adults with Hearing Loss

If hearing loss is severe enough in both children and adults, it will affect voice as well as have obvious effects on speech (prosodic and phonologic changes). Severe hearing loss will impact on language acquisition and usage in young children. Congenital hearing loss takes the greatest toll on voice. Having never heard spoken language like their normal hearing peers, severely hard-of-hearing children (often classified as deaf) will show severe voice–speech symptoms characterized by elevated F_o's (Boone, 1966A; Gilbert and Campbell, 1980); greater than normal pitch variability (Monsen, Engebretson, and Vernula, 1979; Subtelny, Whitehead, and Klueck, 1989); cul-de-sac resonance (Boone, 1993; Monsen, 1976); and nasality variations (hyper- or denasal). In addition to these voice abnormalities, the severely hard-of-hearing person will often speak at a slower rate of speech and show some variation in the melodic prosody of spoken language. The earlier the hearing loss in acquired deafness, the greater the severity of the above symptoms. Similarly, the longer the child or adult has had normal hearing, the less impact severe acquired hearing loss will have on voice pitch and voice quality.

There is a growing number of children and adults who, after a life time of severe hearing loss, have their hearing partially or wholly restored by successful cochlear implants (Iskowitz, 1998). However, the faulty voice–speech behaviors do not disappear immediately after cochlear implant, but the individual can make accelerated progress using the "new" hearing function to change faulty patterns of voice. Similarly, the severely hard-of-hearing child or adult who is well-fitted with a hearing aid does not experience a sudden improvement in voice, but now has the tool (the hearing aid) for developing more adequate voicing patterns with special clinical help. Conversely, children and adults who suddenly acquire a hearing loss greater than 70 dB in the speech range (500, 1K, 2K Hz), after normal language–speech–voice have been established, may gradually show some deterioration of voice and articulation.

Both elevated pitch and excessive pitch variability are two voice abnormalities that can be modified by direct voice therapy. The higher voice pitches found in the speaking voices of both prepubertal and postpubertal hard of hearing children (Gilbert and Campbell, 1980) suggest that not hearing the voices of others in their environment leads to using higher voice pitches than their age peers. The anatomical and physiologic characteristics of the larynx and vocal folds are the same in both hearing and hard-of-hearing children. Accordingly, the hard-of-hearing child will profit from developing an awareness of other voices, as well as developing ongoing awareness of his or her own voice pitch level, by using amplification and instrumental visual tracings of pitch. Lacking an adequate auditory model for his or her pitch target, the deaf child must rely on various visual feedback devices (Visi-Pitch or Phonatory Function Analyzer are examples) for providing visual evidence of both pitch and pitch variability. Oscillographic display panels or displays on a computer screen can isolate for the child the fundamental frequency he or she is using. Most clinical publishing catalogs contain the descriptions of many computer-assisted voice programs that can give immediate visual feedback specific to pitch and pitch variability. Such computer programs can also provide immediate, real-time feedback relative to excesses in voice loudness (too loud or not loud enough). The child's task in both pitch and loudness is to produce voice within some specified "desired" boundaries developed by the clinician.

Innovative clinicians have found several effective ways of making the child or adult aware of pitch level and possible pitch variability. One useful device for altering a deaf person's pitch level is to provide "cue arrows" pointing in the desired direction of pitch change. For example, for a typical deaf child attempting to lower the voice pitch, cards should be printed with an arrow pointing down. These cards should be placed wherever possible in the child's environment—in the wallet, on the bureau or desk, and so on. Also, the classroom teacher and voice clinician can give the child finger cues by pointing toward the floor. Another method for developing an altered pitch level is to have the child place his or her fingers lightly on the larynx and feel the downward excursion of the larynx during lower pitch productions and the upward excursion during higher ones. The ideal or optimum pitch is produced by minimal vertical movement of the larynx. Any noticeable upward excursion of the larynx, except during swallowing, will immediately signal that the child may be speaking at an inappropriately high pitch level. Once an appropriate pitch level has been established, the child may read aloud for a specified time period, placing the fingers lightly on the thyroid cartilage to monitor any unnecessary vertical laryngeal movement.

The typical voice of a deaf child who has had no training in developing a good voice is characterized by alterations in nasal resonance, often accompanied by excessive pharyngeal resonance, which produce a cul-de-sac voice. The major contributing factor to these resonance alterations is the excessive posterior posturing of the tongue in the hypopharynx, which markedly lowers the second formant (Boone, 1966A; Monsen, 1976). The tongue is drawn back into the hypopharynx and creates the peculiar resonance heard in deaf speakers; this back resonance sounds similar to the resonance sometimes heard in speakers with athetoid cerebral palsy, or oral verbal apraxia. The cul-de-sac voice has a back focus to it. In addition, the hearing-impaired child or adult may demonstrate marked variations in nasal resonance—too much nasal focus (hypernasality) or insufficient nasal resonance (denasality); such nasal resonance variations may be due in part to the posterior carriage of the tongue, as well as to the inability to monitor acoustically the nasalization characteristic of the normal speaker.

Altering the tongue position to a more forward carriage and tongue protrusion (see Chapter 5) can contribute greatly to establishing more normal oral resonance in the voice of a deaf speaker. In addition to the procedures outlined in Chapter 6 for altering tongue position, more detailed procedures and therapy materials for both children and adults are available in *The Boone Voice Program for Children* (1993) and *The Boone Voice Program for Adults* (1982). Once the tongue has been placed in a more "neutral setting" (Laver, 1980), the deaf patient needs to practice making vocal contrasts between back-pharyngeal resonance and normal oral resonance. The deaf patient needs to develop an awareness of what it feels like to use the lips, the tongue against the alveolar processes, the tongue on the hard palate, and other front-of-the-mouth postures. Such front focus seems to develop only after intensive practice doing tasks that encourage anterior tongue carriage.

The deaf speaker must also work to eliminate hypernasality, if it is present. The patient first needs to become aware of excessive nasal resonance by reviewing feedback from various instruments that measure airflow in acoustic output simultaneously from both the oral and nasal cavities. How much of the perceived voice is oral and how much is nasal can be determined by the Nasometer. The Nasometer is a microcomputer-based system that can make an acoustic analysis of the relative amount of nasalance in a voice signal. The patient produces voice that is directed into two microphones that are separated by a nasal-oral separator. The computer screen provides real-time feedback about the relative acoustic output between the two channels. The Nasometer provides the same kind of nasal resonance feedback in therapy as the Tonar II (Fletcher & Daly, 1976); both instruments provide valuable visual feedback about vocal resonance for the deaf speaker.

The Voice of Professional Voice Users

Track 6

The professional user of voice puts unusual demands on respiration–phonation–resonance. We use the term *professional voice* for the voice of the actor, singer, teacher, minister, salesperson, telemarketer, politician, broadcaster—those people whose primary occupational competence (and probable success) is dependent on their voices. Some professional users of voice seek the help of vocal coaches or singing teachers, while others develop vocal problems that may require the services of the otolaryngologist or speech–language pathologist. In the first edition of this book (Boone, 1971), the professional act of singing or speaking was well described:

> Speaking and singing demand a combination and interaction of the mechanisms of respiration, phonation, resonance, and speech articulation. The best speakers and singers are often those persons who, by natural gift or training, or by a studied blend of both, have mastered the art of optimally using these vocal mechanisms (p. 1).

One of the obstacles we experience in working with the professional voice user is the relative "performance innocence" of the teacher or clinician. The professional uses his or her voice often beyond the normal limits we generally associate with heavy voice use. The teacher or voice clinician who has never performed beyond these supposed limitations may experience difficulty convincing the performer about what to do to correct a voice problem. Similar to the voice clinician who wants to communicate with the voice scientist or the scientist who likes to dabble clinically, once we stray beyond our swath of training and competence, our "performance naivete" shows to the performance expert.

Another obstacle to working successfully with the professional voice user is the lack of meaningful language between the performer and the clinician. For example, the actor or singer may have been taught a way of breathing for performance that is at variance with new voice science findings specific to respiratory physiology (as presented in Facilitating Approach #21, in the last chapter). Imagery abounds with performers. Yet the clinician cannot take away this imagery without replacing it with descriptions that will enhance performance, as well as encourage using vocal mechanisms in a healthy manner. The skillful clinician can often use performers' imagery about what they are doing, not attack it directly, but modify it by demonstration of less muscle effort producing similar vocal output. Excesses in muscle tension while performing have been categorized by Koufman and others (1996), finding that much unnecessary muscle tension occurs supraglotally, particularly among "bluegrass/country and western and rock/gospel singers." When excessive muscle tensions appear in the clinician's judgment to cause laryngeal problems, voice therapy directed toward decreasing these excessive glottal and supraglottal muscle tensions can be effective. Excessive muscle tension can be reduced by using such clinical approaches as auditory feedback, change of loudness, chant talk, chewing, counseling, focus, changing glottal attack, laryngeal massage, open-mouth approach, relaxation, and yawn–sigh.

One of the best methods of improving voice for the teacher, salesperson, or preacher is using loop auditory feedback (Facilitator, 1998). One way of using loop feedback is for the clinician to provide a voice model that the client "matches" with a response. On the Facilitator, once the recording is stopped, the playback button is pushed and the client listens immediately on earphones to what was just said, and the clinician and client evaluate the response. Subsequent recordings can be made until client response meets some evaluative criteria. Having the client match an auditory model (his or hers or that of the clinician) enables the client to use the vocal mechanisms holistically, which avoids breaking down motor response into separate components (such fragmenting of response should be avoided when possible).

Perhaps among the subgroups of professional voice users, teachers experience the most vocal symptoms (Sapir, Keidar, and Mathers-Schmidt, 1993; Smith and others, 1997). There are heavy vocal demands on teachers; consequently, teachers may profit from a general vocal hygiene approach as well as having their individual vocal situations analyzed for possible vocal abuses and misuse. Specific voice therapy approaches might be taught to minimize excessive muscle tension and to encourage healthier vocal performance under difficult conditions (long, continuous voice usage, often against competing classroom noise). Because the teaching conditions cannot usually be changed, the teacher may well profit from some use of amplification in the classroom as well as from instruction on how to use the voice more efficiently.

One of the most comprehensive texts on management and possible voice therapy for the professional voice user is the text edited by Sataloff, *Professional Voice, The Science and Art of Clinical Care,* 2nd Edition (1997), including sixty-eight chapters written by physicians, voice scientists and voice clinicians, performers, and other voice professionals. Clinicians will find much information of great clinical relevance. For example, Chapter 19, "Endocrine Dysfunction," presents a meaningful summary of the hormonal influences on voice, giving special attention to thyroid influences and sex hormonal determinants of vocal function. There are many other chapters that offer hints and suggestions specific to voice management and therapy for the professional user of voice.

The Voice of Transsexuals

The voice clinician will encounter patients who are experiencing gender reassignment, more often male-to-female, but occasionally female-to-male. While the most obvious voice symptom in the transsexual patient is inappropriate pitch, there may be other voice problems related to voice inflection and voice quality. Inappropriate pitch, however, appears to be the most common initial voice symptom and primary concern of the patient. In the female-to-male transsexual person, a lower pitch can be achieved through hormonal therapy; testosterone has the effect of thickening the vocal folds (resulting in a lower voice pitch) among other virilizing changes, such as increasing facial and body hair and increasing definition of skeletal muscles. The male-to-female patient experiences feminizing effects from taking estrogen, such as experiencing breast enlargement and some softening of muscle definition; however, there are no feminizing effects on vocal folds with pitch level remaining at adult male levels. Although voice therapy aimed at directly elevating pitch can be effective for the speaking voice, the larger vocal folds still produce low-pitched phonation when coughing, laughing, crying, or producing any kind of emotional phonation. Some male-to-female transsexuals report severe reaction from listeners who were startled by the sudden presence of male phonation. It would appear that some forms of vocal fold surgery, such as longitudinal incision of vocal folds or some form of thyroplasty (Blaugrund, Isshiki, and Taira, 1992), can make possible higher-pitched voice in all situations. Even after surgical revision of the vocal folds, the male-to-female transsexual will profit from voice therapy.

Voice quality is more difficult to modify. The altered pitch level still must resonate in the oral pharynx. One of this book's authors (DB) remembers being sent a female patient (who DB did not know was a male-to-female transsexual). Her pitch level was appropriate for her new gender, but the quality of her voice sounded "different." She possessed a very large pharynx (the diameter of the pharynx is dictated by the distance between the two superior horns of the larynx, the insertion points of the lower pharyngeal constrictors) that gave her higher-pitched voice a "male quality." No matter what we did, she still sounded like a male using a higher pitched voice.

There are several vocal postures that can be taught successfully that are consistent with one's desired gender. Females tend to use greater pitch inflections than males do. For example, the normal female voice tends to have a rising pitch inflection toward the end of an utterance; the patient wanting to sound more feminine should work toward an upward inflection of pitch while the person wanting to sound more masculine would practice a dropping inflection (Boone, 1997). The female voice is also characterized by some breathiness with vowel prolongation. Beyond voice per se, Case (1996, p. 257) says that females communicate with greater articulation precision and use "more modal constructions (can, will, may, shall, *must*)." There are gender-biased somatic postures that can be imitated, such as body carriage, head position, style of gait, hand gestures, and facial expressions.

The speech–language pathologist must look at the transsexual patient from a counseling perspective and the need to offer strong psychological support, as well as employing the voice–speech–language evaluation and therapy skills that may be needed.

Management–Voice Therapy for Faulty Voice Usage

Abductor Spasms (Phonation Breaks)

In this particular section, we are talking about functional abductor spasms (not abductor spasmodic dysphonia as presented in Chapter 4), in which the vocal folds suddenly abduct, causing temporary phonation breaks. The patient may be speaking with normal voice when the vocal folds suddenly separate, producing a fleeting aphonia. Shipp, Mueller, and Zwitman (1980) used the term *intermittent abductory dysphonia* to label these annoying and continuing aphonic breaks.

A *phonation break* is a temporary loss of voice that may occur for only part of a word, a whole word, a phrase, or a sentence. The individual is phonating with no apparent difficulty when suddenly a complete cessation of voice occurs. Such a fleeting voice loss is usually situational and it usually happens after prolonged hyperfunction. Typical patients with this problem work too hard to talk, often speaking with great effort, and suddenly experience a complete voice break. Such patients usually struggle to "find" their voice by coughing, clearing their throat, or taking a drink of water. In most cases, phonation is restored and remains adequate until the next phonation break, which may occur in only a few moments or not for days. Other than continued vocal hyperfunction, no physical condition seems to cause these phonatory interruptions. They may result from a variety of physiological sources, ranging from reduced subglottal air pressure near the end of a phrase to the "loading" of the true vocal fold by the ventricular fold or mucus on the true fold. Many times these breaks result from excessive laryngeal muscle tension and inappropriate adjustments of the otherwise normal mechanism. The best management of the problem seems to come from reducing overall vocal hyperfunction. If hyperfunctional behaviors can be identified and reduced, the phonation breaks are usually minimized. For example, a local hard-rock disc jockey suffered from phonation breaks when he was attempting to give the news "straight" for 5 minutes on the hour. It was soon discovered that his broadcasting style away from the news was extremely "hyper" and false and thus produced obvious strain on his vocal mechanism. Voice therapy was directed toward producing a disc-jockey style that was less aversive. The happy result was that he was able to read the news copy free of phonation breaks. Such intermittent losses of voice during voicing are usually the result of prolonged vocal hyperfunction. Once the hyperfunction can be reduced, the phonation breaks usually disappear. Facilitating approaches described in Chapter 6 that have been found useful for eliminating abductory spasms might include counseling, ear training, elimination of hard glottal attack, the open-mouth approach, relaxation, developing greater respiratory efficiency, and the yawn–sigh.

Diplophonia

The diplophonic voice is usually produced by two distinct voicing sources, each phonating simultaneously with the other. Occasionally, diplophonia is produced by the true folds—if one of the folds has a different mass and tension from the other one. For example, in persistent paralytic dysphonia, the patient's voice may sound diplophonic as the paralyzed fold vibrates faster because of its thinner mass (as a result of lower motor neuron atrophy). Laryngeal webs sometimes phonate in the airstream, producing a high-pitched squeal that joins the vocal fold vibration (altered because of the shorter segments posteriorly beyond the edge of the web) and thus a double voice. The epiglottis may also produce a sound that, when added to the true fold vibration, produces a diplophonic voice.

The first step in treating a diplophonia is to identify the double-voice source. Video nasoendoscopy has been an excellent tool for examining the vocal tract, attempting to identify an extra phonation source. Occasionally, vigorous aryepiglottic muscle activity produces a tight pursing of the superior larynx, which may prevent the viewer from looking underneath. The aryepiglottic muscles can be the second sound source with the true folds vibrating underneath. The ventricular folds sometimes occlude from view the true folds underneath; in fact, the most common diplophonic voice sources identified are the ventricular folds, vibrating against the true folds. Any additive lesion to the vocal folds, particularly a unilateral lesion, can change the vibratory characteristics of the folds and produce a diplophonia.

The first consideration in the treatment of diplophonia is whether or not the second sound source can be reduced or eliminated. Surgical eradication of a unilateral additive lesion, for example, might bring the two vocal folds into size compatibility so that their vibratory characteristics are basically the same, eliminating the double voice. Symptomatic voice therapy can often be effective in reducing diplophonia. For example, inhalation phonation (see Chapter 6) is produced by true fold vibration. The voice on inhalation is usually a high-pitched, single voice. Once the single voice is established on expiration, the clinician can usually expand the single phonation into other voicing tasks. The yawn–sigh approach (see Chapter 6) is an excellent way to develop an open, supraglottal airway. As the patient produces a phonated sigh, the supraglottal larynx and pharynx are maximally dilated, which might well eliminate any supraglottal structure, such as the aryepiglottic folds, from vibrating and producing the double voice. Other facilitating approaches from Chapter 6 that might be helpful in searching for a clear, single voice include auditory feedback (in particular loop feedback), focus, glottal fry, and masking.

Track
6 & 13

Functional Aphonia

As in previous editions of this text, the authors take a much more aggressive, frontal approach to the treatment of functional aphonia than do some other textbook authors (Aronson, 1990; Case, 1996; Colton and Casper, 1996). We recommend treating functional aphonia with direct symptomatic treatment coupled with psychological counseling and support. The previously cited authors tend to give more priority to psychological support and therapy, sometimes followed by symptomatic voice therapy.

The diagnosis of *functional aphonia* is made when, on endoscopic examination, the patient is asked to phonate a vowel, such as /i/ or asked to say a word, and the vocal folds are found to be in the paramedian position or even extended further apart. When asked to whistle, if the patient can whistle, the vocal folds make the postural adjustments of near-approximation for the whistle and abducting for breath renewal. The lack of voice is related to lack of adequate vocal fold approximation for no organic reason or lack of neural innervation (see Chapter 3). Sometimes, on flexible endoscopic examination of the patient with functional aphonia, we see severe pursing of the supraglottis, with no view possible of the vocal folds underneath. In functional aphonia, innervation is normal and both vocal folds move quickly to and away from the midline for the whistle, for coughing, for crying, but not for communicative voice. We do not use the term *conversion aphonia* to label this lack of voice, as do Aronson (1990) and Case (1996), because in our experience most of these patients experience a total return of functional voice (with no migration of other symptoms) in one to three voice therapy sessions.

We recommend using the term *functional aphonia*, which implies that there is no physical cause for the voicelessness, and, more often than not, that the patient is ready to "release" the symptom and experience an immediate return of normal voice. In fact, functional aphonic patients as a group present excellent prognoses. As stated in Chapter 3, functional aphonic patients are easily conditioned to continue to speak without voice. Whatever the original cause, the behavior is maintained by the reactions of the people around the patient. Such patients soon develop a *no voice* set toward speaking, and they establish habitual responses; they speak this way today because they spoke this way yesterday. Most patients with functional aphonia express a strong desire to regain their normal voice. (A few patients are served well by their aphonia, and they resist all therapeutic attempts at voice restoration.) The bias of the writers, developed from following aphonic patients over time, is that symptomatic voice therapy is usually effective in restoring normal voices in these patients. Once phonation is reestablished, it remains, and the patient does not develop substitute symptoms to take the place of the previous aphonia.

Successful voice therapy for functional aphonia must begin with the clinician's explaining and discussing the problem with the patient. In the physiological description of the aphonia, the clinician must avoid implying that the patient could phonate normally if he or she wanted. Rather, a description of what the patient is doing ("keeping the vocal cords apart") will make it clear that the clinician knows what the problem is. Following the physiological description, the clinician should say something like, "We will do things in therapy that will bring the cords together again to produce normal voice." The clinician should not (at the first session, at least) ask or show undue interest in *why the* patient is not phonating. After the explanation and discussion of the problem, the clinician should evaluate whatever nonverbal phonations the patient may have in his or her coughing, grunting, laughing, and crying repertoire, and then describe them to the patient as normal phonatory activities "in which the vocal cords are getting together well to produce these sounds." These nonverbal phonations should then gradually be shaped into use for speech, at first confining any speech attempts to nonsense syllables, and then moving on to single words, but with no early attempts at phonating during real communication. Attempts at phonating in conversational situations (i.e., in the real world of talking) should be deferred until good, consistent phonation has been reestablished under laboratory, practice conditions.

Steps to be followed in a symptomatic voice therapy program for functional aphonia might include the following:

1. *Counseling.* Point out to the patient that even though the vocal folds are normal, the problem appears to be an inability to "get them started producing voice." Focus the explanation on the *vocal folds* and not on the *patient.* Perhaps show a brief videotape depicting normal phonation.

2. *Coughing.* Ask the patient to cough. By definition, patients with functional aphonia are able to use the laryngeal mechanism for coughing. Take care to ask the patient to cough, not to ask, "Are you able to cough?" Most aphonic patients can cough. If the patient coughs, then ask him or her to prolong the cough with an extended vowel. If this phonatory prolongation can be done, then ask the patient to make a series of cough-initiated phonations, using the vowel /i/. If the patient cannot immediately extend the phonation, go to step 3 after the cough.

3. *Inhalation phonation.* This facilitating approach (see Chapter 6) uses true vocal fold phonation. The high-pitched phonation is always produced by true folds. If a patient can match the high-pitched inhalation with the same sound on expiration, ask him or her to prolong the phonation, as in step 2. Once the expiratory high-pitched phonation is established, introduce monosyllabic words beginning with vowels and /h/ for voice practice.

4. *Masking.* This approach is designed to reestablish phonation in patients with functional aphonia. Ask the patient to read a passage aloud in his or her whispered aphonic voice while wearing headphones attached to some kind of noise generator (such as speech range masking on The Facilitator). As the patient reads, introduce loud masking at selected intervals. The patient will often reflexively use voice under the masking conditions. Then play back a recording of the patient's reading attempts, which can often reveal true phonation for the patient. (See procedural details of the masking approach in Chapter 6.)

5. *Pacing.* Patients with aphonia should not be pushed too fast. Once normal voice is achieved, often by following one or more of the preceding steps, practice should stay at a single-word (using word lists) level. Making such statements as "Your vocal folds are coming together now" is helpful because they put the "blame" on the folds rather than the patient (Boone, 1966b).

6. *Progression.* Once voice is established by using single words beginning with vowels or /h/, single-word lists using any consonants or vowels can be used. The therapy steps in Facilitating Approaches 10 and 17 will be helpful. Then progress to polysyllabic words, phrases, and sentences, but defer interactive conversation with the patient until voicing appears consistently.

If the voice clinician has any doubt about the patient's general emotional stability, as indicated perhaps by the patient's continued inability to produce some phonation, he or she should refer the patient for psychological or psychiatric consultation. Sometimes the aphonic patient profits most from symptomatic voice therapy concurrent with psychotherapy. If psychotherapy is needed, however, the typical case involves a fairly rapid recovery of voice with relatively brief voice therapy and a much longer period of psychotherapy.

Functional Dysphonia

In Chapter 1 of this text, we looked at three causal factors of voice disorders: organic, neurogenic, and functional. As we have seen throughout this book, these causal factors are highly overlapping. For example, an organic problem like laryngeal web will contribute to dysphonia in different patients in different ways; how the patient *functionally* uses the altered mechanism will play a primary role in how the patient's voice sounds. Similarly, two male patients with unilateral vocal fold paralyses in the paramedian position may have voices that are distinctively different from one another. By functional, we place our emphasis on the physiology of phonation, or *how the patient uses voice*.

We view functional dysphonia as a voice that is produced in a faulty manner. More often, the patient voices with much vocal abuse and misuse, usually with excessive muscle tension or *vocal hyperfunction* (excessive muscular effort). The problem may exist with no organic component, or, perhaps, over time the continued vocal hyperfunction has led to tissue change along the glottal margin, producing vocal fold thickening or vocal nodules. The use of the more descriptive *muscle tension dysphonia* (MTD) in *The Management of Voice Disorders* (Morrison and Rammage, 1994) seems to be a useful approach for considering vocal hyperfunction.

The patient is evaluated initially by endoscopy or stroboscopy and found to have no identifiable organic or neurogenic cause of the dysphonia. Reactive tissue changes, if present, such as nodules or a polyp, are noted. The physiology of the patient's phonation is observed, which may reveal faulty vocal fold approximation (lax or compressed), a compromised mucosal wave, excessive supraglottal activity, high laryngeal carriage, and other symptoms related to vocal hyperfunction as discussed in Chapter 3.

The first step in treating functional dysphonia related to vocal hyperfunction is to identify contributing vocal abuse and misuse. The clinician must give priority to such abuse–misuse identification and develop strategies to reduce its occurrence. For example, the nine-year-old boy with vocal nodules who controls his playground mates by yelling and making "funny noises" has to be taught how to reduce his aversive noise, perhaps in part by teaching him some other ways to produce "healthier" noise (Andrews, 1995; Boone, 1993). Once vocal abuses and misuse have been identified and reduced, direct symptom modification for functional dysphonia can begin.

We often begin our symptomatic therapy by working with the patient to appreciate how he or she sounds. The patients wear headphones and listen to their own voices with real-time amplification, developing an awareness of their voices. If the voice is dysphonic, we may introduce speech–range masking. For example, the patient is asked to read aloud (or count); about ten to fifteen words into the reading we introduce the masking, recording all of the oral reading on an audiocassette. In functional dysphonia, patients' voices are often better when they cannot auditorily monitor what they are voicing (Boone, 1998). If a better or "target" voice is recorded under masking, we use that recording as a therapy model. We can then use a loop-feedback recorder, letting the patient hear the model and see if he or she can "match" it; we record the model and the patient response, stop the recording, and listen immediately to the playback. The clinician helps the patient make the comparison and perhaps shape the next response attempt.

Often, in vocal hyperfunction, the patient demonstrates inadequate breath support, running out of air toward the end of an utterance, often "squeezing" out the last word or two. Respiration training, Facilitating Approach #21, can be helpful. Most of the twenty-five facilitating approaches presented in Chapter 6 are designed to be used in cases of excessive muscle tension or vocal hyperfunction. Whenever possible, in modifying the hyperfunctional voice, the authors recommend using a *gestalt* (holistic approach) with counseling or modeling or auditory imitation, rather than fractionating voice performance by working separately on breathing, open mouth, posture, head position, tongue position, and other components. We do the voice patient a disservice when we work separately on many components and then "try to assemble them together again."

Track 3

Pitch Breaks

As we discussed in Chapter 3, there are two kinds of pitch breaks. First, the upward pitch break experienced by some adolescent boys must be considered as a temporary developmental vocal inconvenience and not a voice problem per se. During the last months of puberty, some boys experience a one-octave pitch break (the voice breaks upward) as they are using conversational voice. There is no need for voice therapy, because this kind of pitch break is temporary. As the laryngeal mechanism reaches full development, the pitch breaks disappear as suddenly as they first appeared. An occasional boy (or his parents) may need brief counseling about the temporary nature of the problem. This counseling is about the only role required of the speech-language pathologist to deal with such adolescent pitch breaks.

The second kind of pitch break is related to continuous vocal hyperfunction, particularly prolonged speaking at an inappropriate pitch level (Boone, 1997). The voice breaks either one octave upward or one octave downward. Occasionally, patients experience two-octave breaks. The voice breaks in the direction (down or up) where it "would like to be." Although we have well established in previous chapters that there is no such thing as an absolute optimum voice pitch, speaking at the very bottom or top of one's range for extended periods of time may contribute to vocal strain. Pitch breaks are a symptom of that strain. The primary focus of voice therapy for pitch breaks is establishing a new pitch, raising or lowering the fundamental frequency one or two notes. Upward pitch breaks, the most common form of pitch break, is usually related to speaking at the very bottom of one's pitch range.

Elevating pitch one or two notes usually eliminates the problem. With the new pitch level, the patient might profit from developing a voice legato with chant talk, using a relaxed voice with chewing, practicing yawn–sigh, eliminating hard glottal attack, and attempting the open-mouth approach (see Chapter 6). A downward pitch break, observed more often in adult women, can usually be corrected by developing a lower voice pitch and using the other facilitating approaches recommended for lowering the pitch level. The final step in eliminating pitch breaks is developing an overall easy, open vocal style as the result of ear training, matching one's voice with target voice models previously tape recorded by the patient and the clinician.

Puberphonia

The high-pitched voice in a young man who has already completed puberty is known as *puberphonia.* The voice may be either at the end of the normal, chest register or in the falsetto register. It is thus sometimes called *mutational falsetto.* The fundamental frequency of the voice is often in excess of 260 Hz (or at middle C in the singing range). The social penalties for men who speak at such high-pitched levels are obvious; an individual who does so is often judged to be effeminate and perhaps inadequate. It is difficult to find the original physical or psychological factors that may have caused puberphonia. The large majority of young men with inappropriately high voices have excellent voice therapy prognosis; many achieve normal pitch levels and vocal quality after only brief exposure to voice therapy.

In previous editions of this book and in the writings of Aronson (1990) and Case (1996), the primary voice therapy for puberphonia begins with the speech–language pathologist asking the patient to cough. If the patient is past puberty, the cough will be the typical low-pitched, abrupt cough of the adult male. The clinician explains to the patient that the vocal folds are able to produce an adult male voice, and then demonstrates a cough, holding on to the phonation, indicating the desirability of the prolonged phonation. The patient is then asked to cough again.

If the cough is not successful in uncovering the young man's natural pitch, we have had good luck using masking. We recommend using speech–range masking rather than white or pink noise, as the masking effect can be achieved at much lower intensity levels. We ask the patient to begin oral reading, recording his reading; near the tenth word, we introduce masking. Using the Lombard effect with the introduction of masking noise, the voice will break into a louder, lower pitch. Recording the oral reading tasks provides a voice model for the patient to hear. At this point, a sensitive clinician supports the patient by saying something like, "It sounds like you have the option now of choosing one of two voices." The typical puberphonic patient is obviously "thrilled" with hearing his lower-pitched speaking voice.

Once the patient can produce a natural lower pitch, the use of a loop recorder is helpful, letting the patient hear the immediate playback of words or phrases he has just said using his new voice. If the lower, natural voice has not been established by using either the cough or masking, digital pressure against the thyroid cartilage is often helpful for demonstrating a lower pitch. The patient is asked to say and extend a vowel, such as /a/ or /i/; as he prolongs the vowel, the clinician applies light digital pressure against the thyroid cartilage, which shortens and thickens the vocal folds, producing a lower-pitched voice. The patient is then asked to see if he can maintain the same low pitch without the pressure. The glottal fry approach (see Chapter 6) has also been found useful for finding lower-pitched phonation in this group.

The typical puberphonic patient experiences a functional lower voice in the first evaluation–voice therapy session. The patients as a group are highly motivated to use their newly discovered voices and usually do not require follow-up counseling or psychological therapy. The speech–language pathologist, however, might schedule the young man for a follow-up visit to determine how he is doing, both from a vocal and emotional perspective.

Track 11

Ventricular Phonation

Ventricular phonation, sometimes called *dysphonia plicae ventricularis,* occurs in its pure form when a patient uses the ventricular or false folds for phonation. Such substitute phonation is characterized by a low-pitched voice related to the relative thickness of the ventricular folds as compared to the true folds. Because of this relatively large tissue mass, there is little chance for subtle changes in mass and thickness (certainly as compared to the normal vocal folds); the result is a monotonous pitch level with minimal frequency variation. A patient who, on laryngoscopy, appears to have a structurally normal larynx and yet speaks with an inappropriately low-pitched, monotonous voice might well be using ventricular phonation.

Nasoendoscopy of patients with harsh functional dysphonia often shows the ventricular folds coming together as part of a total laryngeal shutdown; the overall laryngeal aditus is closed by sphincteral closure of the aryepiglottic folds, which pull the cuneiform prominences seemingly together (Pershall & Boone, 1986). As this total laryngeal closure begins, first the true folds adduct and then the false folds come together. The aryepiglottic folds then cover over the open larynx, and neither true nor false folds are visible. Ventricular phonation may be part of such a strained phonation, although it is difficult to single out a particular closure site.

The clinical management of such total laryngeal closure is facilitated by using the yawn–sigh approach (described in Chapter 6). Under conditions of the sigh, using a prolonged /i/ vowel, supraglottal structures open up, revealing on endoscopy the approximation of the true folds. From the sigh-produced /i/, the clinician can extend the number of sounds and words that the patient can say with the open larynx. Glottal fry, inhalation phonation, and tongue protrusion /i/, described in Chapter 6, are also helpful techniques for eliminating ventricular phonation.

Management–Voice Therapy for Respiratory-Based Voice Problems

The voice problems of children and adults cannot always be solved by voice therapy. In particular, patients with severe respiratory problems may manifest voice problems among many other symptoms associated with a particular respiratory disease. The speech–language pathologist working with patients with breathing abnormalities needs to work closely with other specialists, such as the pulmonary medicine physician or the respiratory therapist. Let us consider separately some respiratory diseases and their overall management, including possible voice therapy.

Asthma

In asthma, the patient experiences a narrowing of airway tubes, particularly in the bronchi and bronchioles, which limits the free passage of air. Spasms of the airway can be caused by the external smooth muscles going into spasm, causing a narrowing of the opening (Berkow, Beers, and Fletcher, 1997). This causes the inner lining of mucosa tissue to become compressed and inflamed, resulting in some mucosal swelling and irritation, causing some production of mucus (which further obstructs the passageway). The patient struggles to take in a breath. The asthmatic spasms can be triggered by such stimuli as pollens, dust mites, animal dander, cold air, smoke, and exercise. The asthmatic symptoms may be chronic (they come and go) or part of a sudden and severe reaction that may require immediate medical intervention.

The speech–language pathologist does not usually encounter the patient during severe respiratory obstruction. Rather, most people with asthma are free of symptoms most of the time, experiencing occasional bouts of wheezing and shortness of breath. Depending on the frequency and severity of respiratory struggle, some patients experience some hoarseness and breakdown in normal voicing prosody. Such patients may seek the help of the voice clinician.

The speech–language pathologist must first differentiate true subglottal asthma from parodoxical vocal fold movement, as described by Blager (1995). (See our discussion of paradoxical vocal fold movement later in this chapter). In the asthmatic patient, the primary management step is treating the spasms and inflammation that interrupt the patient's natural breathing. Oral corticosteroids (Djukanovic et al., 1997) appear to be the most effective treatment for asthma symptoms and airway inflammation; these authors concluded that "a moderate dose of oral corticosteroids leads to a marked reduction in airway inflammation...resulting in reduced airway hyperresponsiveness" (p. 831). Another form of steroid application is the use of aerosolized albuterol (Strauss, Hejal, Galan, Dixon, and McFadden, 1997), which appears to reduce airway inflammation experienced by the asthmatic patient. Reduction of airway inflammation appears primary for increasing airway dilation, allowing a greater passage of air into and out of the lungs.

When respiratory symptoms are under some control, the voice clinician may help the patient develop and use a functional voice. Phonation can often be helped by reducing the number of syllables the patient says on one breath. A baseline measurement should be taken. The patient should then be instructed to cut the total number in half. For example, if a patient says twenty syllables on one expiration, the patient should be instructed to limit utterances to half that number, or ten syllables per breath. This seems to prevent vocal fold squeezing, which makes the last words of the phrase or sentence sound squeezed or dysphonic. Help the person to develop methods of renewing breath while speaking (see Chapter 6). Good posture with the head not tilted upward or downward, the open-mouth approach, vocal hygiene, and the yawn–sigh approach have all been found helpful for the asthmatic patient who wishes to improve vocal efficiency.

Emphysema

Among various chronic pulmonary diseases experienced by the adult population, emphysema is the most common. The primary cause of emphysema is smoking or from continuous exposure to smoke-laden dust. The continuous smoke exposure in the lungs causes the alveolar walls to lose their elasticity, collapsing on pulmonary expiration (Berkow, Beers, and Fletcher, 1997). This collapse of the alveoli in turn causes the bronchioles (the airway conduits to and from the alveoli) to collapse. The result of this alveoli–bronchiole collapse is difficulty in emptying the lung during expiration (Sataloff, 1997). Consequently, the high residual air volumes preclude taking in adequate oxygen renewal on inspiration. The patient with moderate to severe emphysema struggles to get sufficient breath to sustain his or her life. Voice abnormality is of secondary concern.

About 14 million people in the United States suffer from an emphysema-related illness, making it "second only to heart disease as a cause of disability that makes people stop working, and is the fourth most common cause of death" (Berkow, Beers, and Fletcher, 1997, p. 177). Because the primary cause of emphysema is cigarette smoking, the first mandatory treatment step is to stop smoking. Mild emphysema can begin to show after only five or seven years of continuous, heavy smoking. It is the mildly involved patient, often a professional user of voice, whom we often see with a voice problem who seeks the clinical help of a speech–language pathologist.

Voice management can only begin after the patient stops smoking. Formal respiratory therapy for these patients is better left in the hands of the respiratory therapist or other pulmonary specialists. However, the voice clinician often begins by taking voice measurements specific to air volume and available pressures for voicing, measures of duration, and sound pressure level of the voice. Observation of the patient during speaking, oral reading, and singing tasks may also reveal some unnecessary postural–skeletal behaviors the patient is using to maintain breathing, movements that may be inefficient and counterproductive to good voice control.

Some directed practice in diaphragmatic–abdominal breathing in the sitting or standing (vertical) position may be useful, as well as practice in counting syllables per utterance in an attempt to become more aware of when to renew breath. Shortening the length of phonation can help the patient have more control over voice loudness. Using a loop-feedback instrument like the Facilitator can provide direct training with feedback in breath renewal and its direct effect on voice loudness. The emphysema patient can sometimes improve voice quality by speaking at a slightly higher voice pitch. Other facilitating approaches might be tried in the search for a stronger functional voice, such as focus, glottal attack changes, masking, and pitch inflections.

Faulty Breath Control

Many children and adults appear in the clinic with faulty breath control, either caused by some organic disease or from functional causes, or both. That is, there may be a functional overlay to an organic respiratory disease that can be directly treated, improving overall respiratory function as well as providing better breath support for voice. There are an endless number of respiratory diseases, most of which may have some impact on voice. The speech–language pathologist who works with voice patients soon learns to consult with physicians and therapists who work with patients with respiratory diseases, as well as becomes familiar with journals such as *American Journal of Respiratory and Critical Care Medicine* or the Voice Foundation's *Journal of Voice,* or reference books like *Textbook of Respiratory Medicine* (Murray and Nadel, eds., 1994) or *Professional Voice: The Science and Art of Clinical Care* (Sataloff, ed., 1997). Such reference sources not only provide information about the medical treatment of various respiratory diseases, but often contain detailed references about possible management and voice therapy for these patients.

What we do with voice problems with respiratory problems must be consistent with the limitation imposed by various respiratory diseases and the treatments the patient may be receiving from other professionals. The clinician should not be preoccupied with the presenting disease problem, but face the patient more generically, as a person with a voice disorder that shows itself in various pitch–loudness–quality dimensions. In fact, faulty breath control may show itself more as a functional problem than as an organic one. For most patients, the voice clinician should assess respiratory–voice function following many of the evaluation procedures presented in Chapter 5, The Voice Evaluation. The voice evaluation should supplement any other respiratory assessment information. We use the management and therapy suggestions developed in Facilitating Approach #21, Respiration Training, in Chapter 6 for developing better breath support for voice with patients with faulty breath control.

Airway Obstructions

The voice clinician may encounter a number of children and adults with voice problems that are related to airway obstructions. Although obstructive airway problems require medical–surgical intervention and management, the speech–language pathologist may play an important part in both identification and management of the disorder. There are basically two contributing causes of airway obstruction (O'Hollaren, 1995): structural and lesion mass airflow interference and abnormal laryngeal movement interference.

There are both infectious and noninfectious causes of laryngeal-mass obstruction to airflow. Severe involvement of the epiglottis and supraglottal structures is almost always the result of a bacterial infection, treatable with appropriate antibiotic therapy. Depending on the size of the supraglottal swelling, inspiratory and expiratory breathing can be seriously compromised. Subglottal obstruction from disease is most often seen in croup, a viral disease, usually characterized by inhalation stridor. Once croup is differentiated from such problems as paradoxical vocal fold dysfunction (which is often confused with asthmatic stridor), effective treatment includes "hydration, humidification, racemic epinephrine, and corticosteroids" (O'Hollaren and Everts, 1991). Airway obstruction can be caused by tumor mass related to such space-occupying lesions as papilloma, granuloma, carcinoma, or large cysts; once such lesions are identified as compromising the airway, effective medical management may include radiation therapy to reduce the lesion size or surgical reduction or removal of the lesion. The obstructive lesion is watched closely and, when it becomes too large, such as is often observed in juvenile papilloma, a surgical approach restores required airway competence. The voice clinician often plays an important role with the postsurgical, mass-lesion patient, establishing the best voice possible with voice therapy (despite a scarred and abnormal glottal margin).

The most common laryngeal movement obstruction to in and out air movement within the airway is laryngeal paralysis, unilateral or bilateral. In Chapter 4, Neurogenic Voice Disorders, we looked at the multiple possible causes of vocal fold paralyses, and their surgical and voice therapy management. While unilateral vocal fold paralysis contributes to some compromise of the open airway, bilateral abductor paralysis produces a life-threatening obstacle to air passage, requiring immediate surgical intervention. The procedures for management of vocal fold paralysis are presented in Chapter 4 and need not be repeated here.

Even though Jackson and Jackson (1942) described spasmodic closure of the glottis during inspiration, it was not until the observations of Rogers and Stell (1978) that the diagnosis of "paradoxical vocal fold movement" was made for a condition previously misdiagnosed as "bronchospasm." The speech–language pathologist today will find a varied literature describing the causative factors of *paradoxical vocal cord dysfunction* (PVCD), which masks as inspiratory asthma. Case (1996) presents an excellent description and photograph of the larynx during a PVCD inspiration, showing the membranous portion of the folds adducted on inspiration with a posterior triangular glottal chink. The relative smallness of the glottal chink does not permit enough open space for a normal inspiration. Trudeau (1998) suggests three possible etiologies of PVCD: psychogenic, as in conversion reaction; visceral, related to irritation from gastroesophageal reflux; and/or neurological, a form of laryngeal dystonia.

Because strenuous exercise is often identified as a "trigger" of PCVD symptoms, it is helpful in establishing the diagnosis to use monitoring during physical activity with a "flow–volume loop" (Gallivan, Hofman, and Gallivan, 1996). Endoscopy should be attempted during (usually not possible as the patient is struggling) and shortly after inspiratory laryngospasm.

Unlike most descriptions of PVCD found in the literature, Trudeau (1998) does offer a laryngeal control program that can be initiated by the speech–language pathologist. Like Blager (1995) and Case (1996), he places emphasis on helping the patient become aware of aberrant and normal vocal fold posturing during inspiration and expiration. The present authors, also, use extensive videoendoscopy of correct and abnormal vocal fold postures for both phonation and quiet respiration for the PVCD patient to both observe and produce. Patients become aware of how to produce vocal fold configurations in their own larynx, showing them what to do to "open the airway when you take in a breath." The authors have found the use of the yawn–sigh a useful technique for opening the vocal folds and creating a more open airway. Other therapy procedures described by Trudeau (1998) include nasal inspiration, working on /s/ duration (not to maximum levels), and the use of diaphragmatic–abdominal breathing. The present authors also attempt to locate other patients with PVCD and have them meet together for the obvious support they may derive from listening to one another.

Management–Voice Therapy for Vocal Fold Lesions

There are a number of possible vocal fold (VF) lesions among patients evaluated by the speech–language pathologist. In most cases, these lesions produce various forms of dysphonia, some of which primarily require the services of the physician, or sometimes primarily voice therapy with an SLP, and often the services of both. Let us look separately at a few vocal fold lesions and their management–therapy.

Cysts

Submucosal lesions of the vocal folds, such as cysts, are found anywhere on the vocal folds (glottal margin or on inferior or superior fold surfaces) or anywhere on the ventricular folds. The speech–language pathologist who identifies any kind of laryngeal lesion should refer the patient to an otolaryngologist. This is especially true for cysts because their management requires surgical excision rather than voice therapy per se. Courey, Shohet, Scott, and Ossoff (1996) studied forty-one benign laryngeal lesions (nodules, polyps, cysts, and corditis) and identified seven squamous cysts and seven mucous cysts. All fourteen cyst lesions were found on histological examination to be benign. Depending on the site of the lesion, the patient may or may not experience dysphonia. Sataloff (1997) writes that, because cysts rarely resolve spontaneously, they should be removed surgically using a small, superficial incision along the superior edge of the vocal fold, without disrupting the glottal margin. Voice therapy postsurgically is usually confined to helping the patient eliminate any voice compensations (such as increased glottal attack) that may have been used to minimize negative voice effects caused by the cyst.

Granuloma

Laryngeal granuloma may or may not contribute to vocal symptoms, depending on the site and type of granuloma. Granulomas in the larynx are composed of rough, granulated tissue that usually develops reactively to some kind of epithelial irritation. There are different types of laryngeal granuloma, which are related to different kinds of tissue trauma: posterior arytenoid granuloma, vocal process granuloma, surgical irritation granuloma, and those developing from irritated tissue from infectious diseases.

Tracheal intubation often leads to the formation of postintubation granuloma (Balestrieri and Watson, 1982), more prevalent in females than males (believed to be the result of smaller airway openings in females during surgical intubation). Such granuloma lesions are usually in the posterior glottis and arytenoid areas. Similarly, children with smaller airway openings may experience laryngeal trauma from intubation, producing postintubation granuloma. Certainly, children and adults who have been intubated for whatever reason should receive a postintubation laryngeal examination. Any change in postsurgical voice should be investigated to see if there has been intubation trauma with resulting irritation and granuloma. These complications from intubation may not appear immediately but develop over time (McFerran, Abdullah, Gallimore, Pringle, and Croft, 1994). No voice therapy should be initiated until a laryngeal examination is completed. If postsurgical granulomas are identified along the posterior glottis, medical–surgical treatment will promote healing and preserve the airway.

Vocal process granulomas are often related to excessive and continuing gastroesophageal reflux, with the patient often using hard glottal attack as a vocal compensation. Excessive throat-clearing is often evident. Many patients with posterior vocal process granulomas are relatively free of dysphonia. The primary cause of vocal process granulomas appears to be continuing reflux. We will discuss management of reflux later in this section.

Surgery on the vocal folds will sometimes produce a reactive tissue irritation leading to the formation of granulomas. The most common reactive lesion is Teflon granuloma of the larynx (Varvares, Montgomery, and Hillman, 1995), usually caused by possible "overinjection, injecting too close to the vocal fold margin, or injecting too deeply." Teflon injection is usually reserved to give greater bulk to the paralyzed vocal fold in unilateral adductor paralysis, permitting better approximation of the normal fold with the paralyzed fold. This results in a better-sounding voice. However, if the voice begins to deteriorate several months after injection, the possibility of Teflon granuloma should be investigated. Other surgical traumas, such as removal of cysts or altering the glottal margin, have as a possible side effect the development of reactive tissue granuloma. From the perspective of the speech–language pathologist, if surgical revision of the larynx has resulted in a better voice, and then months or years afterwards the voice deteriorates, the larynx should be reexamined using endoscopy or stroboscopy in an attempt to identify possible reactive granuloma. Surgically-induced irritation with resulting granuloma require medical/surgical resolution of the problem.

The speech–language pathologist should be alert to the fact that any inflammatory disease of the larynx, such as tuberculosis, syphilis, or sarcoidosis, can lead to granulomatous tissue changes (Pillsbury and Sasaki, 1982). Such tissue changes may produce voice symptoms. The overall management of voice problems related to inflammatory disease lies in the hands of the physician.

Track
2, 4 & 10

Nodules–Polyps

Vocal nodules in both children and adults are the most common benign lesions of the vocal folds. Continuous vocal abuse and misuse of the vocal mechanisms characterized by hyperfunction and excessive muscle tension appear to be the primary causes of vocal nodules. Accordingly, in the successful management of nodules, both speech–language pathologists and otolaryngologists agree that primary attention must be given to identification of abuse/misuse with management strategies to reduce their occurrence. Yelling and screaming appear to be behaviors that can lead to nodules in children, while speaking in noisy environments and excessive throat-clearing are identified by Case (1996) as common etiologic factors in the development of vocal nodules.

Polyps are more often unilateral lesions (softer and less fibrotic than nodules) and are often caused by a focal, single vocal trauma, i.e., screaming at an accident or unusual yelling at an athletic contest. A polyp may form out of the traumatized vocal fold cover, eventually adding mass and becoming fluid filled. Once a polyp begins, any excessive vocal abuse/misuse can contribute to its continued growth. The vocal symptoms from the single polyp can be more severe (Colton, Woo, Brewer, Griffin, and Casper, 1995) than the voice symptoms of patients with nodules. For example, diplophonia may be heard in the voice of the polyp patient, who typically has one normal vocal fold vibrating against the polyp-laden fold, producing asynchrony of vibration.

Nodules are generally bilateral, appearing most often on the anterior–middle third junction of each fold. This site is on the cover of the midpoint of the ligamentous–muscular section of the glottis (middle of the anterior two thirds of the vocal fold). In comparing stroboscopic findings of eighty patients with benign vocal fold lesions (Colton, et al., 1995), the most common glottal configurations of patients with vocal nodules were an hourglass configuration (openings on each side of the nodules) and a posterior glottal chink. These glottal openings seem to produce compromised glottal approximation, contributing to higher airflow rates with corresponding lower pressures. The mass of the nodules results in a lowering of fundamental frequency and asynchronous vocal fold movements that contribute to the patient's hoarseness.

Children and adults with vocal nodules and polyps are observed to clear their throats continually, reporting that they often feel that they have excessive mucus or "something" on their vocal folds. Excessive throat-clearing (Boone, 1997) is often identified as a vocal abuse, which may lead to further enlargement or further hardening of the nodule mass or to enlargement of the polyp. In the daily cycle of voice use, other abuses are added to the constant throat-clearing, often resulting in a deteriorating voice as the day goes on. However, Hall (1995) found that, of ten women with vocal nodules and ten women with normal larynges, there were no time-of-day differences between the two groups. Clinically, we observe that the voice of the nodule or polyp patient remains more functional throughout the day by avoiding abuse–misuse behaviors and by employing a few good voice techniques, such as renewing breath more often, lessening glottal attack, using greater mouth opening while speaking, and several of the other facilitating techniques described in the last chapter.

Voice therapy for reducing vocal nodules or vocal polyps is the primary choice of treatment. The nodule patient needs to identify and reduce continuing vocal abuse, particularly those abuses that have been found to be causative of the nodule formation. The polyp patient can usually identify the past precipitating event, which is likely to be no longer present. However, the polyp produces enough voice symptoms to which the patient begins to use reactive vocal abuses, such as excessive throat-clearing. Therefore, for each patient group, child or adult, the primary thrust in voice therapy is to identify possible abuse–misuse and develop programs to reduce it (children: Andrews, 1994; Boone, 1993; Johnson, 1996; adults: Andrews, 1994; Boone, 1982; Koschkee and Rammage, 1997).

While reducing vocal abuse–misuse is a continuing management need in treating vocal nodules or polyps, there are some general clinical guidelines for this group of voice patients. Optimizing vocal fold approximation can be achieved by providing electroglottogram feedback and using such facilitating approaches (see Chapter 6) as chant-talk, chewing, elimination of abuses, glottal attack changes, open-mouth approach, and the yawn–sigh. Voice improvement should rely heavily on auditory feedback, letting the patient evaluate different voice forms by listening critically to his or her productions on a loop-feedback recorder (see Auditory Feedback in Chapter 6). For example, record some voicing, stop and play back what the individual just said, evaluate the production, and produce new voicing. Vocal function exercises presented by Stemple, Gerdeman, and Glaze (1994) are helpful for both children and adults who want to develop more efficient voices with less laryngeal strain. Many of the facilitating approaches in Chapter 6 should be used as diagnostic probes. That is, if they appear to be facilitative of a target voice (a voice the clinician and the patient both want), that approach should be used as practice in therapy.

Papilloma

Papilloma is one of the most common benign but recurring lesions in the larynx. The age of onset seems to have a bimodal distribution with peaks occurring before age five (juvenile onset) and in young adults over the age of 20 (Élö, Hídvégi, and Bajtai, 1995). These wartlike, virally-caused growths can reproduce rapidly in the dark crevices of the airway and in particular within the larynx. Recent development in molecular biology has provided detailed analyses of papilloma virus, isolating many different types of papovaviruses identified as the Human Papilloma Virus group (HPV). The treatment of laryngeal papilloma is both surgical and chemical: (1) excessive papilloma are surgically excised (often by laser) whenever their bodies begin to obstruct the airway, and (2) they are treated via medication, often using varying dosages of interferon.

The speech–language pathologist often plays an early role in the discovery of patients with laryngeal papilloma. The papilloma patient at any age begins to experience some developing dysphonia, often accompanied by some inhalation stridor (particularly while sleeping). On laryngeal examination, the patient is found to have space-occupying lesions within the airway. The patient is then referred to the otolaryngologist, who identifies the lesions as papilloma and then selects particular treatments (interferon, surgery). Because the primary management of the papilloma patient is medical–surgical, voice therapy has no effect in reducing or eliminating the viral tumors of papilloma.

Although the primary role of speech–language pathologists is in finding the problem at the time of voice evaluation, they may be called on during medical treatment or after surgery to help the patient develop and maintain the best voice possible. The laryngeal papilloma patient will usually profit from improving use of respiration to support phonation, perhaps reducing the number of syllables said on one expiration. We have found that loop auditory feedback is a useful therapy mode for helping these patients develop the best voice possible, considering the amount of glottal scarring and structural interference they may be experiencing. The voice clinician should remember, however, that voice therapy for laryngeal papilloma patients is limited to voice improvement with a damaged mechanism, and is not designed to limit the growth of new papilloma or aid in eradicating papilloma that already exist.

Reflux

There is increased evidence that many children and adults with dysphonia have a gastroesophageal reflux disease (GERD) contributing to their voice problem (Gumpert, Kalach, Dupont, and Contencin, 1998; Shaw, Searl, Young, and Miner, 1996). While GERD is the most prevalent designation for acid reflux in the larynx and pharynx, it can also be called *laryngopharyngeal reflux* (LPR) or *laryngopharyngeal reflux disease* (LPRD). The symptoms of acid reflux vary considerably among voice patients, ranging from no symptoms to mild heartburn to extreme burning or choking in the larynx, awakening the patient from a deep sleep. Typical symptoms of GERD may include morning hoarseness, sour taste in mouth with bad breath, frequent throat-clearing and coughing, and severe symptoms occurring when the head is lower than the abdominal area (such as in shoe tying, diving, or tumbling). For a more detailed description of the symptoms and pathology involved in reflux, the reader may wish to review the consensus conference report on laryngopharyngeal reflux (Koufman, Sataloff, and Toohill, 1996).

Among the physical findings on laryngeal examination are posterior glottal redness, contact ulcers, pharyngeal irritation, and arytenoid hyperplasia with possible granuloma. The patient on questioning may be unaware of any symptoms related to GERD; this is especially true among children (Gumpert and others, 1998). If, on examination of either a dysphonic child or adult, there are obvious signs of GERD, the diagnosis of reflux should be pursued. Among the most definitive diagnostic tests is twenty-four-hour pH monitoring to determine the presence of acid in the lower pharynx or posterior larynx. The treatment of reflux includes elevating the bed headboard, using antacids, avoiding activities that compress the abdomen, taking H2 blockers to reduce acid production (particularly at night), and reducing exposure to spicy foods, tobacco, alcohol, and caffeine products. Following these management suggestions for reflux can bring about a dramatic lessening of symptoms, both in voice and pharyngeal–laryngeal mucosal irritation.

The speech–language pathologist usually encounters the dysphonic patient with GERD initially at the time of the voice evaluation. If the signs of posterior laryngeal irritation are present, the patient is referred to the otolaryngologist. They will work as a team to plan a successful reflux management regimen and a voice therapy program that can produce optimal vocal function. Helping the patient reduce throat-clearing and nonproductive coughing (more often habit than mucus-expectorating), developing easy glottal attack, changing throat focus to facial mask focus, and sometimes elevating voice pitch one or two half-notes are among the facilitating approaches that help the GERD patient maintain a good, functional voice.

Sulcus Vocalis

Although Ford and others (1996) cite the earliest mention of sulcus vocalis in the literature (Giacomini, 1892), there has been a lot of clinical confusion over the years as to both the etiology and description of the disorder. *Sulcus* is a generic term that means "furrow" or "indentation." In sulcus vocalis, on endoscopy or stroboscopy we see a furrowed medial edge of the vocal fold, usually bilaterally symmetrical, with the entire length of the vibrating folds in a spindle configuration. The patient presents clinically with some degree of dsyphonia, often referred with a confusing array of previous diagnoses such as bowing, presbylaryngis, paralysis, or thyroarytenoid atrophy (Hirano, Yoshida, Tanaka, and Hibi, 1990).

One of the more definitive studies of sulcus vocalis was done by the Wisconsin group (Ford and others, 1996), which included two studies (normative and clinical), finding that sulcus vocalis can be seen in three forms. They first identified among 116 control subjects nine subjects who displayed *physiologic sulcus,* an indentation of the vibrating fold without "histopathologic change in the lamina propria." Although these subjects showed some fold indentation, their voices were judged as normal. Among twenty clinical cases with a diagnosis of sulcus vocalis, they found two other distinct types (congenital or acquired from irritation) with clear involvement of the lamina propria with spindle or posterior gaps between the two involved folds. All of these clinical cases showed some compromise in mucosal wave, resulting in audible dysphonia of varying degrees.

The speech–language pathologist today sees more patients with sulcus vocalis than in former years. With mirror examination, many of these abnormalities were missed. However, videostroboscopy permits close examination of vocal fold cover abnormalities; with sulcus vocalis, when the folds are abducted, we can often identify the fold furrow; on adduction with phonation, we can see the compromised mucosal wave produced by the stiff, compromised lamina propria.

If sulcus vocalis is identified, the treatment is primarily surgical followed by voice therapy to develop optimal phonation. There appear to be three surgical approaches that have been found to improve glottal function: intracordal injection, medialization by thyroplasty, or multiple small incisions across the sulcus (Pontes and Behlau, 1993). After surgery, glottal function needs reassessment by the speech–language pathologist. Improved function may still require that old habits of the patient need to be identified and corrected, particularly in reducing vocal hyperfunction. Although voice therapy after surgery for sulcus vocalis is highly individualized, reducing effort associated with breathing and phonation often results in a better-sounding voice. Auditory feedback with real-time amplification has been found useful in establishing easy-onset phonation after surgery with this patient group.

Summary

In this Chapter, we have looked at particular kinds of voice problems with an emphasis on the speech–language pathologist's perspective. We found that there was often an organic component to the voice disorder that requires some acknowledgment of the limitations that contribute to the voice problem. Voice therapy by itself is not always appropriate. Likewise, medical or surgical treatment by itself may be too limited. Rather, for many of the special voice problems described, the best management is a team effort between medical–surgical specialists and the speech-language pathologist.

8 Voice Therapy Following Treatment for Laryngeal Cancer

The first consideration when the diagnosis of laryngeal cancer is made is how to best cure the disease and preserve the patient's life. After the best treatment of the disease is selected, one can turn attention to the best means of restoring the voice following cancer treatment. Treatment of laryngeal cancer is generally by means of irradiation, surgery, or chemotherapy or combinations of these modes of treatment. The selection of method or methods will be made by the physician (oncologist) and the patient based on the type, location, and extent of the disease process. A brief discussion of these considerations is presented by Hall and Merricourt (1995). There is more than one type of cancer and not all respond in the same way to a given mode of treatment, such as chemotherapy or irradiation.

Modes of Cancer Treatment

Each of these cancer treatment modes presents some complications to voice therapy. For example, irradiation can cause swelling in the early stage of treatment and dryness and stiffness of the vocal fold cover later. As we discussed in Chapter 2, a flexible vocal fold cover is important to the production of a mucosal wave, which in turn gives rise to phonation. Surgery can leave a tissue deficit where a tumor was excised and stiffness due to scarring following healing. The tissue deficit also may leave a gap in the glottal area when the folds are approximated. This gap may cause air wastage and a breathy vocal quality and may result in inadequate vocal loudness and a short phonation time. Dryness may add to the susceptibility of the vocal fold cover to vocal abuse and a strained vocal quality that may produce larger than normal shimmer measures as noted in Chapter 5. Thus dryness, inadequate tissue mass, irregular vocal fold edges, and stiffness can all make vibration of the vocal fold cover, as discussed in Chapter 2, extremely difficult or impossible. This will render the voice abnormal in one or more vocal parameters.

Case Examples

The picture of a larynx in Figure 8.1 shows a lack of tissue mass due to surgery for removal of a laryngeal cancer. There is a gap between the vocal folds even in full adduction. The voice is breathy, low in loudness, and rough in quality. The breathy quality results from the air wastage through the glottal gap, while the low

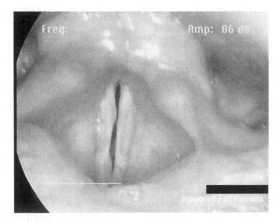

FIGURE 8.1 *Lack of tissue mass in right vocal fold after surgical removal of laryngeal cancer.*

loudness level is due to inadequate medial compression required for louder voice production. The rough vocal quality is due to two factors: unequal mass between the right and left vocal folds and, thus, an irregular vocal fold vibrator pattern; secondly, an attempt to compensate for the excessive glottal gap by hyperactivity of the false vocal folds, which weight the vocal folds unequally. A third factor whose effect is difficult to estimate, is the scarring following surgery. On stroboscopy the vocal folds appear unevenly stiff, which is likely due to the formation of scarring, which produces adynamic segments in the vocal folds in the area where tissue has been excised. In voice therapy, for this patient, we need to first eliminate the excessive vocal effort thus reducing the false fold activity. This was accomplished by inhalation phonation, which retracts the false folds (discussed in Chapter 6). We gradually shifted from inhalation to exhalation phonation using the /i/ vowel because it is produced with the root of the tongue elevated and out of the hypopharynx. The next step in voice therapy was to use an upward pitch shift to slightly increase vocal fold tension and gain slightly better approximation (reducing the glottal gap) of the postsurgical vocal folds. The upward pitch could be only slight due to some vocal fold scarring. Greater shifts upward produced too much tension of the vocal folds and phonation breaks occurred due to stiffness of the vocal fold cover. A shift of 20–25 Hz was desirable in this case. The improved approximation from increased vocal fold tension during pitch shift increased vocal loudness. Subglottic air pressure was increased slightly as well. This case demonstrates how the treatment (surgery) for cancer produced a dysphonia as a byproduct of treatment for the disease. Voice therapy was based on achieving the necessary vocal adjustments using facilitation techniques that would alter the effects of postsurgical anatomy and physiology of the larynx and also counter the **inappropriate** compensatory behaviors the patient had developed.

In a second case in which the stiffness of the vocal fold cover is due to postirradiation treatment for cancer, we shifted pitch downward to take advantage of the greater mucosal wave that occurs in lower pitches and also decreased subglottic air pressure so the folds were not overdriven. We used this therapy approach in a patient who had irradiation treatment for a superficial cancer of the vocal fold cover, bilaterally. He was able to return to teaching with a much improved voice and a voice that would last throughout the teaching day. The pretherapy voice was very weak, extremely breathy, and was of very short duration of phonation. This was due to a more or less uniform stiffness of the entire vocal fold area, bilaterally. The effect is very much like that produced by surgical stripping of the vocal fold to remove superficial vocal fold cancer.

A third case illustrates another role of the speech pathologist in the follow-up and management of patients being treated for laryngeal cancer. A twenty-six-year-old female was seen for evaluation of voice following surgical removal of superficial squamous cell cancer. Of interest, the patient is a nonsmoker, does not use alcohol, is a vegetarian, and a marathon runner. She is in excellent shape but has cancer of the larynx. The cancer has returned three times in less than two years and has been removed three times. The decision of a team of ENT physicians is to continue to monitor the return of the cancer and remove it before it becomes deeply embedded in the vocal folds. The speech pathology clinic is to evaluate the patient every four to six months along with evaluations by the ENT team. The speech pathologist provides videostroboscopic monitoring of the larynx and acoustic evaluation of the voice as a means of tracking the cancer regrowth. Figure 8.2 is a picture of the larynx of this young adult female patient with laryngeal cancer. In addition, the speech pathologist provides ongoing voice management so the patient is using the larynx optimally and does not engage in vocal abuse, which may make the voice poorer in quality and contribute to edema, a condition that can make obtaining an accurate status of the cancer more difficult. While this is a very unusual case, the monitoring role of the speech pathologist is not unusual and has been applied in cases of contact ulcer, papilloma, and of polyps and polypoid cord degeneration.

Facilitation Techniques

Our clinical experience with postsurgical and postirradiation treatment dysphonias has demonstrated some success using the following techniques from Chapter 6:

1. Inhalation phonation using the vowels /i/, /u/, and /o/
2. Pitch shifts upward and downward based on patient's vocal response
3. Glottal fry if vocal fold stiffness is not too great
4. Nasal glide stimulation

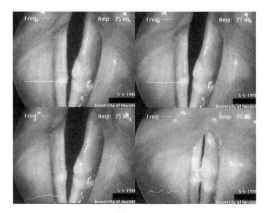

FIGURE 8.2   *Four views of the larynx of a 26-year-old female with recurring squamous cell carcinoma, followed over a two-year period.*

5. Head turned to the side and lateral digital pressure to the thyroid cartilage
6. Loudness changes, usually lower
7. Tongue protrusion /i/
8. Glottal fry to tone

Patients with postsurgical and postirradiation dysphonias are a challenging vocal population. The critical factor in success with voice therapy in postsurgical or irradiation patients is the degree to which mucosal wave has been preserved. We have more often than not been able to improve the voice of these patients through voice therapy, but we have not always been successful due to too much vocal fold stiffness or scarring or the absence of tissue (postsurgically), creating irregular vocal fold medial edges. These patients may also have difficulty swallowing and thus may benefit from swallowing therapy.

Vocal Hygiene

In addition to the techniques listed above to improve the voice we have also noted the need for additional attention to vocal hygiene, such as avoiding excessive strain in trying to talk over noise and increasing water intake. Increased hydration is a key component in these often dry patients. Reduction of alcohol intake, which also is drying, and substitution of silent cough and sniff swallow (Zwitmah, 1973) for voiced coughing and throat clearing are crucial for these patients. Because their anatomy and physiology is often altered by treatment of the disease, they have less latitude or tolerance for vocal abuse and their mode of vocal fold vibration is less robust.

Counseling and Support

Some attention to family support and the supporting and counseling role of the speech–voice pathologist is warranted with these patients. The disease may result in increased stress due to loss of income and added medical bills as well as the impact of having to deal with one's mortality due to the diagnosis of cancer.

It is even more critical when the patient has undergone total laryngectomy. It must be remembered that a laryngectomy is an amputation and that the resultant loss of voice immediately following surgery has profound effects on the psychological well-being of the patient and the family.

Laryngectomy

When surgery is the method of treatment, the extent and location of the tumor will dictate the extent of the surgery. If the tumor crosses the midline, then total laryngectomy (or near total or subtotal laryngectomy) may be indicated; if the tumor is on one side of the larynx then hemilaryngectomy or other partial laryngectomy may be an option. If the tumor is above the level of the vocal folds then supraglottal laryngectomy is an option. The type and extent of surgery will dictate the remaining tissue and a careful evaluation by the speech–language pathologist will be required to assess the approach for the voice rehabilitation program. One will need to address the type of approximation of the remaining vocal folds or the type of neoglottis remaining after surgery. Treatment for voice rehabilitation in the case of cordectomy or modified total laryngectomy is a highly individualized process. The techniques that produce the most consistent voice production will be selected and, later in the therapy process, the loudness, quality, and pitch aspects of voice may be addressed. Consistent voice production is the key initial goal of voice reinstatement.

The first meeting of the speech–language pathologist and the laryngectomee patient will be important to developing a good working relationship. It is of advantage to see the patient prior to surgery if possible. A preoperative visit should include encouragement of the patient and family. It should include a brief assessment of all aspects of speech. Information should be provided about the various speech–voice options and general encouragement about the various successful methods of alaryngeal voice. It may be helpful to have a laryngectomee attend with the SLP if the laryngectomee has good alaryngeal speech. It can be encouraging to see and hear a person who has successfully been rehabilitated following treatment for laryngeal cancer.

The Artificial Larynx

We frequently encourage the use of an artificial larynx during the first few days following surgery. When healing is still incomplete and swelling may be significant, we may introduce the patient to a Cooper-Rand intraoral electrolarynx. This device is shown in Figure 8.3 with other artificial devices. The Cooper-Rand does not require pressure to the neck like other handheld devices and thus works when fistulae or swelling are problems. Some neck-type electrolarynges may be converted to intraoral devices with a converter such as the Neovox. Watterson and McFarlane (1995) discuss the various types of devices available and their use in a chapter in a current monograph. In a recent study, Watterson, Cox, and McFarlane (1998) investigated the speech intelligibility (for vowels and sentences) of four different electric neck larynges. Among other findings, the vowel /a/ was most intelligible and /u/ was the least intelligible. On a scale of 1 to 5 (5 being highly intelligible) the mean sentence intelligibility rating for all artificial larynges combined was found to be 2.98. Even if the laryngectomee uses T-E puncture (TEP), the use of an electrolarynx is a good alternate mode of phonation should the other mode fail or the external environmental factors (e.g., background noise) dictate a shift to another mode of speech. In looking at alternative types of artificial devices, one should not overlook the various pneumatic types (two examples may be seen in Figure 8.3) of artificial devices. These are simple and easy to use, while remaining quite affordable. They produce a satisfactory form of alaryngeal speech. Indeed, we have had such professional voice users as a preacher and athletic coach who used the pneumatic type of artificial larynx quite successfully. We recently saw a laryngectomee who began her postsurgical speaking with a Western Electric neck device (Figure 8.3), which she managed very well. She then wanted to switch to a TEP voice, which she mastered well and was well understood. She, however, did not like to change the prosthesis and did not want to go to an indwelling prosthesis. She is now using an Ultravoice device embedded in her upper dental plate (Watterson & McFarlane, 1995). She is also well understood with this device. This patient now has three methods of a laryngeal voice: Neck Electrolarynx, TEP prosthesis, and the Intraoral Ultravoice. At her last visit she said she "may try the indwelling device."

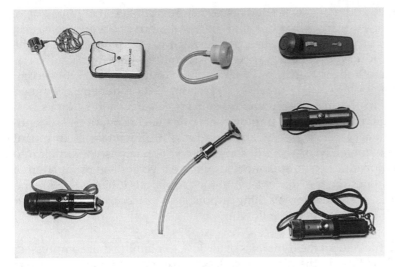

FIGURE 8.3   Seven Artificial Prostheses Top left: *Cooper-Rand intraoral electronic larynx;* Top center: *Memacon artificial larynx DSP8 pneumatic;* Top right: *Western Electric neck device;* Bottom left: *Park Jed-Com electrolarynx;* Bottom center: *Tokyo reed-type pneumatic artificial larynx;* Center right: *Servox neck device;* Bottom right: *Aurex neck-held electrolarynx neovox.*

Traditional Esophageal Speech

While the development of **TEP** speech has made the use of traditional esophageal speech less frequent, the speech–language pathologist should know something about this form of speech and how to teach it if the need arises. At the very least one needs to know where to find information on the teaching of traditional esophageal speech. We provide this information here in this chapter. Also, many of the good techniques for development of traditional esophageal voice are good principles to follow in development of other types of alaryngeal speech.

Teaching Esophageal Speech after Conventional Laryngectomy.   Two methods of teaching esophageal speech may be employed: injection and inhalation. We usually begin with the injection method, which is the easiest to teach and is quite compatible with the articulation practice the patient may have used with the artificial larynx.

Both methods, however, employ the same basic principle of compressing air within the oropharynx and injecting this denser air into the more rarefied (less dense) space of the esophagus. Denser air within a body moves in the direction of the less dense body of air whenever the two bodies are coupled together. Some of the compressed air within the oral cavity undoubtedly escapes through the lips, some through the nasopharyngeal port, and some (particularly if the opening of the esophagus is open) into the esophagus. Both methods for esophageal voice bring compressed air into the esophagus; once the air is in the esophagus, external forces compress the air within it and expel it. Hopefully, the esophageal expulsion sets up a vibration of the pharyngo-esophageal (P-E) segment and the patient experiences an eructation or "voice." We consider separately the procedures for teaching the injection method and the inhalation method (sometimes combined with injection).

The Injection Method.   Certain consonants appear to have a facilitating effect in producing good esophageal voice. Individual patients may have their own favorite facilitating sounds, but more often than not these are plosive consonants (/p/,

/b/, /t/, /d/, /k/, and /g/) or affricatives containing plosives (/+ʃ/ or /ʤ/). Stetson (1937) reported many years ago that /p/, /t/, and /k/ were the easiest sounds for the new laryngectomee to use; Moolenaar-Bijl (1953) reported that the same phonemes produced esophageal speech faster in most patients than the traditional swallow method of teaching. Diedrich and Youngstrom (1966) recommended the voiceless /p/, /t/, /k/, /s/, /ʃ/, and /+ʃ/ phonemes as good sounds to employ in the injection method of air intake. Injection of air is best accomplished by using speech that employs some of the consonants just identified. As the patient whispers monosyllabic words with a facilitating consonant before and after the vowel, he or she will sometimes spontaneously inject air into the esophagus and produce an "unplanned" esophageal voice. The production of the consonant facilitates the transfer of air into the esophagus (Shanks, 1995). The injection method is preferred for teaching esophageal voice. Specific steps for teaching injection might include the following:

1. Discuss with the patient the dynamics of airflow, explaining that compressed, dense air will always flow in the direction of less dense, rarefied air. Explain also how the movements of the tongue in the injection method increase the density of the air within the mouth, enabling the air to move into the esophagus. Then demonstrate how the whispered articulation of a phoneme, such as a /t/ or a /k/, is the kind of tongue movement that produces the injection of air into the esophagus. After producing the whispered /t/, demonstrate for the patient an esophageal voice for the words such as *tot* or *talk*.

2. Now ask the patient to produce the phoneme /p/ by intraoral whisper. Care must be taken that the sound is made by good firm compression of the lips, with no need for stoma noise. Make sure that the patient avoids pushing out the pulmonary exhalation or using tongue and palatal–pharyngeal contact as the noise source. The intraoral whisper can be effectively taught by having the patient hold his or her breath and then attempt to "bite off" a /p/ by compressing the air caught between his or her abruptly closed lips. The patient should continue practicing this until true intraoral articulation is clearly grasped. This is demonstrated when he or she is consistently able to produce a precise /p/. Once the patient can do this, he or she should move to the next voiceless plosive, /t/. Here, the tongue tip against the upper central alveolar process is the site of contact, and practice should be continued until the patient can produce a precise, clear /t/. The same procedure should be repeated for /k/, again first demonstrating for the patient the different site of contact.

3. When good intraoral voiceless plosives have been produced, the patient is ready to add the vowel /a/ to each plosive. With /p/, for instance, he or she makes the plosive, and then immediately attempts to produce an esophageal phonation of /a/, producing in effect the word *pa*. If this is successful, the patient may combine the /p/ with a few other vowel combinations before going on to the /t/ and /k/. If the patient fails to produce the esophageal voice at this point, he or she should go back and work for even crisper articulation of the plosive sounds. If the patient is still unsuccessful after increased practice in articulation, he or she should attempt the inhalation method as the primary means of air intake.

4. The average laryngectomee experiences some success with the injection method when using the /p/, /t/, and /k/ phonemes. Therefore, he or she might be provided with about five monosyllabic words for each of the phonemes, for example, for /p/, the words *pat, pip, pack, pot,* and *pop.* The task is now to say each word, one at a time, renewing the esophageal air supply as he or she speaks, which is an obvious advantage of using the injection method. It is through the mere process of articulation that the patient takes in air. After the patient has demonstrated success with these phonemes, introduce their voiced cognates, /b/, /d/, and /g/. The same procedure should be repeated, ending with about five practice words for each new phoneme.

5. Additional phonemes, such as /s/, /z/, /ʃ/, /+ʃ/, /ʒ/, and /ʤ/, may be introduced for practice. As the patient gains phonatory skill with each new consonant, he or she must spend extra time learning to improve both the quickness and the quality of production. Too many patients err in trying to develop functional conversation too early. Considerable practice should be spent at the monosyllabic word level practicing one word at a time and making constant efforts to produce sharp articulation and a good-sounding voice.

6. Practice with basic control techniques is essential for developing successful and fluent esophageal speech. Therefore, we have the patient practice several skills directly in each speech session:

    a. Rapid production (one-half second or less) of esophageal phonation can improve response. If we call for ten productions of the /a/ vowel, the patient must respond with ten productions.

    b. Ability to sustain a tone for two and a half to three seconds or longer.

    c. Ability to interrupt the tone into three or four segments.

    d. Ability to stress the first or second syllable on command (such as in the word *"chipper"* for first-syllable stress, and *above* for second-syllable stress).

    e. Ability to make a soft or loud tone on command.

Each of these skills is practiced for a part of each speech session, much as a serious golfer practices on the putting green and driving range as well as playing in a real game. Patients who are too eager to achieve connected speech and ignore practice may carry bad habits into speech that will detract from their developing good esophageal speech and that are more difficult to correct at a later date.

7. At this point, if the patient has been successful, the inhalation method can be introduced to further improve air intake and esophageal phonation. The patient should produce a normal inhalation and, at the initial moment of exhalation, produce the consonant and say the word. Beyond the single words alone, we often couple the words together in phrases, such as *bake a cake, stop at church, park the black cart,* and so on. Once plosive-laden phrases are mastered, we then use the oral reading materials from voice and diction books, including, when possible, the facilitative consonants we have been using.

The Inhalation Method.   The flow of air in normal respiration is achieved by the transfer of air from one source to another because of the relative disparity of air pressure between the two sources. For example, when the thorax enlarges because of muscle movement, the air reservoir within the lung increases in size, rarefying (decreasing) the air pressure within the lung. Because the outside atmospheric air pressure is now greater, the air rushes in until the pressure within equals the outside pressure. The flow of air is always from the more dense to the less dense air body, and the flow continues until the two bodies are equal in pressure. By this same airflow mechanism the esophagus inflates in the inhalation method of air intake. The patient experiences a thoracic enlargement during pulmonary inhalation, which reduces the compression on all thoracic structures, including the esophagus. If the cricopharyngeus opening into the esophagus is slightly open at the time of the slight increase in the size of the esophagus, air from the hypopharynx will flow into the esophagus. During the exhalation phase of pulmonary respiration, when there is a general compression of thoracic structures, the esophagus also experiences some compression, which aids in the expulsion of the entrapped air. As this air passes through the approximated structures of the lower pharynx–upper esophagus (P-E segment), a vibration is set up, producing esophageal phonation. The advantage of the inhalation method of esophageal air intake is that it follows the patient's natural inclination or pulmonary inhalation followed by exhalation–phonation. Simply to take a breath and then talk is the most natural way of speaking, and for this reason the inhalation method offers the patient learning esophageal speech some early advantages.

In proceeding to the following steps for teaching the inhalation method, remember that the approach is best used in combination with the injection method.

1. Explain and demonstrate to the patient some aspects of normal respiration. Many normal speakers, for example, have never thought much about normal respiration, and many do not know that their voicing has always been an exhalation event. Explain to the patient that when the chest is enlarged by muscle action, the air flows into the lungs, and that, in the laryngectomee's case, the air comes through the stoma opening in the trachea and down into the lungs. Point out that the chest enlarges by muscle action, not by air inflation; thus, the air comes in as the chest enlarges. When the laryngectomee's chest enlarges, a concomitant enlargement of the esophagus usually takes place; when the esophagus is enlarged, there is a greater chance for air to come into it. When the chest becomes smaller, the pulmonary air is forced out, and the air within the esophagus is also more likely to be forced out. If possible, demonstrate esophageal voice using this method.

2. Before attempting to produce voice, the patient should practice conscious relaxation and correct breathing methods. He or she should become aware of thoracic expansion and abdominal distention on inhalation and of thoracic contraction on exhalation. Respiration practice should only be long enough to permit the patient to develop this kind of breathing awareness, because patients do not seem to benefit much from extended breathing exercises per se.

3. Now the patient should attempt to add air into the esophagus during his or her pulmonary inhalation. Diedrich and Youngstrom (1966) recommended that "the patient be told to close his mouth and imagine that he is sniffing through his nose, and to do so in a fairly rapid manner" (p. 112). Even though the sniff is basically a constricted inhalation, it is frequently accompanied by esophageal dilation (the normal person often swallows what he or she sniffs). As an extension of the sniff, the patient should be asked to take a fairly large pulmonary breath (through the stoma, of course). When his or her lungs appear to be about half inflated, the patient should say "up" on exhalation. This procedure can be repeated until the patient experiences some phonatory success.

4. For the patient who does not experience success in step (3), the following variation of the inhalation method sometimes produces good esophageal air: Ask the patient to take a deep breath, and, as he or she begins the inhalation, to cover the stoma. While the muscular enlargement of the thorax continues (despite the patient's lack of continuing inhalation), there will be a corresponding enlargement of the esophagus, perhaps permitting air to flow into the esophagus. For their patient who can get air into the esophagus but cannot produce the air escape necessary for phonation, the same mechanism applies in reverse. Here, the patient takes a deep inhalation and, as he or she begins to exhale, occludes the stoma; as the thorax begins to decrease in size, there will be increased pressure on the esophagus, which might well result in expulsion of esophageal air (and phonation).

5. If esophageal phonation is achieved by either of the last two steps, the patient should proceed from his or her "up" response to single monosyllabic words beginning and ending with /p/, /b/, /t/, /d/, /k/, and /g/. Time should be spent practicing at this single-word level, until the technique is mastered in terms of loudness, quality of sound, and articulation. The patient who masters the basic techniques of air intake and phonation at the single-word level may become the best esophageal speaker.

6. At this level, use steps (4) to (7) from the injection method.

Teaching Esophageal Speech with a Tracheoesophageal Puncture Shunt (TEP)

Today, most laryngectomees are candidates for the **TEP, tracheoesophageal puncture,** and the prosthetic approach to alaryngeal speech rehabilitation. In many patients the TE puncture will be done at the same time as the total laryngectomy (Hamaker and Hamaker, 1995). With the TE puncture completed at the time of laryngectomy it is possible to use the fistula for the feeding tube rather than inserting the NG tube through the nose. This is helpful and more comfortable for the patient. Also, the cricopharyngeal myotomy (weakening the PE segment by surgically cutting all the muscle fibers) often will be done at the time of laryngectomy as well. This is done to create a PE (pharyngoesophageal) segment that will not present too much resistance to the outward flow of air during phonation and will allow for adequate vibration of the PE segment during alaryngeal voice production. If the myotomy is not done at the same time as the laryngectomy, it can be done later as a secondary procedure if a too tight PE segment is indicated by esophageal insufflation testing. Esophageal insufflation testing, in which the patient's own pulmonary air is introduced into the esophagus, can demonstrate the status of the PE segment. This test will provide a prognosis for fluent TEP or traditional esophageal speech production (Blom, 1995). To conduct esophageal insufflation testing the insufflation tube is inserted into the nose and down into the PE segment. The distal end of the testing tube is fitted with a cuff that is placed over the stoma. The patient then forces lung air into the cuff, through the tube into the esophagus. Four responses are noted. The pharyngeal constrictor muscle may go into spasm and the air is difficult to control, with only a burp or single work produced, but control is not possible under the conditions of spasm. The second type of response is the hypertonic pharyngeal constrictor response, which allows the patient to produce phonation but control is still a problem. Phonation is produced effortfully in short uncontrolled segments. A third response to insufflation testing is the desired degree of constrictor tone that allows controlled sustained phonation. This response will allow phonation for eight seconds and the person can be trained to control loudness and pitch for stress purposes. The final type of response to testing is the weak or hypotonic type of constrictor muscle activity, which produces a weak breathy phonation of short duration and too high rate of airflow through the weak PE segment.

Five to seven days following fistula creation, the patient is measured for the proper fitting of the prosthesis. The fistula is dilated and the prosthesis is inserted. A good description and pictures of these procedures is provided by Blom (1995) and in McFarlane and Watterson (1995). The fitting of the correct length of the prosthesis is critical for the best TEP voice result. A prosthesis that is too short may be expelled during forceful coughing. One that is too long will make contact with the posterior esophageal wall, thus interfering with voice production and causing a leak due to malfunction of the one-way valve or fistula enlargement. The correct length is determined by placing the measuring device (Figure 8.4) into the stoma and through the punctured fistula. This will allow one to gauge the distance from the back wall of the pharynx to the opening into the stoma. When the correct prosthesis is selected the TE puncture fistula must be dilated with the dilator (Figure 8.5). Using an inserted device and a gel cap (Figure 8.6), constant firm pressure is applied until the prosthesis slips into place. The gel cap eases the insertion of the prosthesis by reducing friction and providing lubrication for the surrounding skin. The stoma is then occluded by the thumb or the finger and voice

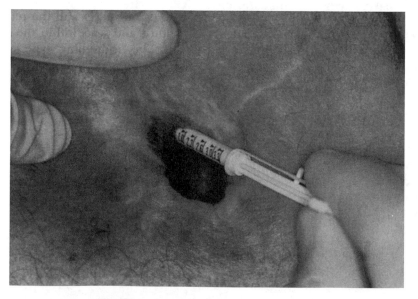

FIGURE 8.4 *Measurement of tracheoesophageal puncture tract length, i.e., distance between the posterior tracheal wall and anterior esophageal wall, using a Blom-Singer® measurement device. Used with permission of E. D. Blom.*

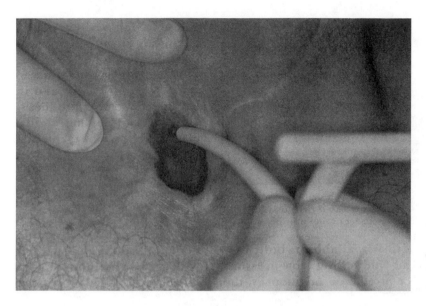

FIGURE 8.5 *A Blom-Singer® tracheoesophageal dilator is inserted through the stoma into the esophageal puncture. (Used with permission of E. D. Blom.)*

production is tested. If the prosthesis is in place and the back wall of the esophagus is not in contact with the prosthesis, then the air will be shunted into the esophagus and the PE segment will be set into vibration.

The patient who has a tracheoesophageal shunt or puncture will generally be able to develop good esophageal voice more quickly than the patient with a conventional laryngectomy. On expiration, by shutting off the open stoma with a finger or by using a one-way stoma valve, the patient is able to divert outgoing tracheal air into the Blom-Singer or other (Bivona) prosthesis, introducing air directly into the esophagus. Being able to do this negates the need for teaching the patient to trap air in the esophagus by either the injection or inhalation methods. Two types of TEP prostheses are shown in Figure 8.7.

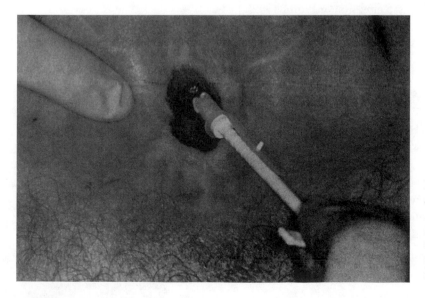

FIGURE 8.6 *Insertion of a lubricated gel cap-tipped Blom-Singer® indwelling low-pressure voice prosthesis on a safety lock inserter. Used with permission of E. D. Blom.*

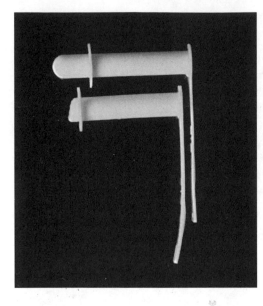

**FIGURE 8.7   Two Blom-Singer
Protheses** *The top larger prosthesis is a
modification of the original "duckbill' prosthesis inserted via a shunt through the trachea into the esophagus. The lower, slightly
smaller prosthesis is the newer low-pressure
voice prosthesis.* (Used with permission of
E. D. Blom.)

The decision must first be made whether the patient wishes to wear a one-
way valve fastened over the stoma. This valve permits air to come in from the outside on inspiration, but shuts off on expiration, allowing air to travel through the
shunt into the esophagus. Fujimoto, Madison, and Larrigan (1991) looked at the
effect of the valve on developing good voice as opposed to using finger closure of
the stoma, finding that there were no real differences in quality of voice between
the two methods. The patient who must use his or her hands in work might profit
from wearing the stoma valve; otherwise, occluding the open stoma when one
wants to speak might be best achieved by using one's finger to close off the stoma.
It does appear, however, that recent research favors the low-pressure prosthesis
(see Figure 8.7) over the duckbill prosthesis for developing the best speaking voice
(Pauloski, Fisher, Kempster, & Blom, 1989).

The teaching steps below are designed for the patient with a tracheoesophageal shunt, using finger occlusion of the stoma to speak.

1. The speech–language pathologist should review the procedures the patient
has had. The chapter by Hamaker and Hamaker (1995) is helpful here because it
summarizes most of the surgical procedures available.

2. A review of how normal voice is produced is helpful for the patient who
may never have realized, for example, that all speech in English is produced on
pulmonary expiration.

3. Practice should be given to producing precise articulation. The patient
should be encouraged to practice intraoral whispers so that the words are distinct
and clearly understandable to listeners.

4. The patient is asked to take in a normal breath, occlude his or her stoma with a
thumb or a finger, and say a monosyllabic word on expiration. It is important that

the patient be counseled to use the thumb or finger only as a diverting body to the airstream. Sending the air through the shunt (or the appliance in the shunt) does not require heavy finger pressure. Only a very light touch is required to divert the air from the stoma on expiration. If voice is achieved on the single word, the patient can go to the next step. If not, the patient should practice the timing of inspiration (open stoma) and expiration (closed stoma) in synchrony with saying one word. Trial-and-error repetitions may be needed here. Most patients can produce an effortless esophageal voice with very little difficulty. It has been our observation that patients who cannot successfully divert tracheal air through the shunt are pushing too hard with their fingers. Only light touch on the stoma opening is needed. Because patients undergo a cricopharyngeal myotomy to weaken the muscle of the PE-segment, only modest air pressure is required to set the segment into vibration.

5. Go from single words to phrases as soon as the patient can do so. It is important to keep the inspiratory breath a normal one. The patient needs no more breathing effort than he or she ever did. It takes some practice to time the inspiratory–expiratory phonation to match the words or phrases one is attempting to say.

6. Once the patient can say phrases, it has been our observation that, by using natural articulation, he or she begins injecting air into the esophagus from above and using the pulmonary air passing out through the esophagus. Therefore, some patients can speak some words and phrases without occluding their stomas, obviously renewing the air reservoir within the esophagus by injection. Extended daily practice of several hours for a week or two is required before a patient with a tracheal esophageal shunt is able to use his or her new esophageal voice conversationally.

7. Review with the patient that the best voice seems to be produced with the least amount of effort; that is, a normal speaking breath, light finger touch, and so on.

8. The patient should be instructed in how to change, clean, maintain, and care for their own prosthesis. This is not a weekly or even monthly task when the prosthesis is an indwelling device (Blom, 1995).

Anyone who is attempting to assist a patient to develop TEP speech should become thoroughly familiar with the devices, procedures, and materials involved. Blom (1995) provides guidance in patient selection, esophageal insufflation testing, indwelling prostheses, and prosthetic fitting. This information is constantly being updated.

Helping the Patient with a Laryngectomy. The patient with a new laryngectomy is facing a number of social obstacles. Research by Blood, Luther, and Stemple (1992) has found that 73 percent of forty-one laryngectomy patients showed good adjustment to their problem. Fear of cancer reoccurrence and some loss of self-esteem are among problems the patients report. The speech–language pathologist working with the laryngectomee must provide some counseling and social guidance for the patient (Renner, 1995; Salmon, 1986). The patient needs exposure to other laryngectomy patients, some participation in laryngectomy clubs, and encouragement to participate again in life activities experienced before the operation.

Successful rehabilitation after laryngectomy is highly related to the patient's overall life adjustment, coping skills, and general well-being.

Summary

In this chapter, we considered the types or modes of cancer treatment (radiation, surgery, and chemotherapy) and their effect on the voice. Some case examples that demonstrate the voice treatment approach used with patients undergoing each method of treatment were considered. Such factors as vocal fold dryness and stiffness as well as absence of tissue posttreatment were discussed. Voice facilitation techniques, which have been successful in producing vocal improvement in patients who have been treated for laryngeal cancer, were listed. These techniques were further discussed in Chapter 6.

The importance of such topics as vocal hygiene and counseling support for patients who have been treated for laryngeal cancer was presented. The treatment approaches for patients who underwent total laryngectomy are provided as well. The methods used and references for further information on these approaches are provided in the material. A variety of artificial larynges are identified and some advantages and disadvantages listed. Methods of traditional alaryngeal speech production are provided as well as up-to-date information on tracheoesophageal puncture speech production. A number of figures are presented that demonstrate laryngeal cancer and devices and procedures used in voice rehabilitation for patients who have undergone treatment for laryngeal cancer.

Therapy for Resonance Disorders

In this text the disorders of resonance are treated separately from the disorders of voice that result from the larynx being misused or from laryngeal lesions. While many of the neurological disorders discussed in Chapter 4 have a hypernasal component or resonance component, these are treated separately in that chapter. The resonance disorders of hypernasality, denasality, assimilative nasality, and oral pharyngeal resonance disorders of stridency, thin voice quality, and cul-de-sac voice will be addressed in this chapter.

The most common resonance disorder is *hypernasality* (excessive nasal resonance). It can be an early sign of a neurological disease, or it can be the result of a congenital disorder such as cleft palate. It can also result from a surgical treatment. The cause of hypernasality must be determined as a prelude to successful treatment. Hyponasality or denasality can be caused by a number of obstructions, such as nasal polyps, allergies, or hypertrophied adenoids. Another nasalance problem, assimilative nasality, must be distinguished from either hypernasality or denasality. Speech–language pathologists play a primary role in the diagnosis and treatment of various nasality problems.

Resonance is selective amplification and filtering of the complex overtone structure by the cavities of the vocal tract after the tone has been produced by the vibration of the vocal folds. Stated another way, **vocal resonance** is the perceptual increase in loudness of the laryngeal tone due to the concentration and reflection of soundwaves by the oral, pharyngeal, and nasal cavities during voice production. The vocal folds provide the source of vibration that gives rise to the complex sound waves. These periodic vibrations, characteristic of the normal voice, are filtered in the supraglottal space of the pharyngeal, oral, and nasal cavities, or the upper airway. Our discussion of resonance in Chapter 2 showed that the *F*-shaped upper airway amplifies and filters the sounds coming into it from the larynx, depending on the frequency of the sound waves and the shape and size of the particular cavity. The pharyngeal cavity constantly changes its horizontal and vertical dimensions by active movement of muscles, which in turn changes its overall configuration (Pershall and Boone, 1986; Watterson and McFarlane, 1990). The open coupling between the pharyngeal cavity and the oral cavity (particularly when the velopharyngeal mechanism is closed) enables the traveling sound wave to be further filtered by the continuous modifications of oral cavity size that occur during speech by the movements of the tongue and jaw. What emerges as voice resonance is the fundamental frequency (laryngeal vibration) modified by the natural resonant frequencies occurring at the various supraglottal sites (above the vocal folds), within the pharynx, and through the oral cavity. When the velopharyngeal port is open, the pharyngeal–oral coupling with the nasal cavity is then possible so that sound waves are further absorbed and filtered as they pass through the chambers of the nasal cavity, as for the production of /m/, /n/, and /ng/ in English. When the pharyngeal–oral cavity and the nasal cavity are inappropriately coupled, structural (e.g., cleft palate) or functional (by habit), this may cause some of the most common nasal resonance problems. We consider the evaluation, management, and therapy of nasal resonance problems in this chapter.

Nasal Resonance Problems

Under the broad heading of nasal resonance fall three types of disorders: hypernasality, denasality, and assimilative nasality. Although individuals listening to speakers with these problems might only be able to say, "the voices all sound nasal," distinct differences among the three types call for differential diagnosis and management and different voice therapy approaches. As a prelude to our discussion of separate approaches, let us define the three terms:

Track 5

Hypernasality

Hypernasality is an excessively undesirable amount of perceived nasal cavity resonance during the phonation of normally nonnasal vowels and nonnasal voiced consonants. Voiced consonants and vowel production in the English language are primarily characterized by oral resonance with only slightly nasalized components being acceptable. If the oral and nasal cavities are tightly coupled to one another by lack of velopharyngeal closure (for whatever reason), the periodic sound waves carrying laryngeal vibration will receive heavy resonance within the nasal cavity. Only three phonemes of the English language should receive the degree of nasal prominence produced by an open velopharyngeal port: /m/, /n/, and /ng/.

Denasality

Denasality is the lack of nasal resonance for the three nasalized phonemes /m/, /n/, and /ng/. In the strictest sense, therefore, denasality could be categorized as an articulatory substitution disorder. Generally, denasality also affects vowels, in that the normal speaker gives some minor nasal resonance to vowels. A voice with this inadequate nasal resonance sounds like the voice of a normal speaker suffering from a severe head cold and stuffed up nose.

Assimilative Nasality

In assimilative nasality, the speaker's vowels appear nasal when adjacent to the three nasal consonants. The velopharyngeal port is opened too soon and remains open too long, so that vowel resonance preceding and following nasal consonant resonance is also nasalized.

Normal English consonants are produced with high intraoral pressures (3 to 8 cm H_2O) with essentially no nasal airflow except for the three nasal consonants, which have low intraoral pressures (0.5 to 1.5 cm H_2O) and high rates of nasal airflow (100 to 300 cc sec), as reported by Mason and Warren (1980). Aerodynamic studies of cleft palate speakers and problems of excessive nasality have provided some needed quantification to help differentiate patients with excessive nasal resonance from patients lacking sufficient nasal resonance (Warren, 1979). From his studies of air pressures and airflow patterns, Warren has estimated the size of the velopharyngeal (VP) port. Although most normal speakers demonstrate tight velopharyngeal closure with no air leakage (Thompson, 1978), speakers with openings as small as 5 mm or less may still have voice quality that is perceived by listeners as normal (Mason and Warren, 1980). Patients with nasal voices who produce high nasal airflow rates are perceived (we stress *perceived* because hypernasality is a perceptual phenomenon that can only occur on voiced sounds) as having hypernasality, whereas denasality is perceived as a speaker with a cold or stuffed up nose and is accompanied by low nasal airflows, due to a plugged nasal passage (e.g., nasal polyps or swollen turbinates) or a closed VP mechanism. Probably no area of voice therapy is more neglected or more confusing than therapy for nasal resonance problems.

Historically, the implication in the early literature was that most problems of nasality (usually hypernasality) could be successfully treated by voice therapy—that is, by ear training, or by blowing exercises (Kantner, 1947), or by the exercises for the velum suggested by Buller (1942), or by the treatment Williamson used for seventy-two cases of hypernasality, which put some emphasis on relaxing the entire vocal tract (1945). Most of these early approaches were developed for functional hypernasality, but were later applied by various clinicians to organically based problems of palatal insufficiency and cleft palate. For most of these structural problems and most neurological disorders, however, such approaches as blowing and relaxation were ineffective. If the velopharyngeal mechanisms were structurally and neurologically unable to produce velopharyngeal closure, no amount of relaxation or exercise could have much effect in reducing excessive nasal resonance by closing an inadequate velopharyngeal port mechanism. Realistic management and therapy for any problem in nasal resonance, therefore, requires that the patient have a thorough differential evaluation, including detailed examination of the VP mechanism, aerodynamic studies, functional speech–voice testing, a detailed acoustical and perceptual analysis of voice, and videoendoscopic studies (McFarlane, 1990; Watterson and McFarlane, 1990; Watterson, 1991).

Evaluation of Nasal Resonance Disorders

There are more similarities than differences between patients with resonance disorders and those with phonation disorders. For this reason, the evaluational procedures outlined in Chapter 5 are equally relevant here. In addition to obtaining the necessary medical data (such as what treatment has already been provided), clinicians must pursue case history information (description of the problem and its cause, description of daily voice use, variations of the problem, onset and duration of the problem, and so on). Clinicians must observe closely how well the patients seem to function in the clinic and during out-of-clinic situations. Considering how subjective our judgments of resonance disorders are, it is crucial that clinicians know how their patients perceive their own voices. A mild resonance problem, for example, can be perceived by a patient and/or others as severe, but a severe resonance problem, at times, may be ignored. Indeed, some consider the popular country and western singers Willie Nelson and George Jones as hypernasal, whereas others think that they sing with an "authentic regional twang."

Track 5

Analysis of Voice in Speech.   An obvious way to begin the evaluation of someone with a nasal resonance disorder is to listen carefully to his or her voice during spontaneous conversation. This can provide a gross indication of what the problem may be (assimilative nasality, hypernasality, or denasality). The perceptual aspect of nasal resonance disorders is extremely important. It is, however, difficult to make a clinical judgment about nasality by listening to someone as he or she speaks; in fact, such a judgment is likely to be wrong. For example, Bradford, Brooks, and Shelton (1964) found that neither a group of four experienced judges nor one of four inexperienced judges could reliably judge the recorded voice samples of children producing /a/ and /i/ with nares open and closed (by digital pressure). This may not be too surprising because both vowels are basically nonnasal in English. The judges were similarly unreliable when judging nasality from conversational speech samples. Although the casual judgment that "something is nasal about the speech" is usually correct, few examiners can quickly and reliably differentiate the type of nasality (hypernasality, assimilative nasality, denasality) on the basis of such a conversational sample alone. Voice quality judgments are more accurate if made on the basis of tape-recorded samples of a patient's conversational speech, his or her vowels in isolation, and his or her sentences (some with only oral phonemes and some loaded with nasal phonemes). Loading sentences with nasal phonemes is helpful for making judgments of denasal speech. The taped sample allows the clinician repeated playback. Focusing on a specific parameter (loudness pitch, quality, nasal versus denasal) on each playback may increase the clinician's objectivity. To counter the "halo" effect—the influence of a speaker's articulation on the judgment of his or her nasality—Sherman (1954) developed a procedure of playing the connected speech sample backward on the tape recorder, thus precluding the identification of any articulation errors. Reverse playback is most helpful in differentiating between hypernasality and denasality. Spriestersbach (1955) found that the reverse playback of speech samples of cleft palate subjects reduced the correlations between articulation proficiency–pitch level and judgments of nasality. We have found that asking patients to repeat or read aloud passages that are totally free of nasal consonants, such as "Betty Takes Bob to the Show" (Boone, 1993), or passages that are loaded with nasal consonants, such as "Many Men in the Moon" (Boone, 1993), helps us differentiate hypernasality, denasality, and assimilative nasality from one another. It is important to note that hypernasality occurs only on vowels, semivowels, and voiced consonants. Using phrases loaded with nasal consonants is used only to demonstrate denasality. The absence of normal nasal resonance on these nasally loaded phrases is diagnostic of denasality or hyponasality.

We have also found that if we use the following simple screening procedures, we get a good, quick clinical classification of the type of resonance disorder present. These quick tests are simple and require no instruments to perform.

First, we have the patient say these two sentences while holding the nose: "My name means money" and "Mary may make many messes." If these sound "plugged" both when the nose is held and when the nose is released, the problem is denasality. In other words, if there is no difference between the nose-held and nose-released conditions, the problem is denasality. If there is a big difference between the nose-held and nose-released conditions then the problem is likely hypernasality.

Another simple clinical technique is called the "snap release /s/." We have the patient sustain a loud /s/ while the nose is held and quickly released. If a "snap" is heard on releasing the nose, this means the VP mechanism is partially open and the problem is probably hypernasality. The actual "snap" is nasal air emission but gives a clue of the status of the VP mechanism. While hypernasality is a phenomenon of voiced sounds only, this technique is using a nonvoiced sound /s/ to test the adequacy of closure of the VP mechanism. This is done because there is more intraoral breath pressure required for a voiceless consonant, /s/, than a voiced consonant.

Next, we have the patient say, "This horse eats grass" and "I see the teacher at church." If we hear any "snorting" back in the pharynx, we can assume that it is probably due to inadequate closure of the velopharyngeal port and that the problem with this speaker's voice is hypernasality.

We next ask the patient to say, "Maybe baby, maybe baby." If there is no difference between the two words (*maybe* and *baby*) and both sound like *maybe* the problem is hypernasality; however, if both words sound like *baby* the problem is denasality.

Finally, we ask the patient to sustain the /i/ and the /u/ vowels, while we gently flutter the nose (**nasal flutter test**) by occluding the nares with the thumb and forefinger. If we hear a pulsing change in the acoustic signal, the problem is hypernasality. Patients with hypernasality often have laryngeal abnormalities, as well. For example, children with velopharyngeal closure problems are reported to have a higher than normal incidence of vocal cord nodules and polyps (McWilliams, Lavorato, and Bluestone, 1973). Therefore, the clinician must not only make judgments about resonance abnormality, he or she must also listen closely to voice quality (for problems of hoarseness, loudness, and breathiness, etc.). The voice sample then should be analyzed for resonance, vocal quality, and articulation. Besides listening to the voice, the clinician must employ stimulability testing (to assess the functional potential for improvement) and other testing techniques.

Stimulability Testing. Although stimulability testing was designed for use with problems of articulation, it is also effective with problems of voice. The basic purpose of stimulability testing, as first described by Milisen (1957), was to see how well the patient can produce an errored sound when he or she is repeatedly presented with the correct sound through both auditory and visual stimuli. One way of distinguishing between true problems of velopharyngeal structure (the mechanism is wholly incapable of adequate closure) and functional velopharyngeal inadequacy (the mechanism has the capability of closure) is to see if the patient can produce oral resonance under stimulability conditions (Morris and Smith, 1962). Obviously, the patient's success in producing oral resonance would be a strong indication that velopharyngeal closure is possible. Shelton, Hahn, and Morris (1968) have observed:

> If repeated stimulation consistently results in consonant productions, which are distorted by nasal emission and vowels which are unpleasantly nasal, the inference can be drawn, at least tentatively, that the individual is not able to change his speaking behavior because of velopharyngeal incompetence (p. 236).

Success in producing oral resonance under conditions of stimulability would be a good indicator for voice therapy. It is also a favorable prognostic sign.

Another simple stimulability test is to hold the patient's velum up with a tongue depressor while fluttering the nose during the patient's production of a sustained /i/ vowel. Next, remove the tongue depressor and repeat the process listening for a difference in resonance. If the difference is dramatic the patient will likely not be able to benefit from voice–speech therapy alone but will require a palatal lift, speech obturator, or surgical management. Watterson and McFarlane (1990) describe five classes of velopharyngeal function based on videoendoscopic observations during speech testing. The classes of VP function are: (1) Normal VP function, (2) Consistent VPI (velopharyngeal incompetency), (3) Task Specific VPI, (4) Irregular VPI, and (5) Abnormal Resonance without VPI.

Articulation Testing.   Articulatory proficiency can provide a good index of a patient's velopharyngeal closure. *Nasal emission,* the escape of air through the nose, is a most common articulation error on plosive and fricative phonemes among subjects with inadequate velopharyngeal closure. Even though a patient may have his or her articulators in the correct position, in relation to their lingual–alveolar–labial contacts, the error occurs because increased oral pressure escapes nasally through the incomplete posterior palatal closure. The presence or absence of nasal emission, therefore, is a most important diagnostic sign of velopharyngeal adequacy. It is important in articulation testing to distinguish between errors that result from faulty articulatory positioning and errors related to inadequacy of the velopharyngeal structure.

An excellent articulation test for assessing competency of velopharyngeal closure is found in the forty-three special test items from the Templin-Darley Tests of Articulation (Templin and Darley, 1980), known as the Iowa Pressure Articulation Test. This test is particularly sensitive for identifying the presence of nasal emission during the production of certain consonants. However, any standardized articulation test is useful for determining those phonemes that are distorted because of inadequate velopharyngeal closure. The clinician must closely assess the identified errors to determine if lingual placements are accurate to make the target phoneme correctly. Many younger children with velopharyngeal problems exhibit sound substitutions and omission errors in addition to the nasal emission and nasal snort distortion they produce because of inadequate velar closure. Older children and adults with nasal emission problems may well have correct articulatory lingual placements, and their distortions are a product of posterior nasal escape of the air stream. Following successful pharyngeal flap surgery or the proper fitting of an appliance, nasal emission sometimes continues until it is modified through speech remediation. The past learning and the muscular "set" for making distorted nasal emission may continue even though the closure mechanism may now be considered normal. It is usually possible, however, to eliminate nasal emission through therapy, once structural adequacy has been achieved.

The sixteen so-called pressure consonants provide the best test of the adequacy of the velopharyngeal mechanism. These pressure consonants—/p, b, k, g, t, d, f, v, s, z, sh, ʒ, ʤ, ʧ, θ, ɤ/—should be included in any testing of the adequacy of the velopharyngeal port mechanism, because these sounds require the greatest degree of VP closure and greatest intraoral air pressure. Denasality in its purest and most overt form would be exhibited on an articulation test with these oral substitutions for the nasal phonemes: /b/m/, /d/n/, and /g/ng/. The sentence "My name means money" would be produced, for example, as "By dabe beads buddy."

Assimilative nasality would be observable only for vowels in words containing nasal phonemes. Nasal emission would be most common in patients with palatal insufficiency in affricates (such as /tʃ/), fricatives (such as /s/), and plosives (such as /p/). Clinicians should be alert to the relatively high number of articulation errors often present in the speech of patients with cleft palate or those with VPI unrelated to cleft palate. In fact, from a speech therapy point of view, there is often more merit in focusing on articulation errors in cases of cleft palate than on resonance per se; as speech intelligibility improves, the hypernasality of these patients interferes less and less with effective communication. The type of articulation test or tasks used to assess articulatory proficiency is a matter of clinical choice. However, with the increasing availability of diagnostic aids for determining adequacy of velopharyngeal closure, clinicians must not abandon their articulation assessments, which may well be among the most valid tools for indirectly diagnosing velopharyngeal inadequacy during speech tasks. In addition to the most obvious articulation errors in the speech of patients with velopharyngeal inadequacy, such as glottal stops and pharyngeal fricatives, errors may include tongue tip sounds made too far back in the mouth, posterior productions of other sounds and weakened plosives, fricatives, and affricates.

The Oral Examination.   It should be stated that oral examination provides the least amount of information about the function and status of the velopharyngeal port mechanism of all procedures that the speech–language pathologist can perform. That is to say that, because the actual closure of the VP mechanism is made behind and above the level of the velum, the port is hidden from direct view through the oral cavity. Thus, viewing with an oral endoscope from below or viewing from above by means of a nasendoscope, or using videofluoroscopy techniques, airflow techniques, or indirect methods, such as articulation testing or nasal flutter testing, will all provide better and more usable evidence of the adequacy of VP function than will direct unaided oral inspection of the velum.

However, by direct visual examination, the clinician can make a gross observation of the relationship of the velum to the pharynx, note the relative size of the tongue, make a judgment of maxillary–mandibular occlusion, view the height of the palatal arch, survey the general condition of dentition, and determine if there are any clefts or open fistulas in the palate. Remember that direct visualization of palatal length and movement provides only a very gross indication of velopharyngeal closure, because the anatomic point of closure is superior by some distance to the lower border of the velum. That is, a lack of velar contact with the pharynx at the uvular-tip end of the velum is not an indication of lack of closure further up, where closure usually occurs. Conversely, the touching of the uvula to the posterior pharyngeal wall is not an indication of adequate VP function and closure. A markedly short palate or a palate with obvious pharyngeal contact can be noted on direct inspection of the oral cavity, and such a notation would be diagnostically important as an indicator of the need for further evaluatiuon of VP function. However, the presence of hypernasalitay is also an indication of the need for further evaluation of the VP mechanism. The less obvious problems of borderline closure cannot be determined by direct inspection and probably require videoendoscopic or fluorographic confirmation, which we discuss in the next section.

Only the **presence or absence** of velar movement can be determined with some validity by directly viewing the soft palate. It is extremely important to know the status of the VP mechanism when crucial management decisions are being made, that is, when it is being decided whether a child should have a pharyngeal flap, an appliance, or speech therapy (which we discuss in the section on the treatment of hypernasality). Direct oral observation is only possible during vowel productions; however, the degree of closure of the velopharyngeal port is more critical on consonants (especially voiceless consonants) and consonant clusters than on vowels. A degree of openness is acceptable on vowels that is not acceptable on consonants. Thus, instrumentation needs to be employed to make accurate observations during the critical production of consonants. Zwitman (1990) describes the use of oral endoscopy for observation of the VP mechanism during vowel production and plosive–vowel production. Watterson and McFarlane (1990) describe the use of nasal videoendoscopy for making valid observations of the VP mechanism during connected speech.

Velar movement is sometimes impaired in what might appear (through oral inspection) to be a normally symmetrical palate; here, the patient has a sluggish palate, sometimes as a symptom following a severe infectious disease (influenza, encephalitis, and so on). It cannot be emphasized enough that adequacy of pharyngeal movement is almost impossible to determine by direct oral examination alone; it is best seen by lateral-view videofluorographic film or with endoscopy (nasal or oral).

In some problems of nasality, particularly those not associated with palatal insufficiency, the relative size and carriage of the tongue may have some diagnostic relevance. For example, some problems of "functional" nasality may be related to inappropriate size of the tongue for the size of the oral cavity, or to innervation problems of the tongue.

The clinician should make a thorough search for any openings of the hard or soft palate that might contribute to an articulation distortion or to some problem of nasal resonance. Some patients have small openings (fistulas) or lack of fusion around the border of the premaxilla, particularly in the area of the alveolar ridge. In some individuals such fistulas may produce airstream noises, creating articulatory distortion (by loss of intraoral air pressure), but almost never will such isolated openings this far forward on the maxilla produce nasal resonance.

The absence or presence of soft-palate and hard-palate clefts should be noted; if such clefts have been previously corrected surgically, the degree of closure should be noted. In the case of a bony-palate defect, for example, sometimes the bony opening has been covered by a thin layer of mucosal tissue, not thick enough to prevent oral cavity sound waves from traveling into the nasal cavity. This same observation applies to the occasional submucosal cleft at the midline of the junction of the hard and soft palates. The major signs of a submucosal cleft are bifid or split uvula, inverted A-shape defect in the velum, lack of a palpable posterior nasal spine, or a thin soft palate (which may appear darker in color) in the midline portion. Any other structural deviations—of dentition, occlusion, labial competence, and so on—should be noted and considered with regard to their possible effects on speech production and nasal resonance.

Evaluation Procedures.   Many instruments available today can help the clinician evaluate various aspects of nasal resonance. These instruments can also be valuable in the process of deciding what to do for a patient with a nasalization problem. We consider separately instruments that provide aerodynamic data, acoustic information, radiographic visualization, and visual probe information.

Aerodynamic Instruments.   Pressure transducers and pneumotachometers are instruments of choice for measuring the relative air pressures and airflows emitted simultaneously from the nasal and oral cavities during speech (Warren, 1979). There are other instruments that measure pressure and flow. As mentioned in Chapter 5, the Phonatory Function Analyzer is a good instrument for airflow measures and can be used with a tube in the mouth or with a face mask. The Aerophone is a device that combines airflow and air pressure measurement capabilities. Pressure and flow data are measured from the two channels simultaneously, which permits relative comparisons. Normal speakers, except during the production of nasal consonants, exhibit relatively no nasal pressure or flow. Speakers with nasality problems show deviations in the relative amount of nasal and oral flows, as is well documented in the work of Mason and Warren (1980) and Warren (1979). The aerodynamic procedures basically provide the clinician information about possible leakage through the nose when the velopharyngeal mechanism should be closed. Manometers have also been useful for measuring relative nasal–oral airflows. Manometers measure the amount of pressure of the emitted airstream and do not measure resonance per se; as we have mentioned resonance is a perceptual event. Two types of manometers are used clinically, the water-filled U-tube and the mechanical pressure gauge. Both of these measure airflow pressure and not nasality; however, in comparing oral with nasal readings, some indication of velopharyngeal competence is given, which may, of course, have some relevance to the judgment of nasality. The water-filled U-tube works this way: A glass U-tube is partially filled with a colored liquid, and one end of the tube is fitted into a rubber hose. The free end of the hose is fitted with a nasal olive. The olive is placed nasally, and any utterance of the patient that is characterized by nasal emission will displace the liquid and thus provide the patient and clinician with some visual evidence of nasal emission. The second type of manometer, a mechanical pressure gauge, is available but it has not proven to be an effective clinical tool for evaluating poor velopharyngeal function. Again, the modern clinician and voice scientist will use instruments such as the Aerophone by Kay Elemetrics and the Phonatory Function Analyzer by Nagashima.

Acoustic Instruments.   Historically, the Tonar II was designed by Fletcher (1972) to provide relative data of the acoustic signal emitted from both the oral and nasal cavities: how much of the perceived voice signal is "coming" through the nose, how much from the mouth? The Tonar II, which is no longer available, provided for a running speech sample and continuous feedback of the oral–nasal acoustic ratio, which was displayed on the instrument display panel. Because the oral–nasal acoustic ratio fluctuates with each utterance, a one-second or ten-second averaging could be set on the instrument by the clinician. The patient was asked to read or repeat a continuous verbal passage, speaking directly into the two separate microphones, one receiving the oral signal and one the nasal signal. The oral signal value was divided into the nasal signal value to yield the actual oral–nasal acoustic ratio, a process that was done automatically at one- or ten-second intervals (depending on the interval set by the clinician) by the Tonar II (Fletcher, 1972). The typical speaker with normal nasal resonance will experience a "top" oral–nasal ratio of under 10 percent. Speakers with severe hypernasality will experience ratios in excess of 80 percent. One advantage of using the Tonar II to analyze relative nasality was that it provided a continuous value specific to relative nasal and oral resonance in running speech.

The Kay Elemetrics Nasometer is a modern instrument that provides both diagnostic and ongoing therapeutic feedback of oral–nasal resonance. A picture of a clinician and patient using the Nasometer may be seen in Figure 9.1. Using the Nasometer in a study of twenty children with normal VP function and twenty children at risk for velopharyngeal insufficiency, Watterson, Hinton, and McFarlane (1996) constructed and tested two novel stimuli for obtaining nasalance measures from young children in an attempt to establish a cutoff score between normal and excessive nasalance. The new passages constructed and studied were the Turtle Passage and the Mouse Passage. The Turtle Passage contained no normally nasal consonants while the Mouse Passage contained about 11 percent nasal consonants. They concluded that "Clinicians should have least confidence in nasalance scores for patients who are borderline normal. Because borderline normal patients are difficult to classify, however, absolute nasalance cutoff scores may never be a reality" (p. 72). Watterson, Lewis, and Deutsch (1998) used the Kay Elemetrics 6200 Nasometer to study nasalance and nasality in low and high pressure speech. They concluded from their study of twenty children with managed clefts and five children without clefts that, "Sensitivity and specificity scores indicated that the Nasometer was reasonably accurate in distinguishing between normal and hypernasal speech samples."

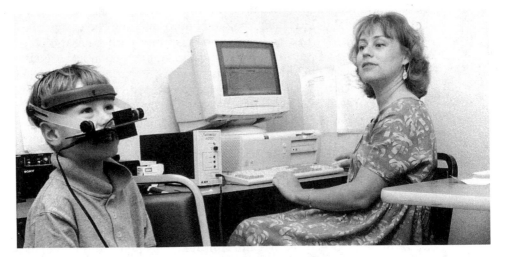

FIGURE 9.1 *A five-year-old boy wears the oral–nasal dual microphones for determining his oral–nasal ratio on the Nasometer.*

Indeed, the **Nasometer** and the **CSL, Computerized Speech Laboratory** by Kay Elemetrics have proven to be very helpful to patients in the hands of skillful and knowledgable clinicians and represent an improvement from the instruments used earlier (Murry and Doherty, 1980; Takahashi and Koike, 1975).

It has been demonstrated spectrographically that speakers with increased nasalization demonstrate more prominent third formants with an increase in formant band width, accompanied by a rise in fundamental frequency. In his acoustic study of nasality using the spectrograph, Dickson (1962), concluded that there was no way to "differentiate nasality in cleft palate and non–cleft palate individuals either in terms of their acoustic spectra or the variability of the nasality judgments" (p. 111). It is doubtful that the visual write-out provided by the spectrograph can provide the clinician with any more information about the type of nasality he or she hears than does listening carefully to the same samples. The spectrograph and CSL can help identify the aperiodic noise of nasal emission, but differentiating between spectrograms of speakers with hypernasality and those with denasality or assimilative nasality is most difficult. As clinicians learn to use the spectral analyses the spectrograph and CSL can provide, however, these instruments may well become most useful tools for studying various parameters of nasality. The CSL may be seen in Figure 9.2 and was discussed in Chapter 5.

The Nasometer is a newer and advanced adaptation of the Tonar II and is clinically very useful. It provides visual feedback on a computer screen for the patient that allows the clinician to set a predetermined level of acceptable nasal–oral ratio. The peak of nasal productions is also demonstrated on the screen. Watterson, McFarlane, and Wright (1993) discuss some of the problems with measurements of nasalance using the Nasometer. Hardin, Van DeMark, Morris, and Payne (1992) also discuss some the cautions in using the Nasometer scores and its data measurements when compared to perceptual judgments. The work of Watterson and others (1995; 1998) discusses nasometer use and its clinically important information.

Radiographic Instruments.   Radiographic studies of the velopharyngeal mechanism during speech provide ready information about structural and physiological limitations of the mechanism in those patients who demonstrate velopharyngeal incompetence. For example, through a lateral-view film we can determine the relative amount of velopharyngeal opening during speech, the length of the velum, relative movements of the velum and the posterior pharyngeal wall, and so on

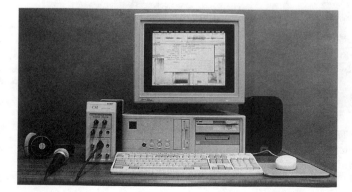

FIGURE 9.2 *The Computerized Speech Lab (CSL) offers hardware specifications and software programs both for voice evaluation and voice therapy. Its accompanying CD-ROM offers excellent patient samples of voice disorders, including many with resonance deviations. Shown here with permission of Kay Elemetrics Corp., Lincoln Park, New Jersey.*

(Bowman and Shanks, 1978). However, there are limitations to the use of lateral views attempting to view closure, because lateral wall movement of the pharynx, which may contribute heavily to velopharyngeal closure, cannot be visualized. Sometimes the patient is asked to swallow barium and, as the barium passes through the pharynx, measurements are made of the relative pharyngeal opening as it relates to the velopharyngeal closing mechanism (Skolnick, Glaser, and McWilliams, 1980). The most useful radiographic views of velopharyngeal closure require the patient to make some speech utterances, including phrases and sentences that include pressure consonants. The speech–language pathologist needs to work closely with the radiologist, presenting the speech tasks as the films are made and "reading" the films when they are completed. Sometimes a radiographic display can demonstrate a problem in velopharyngeal closure that cannot be detected by any other method except for nasovideoendoscopy.

Visual Probe Instruments.   Shelton and Trier (1976) have written that direct measures of velopharyngeal competence through the use of "endoscopes, nasopharyngoscopes, and ultrasound apparatus" offer some advantages in making treatment decisions. The oral endoscope (Zwitman, Gyepes, and Ward, 1976) has been a useful instrument for determining the degree and type of velopharyngeal closure, as shown in Figure 9.3. The body of the oral endoscope is extended above the tongue within the oral cavity so that the lighted tip and viewing window lie just below the uvula and within the oropharyngeal opening. By turning the viewing window up toward the velopharyngeal area, the velum, the lateral pharyngeal walls, and the posterior pharynx may be visualized. Two views of varying degrees of velopharyngeal closure in the same subject are shown in Figure 9.3. One important disadvantage of the oral endoscope is that one can only observe vowel or limited consonant and vowel combinations such as /pa/ of /ba/. This is due to the unnatural introduction of the oral endoscope into the oral cavity and its effect on articulation and connected speech (McFarlane, 1990).

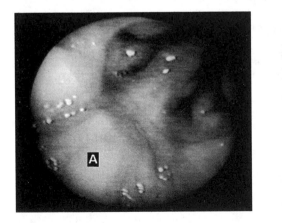
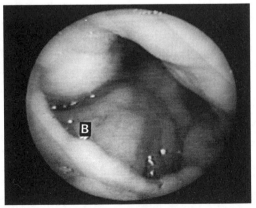

FIGURE 9.3   Velopharyngeal Closure *This oral videoendoscopic view of velopharyngeal closure demonstrates two degrees of closure in a sequence from (A) an open v-p mechanism, through (B) the bulging of Passavant's Pad with posterior and lateral pharyngeal wall movement and the velar movement.*

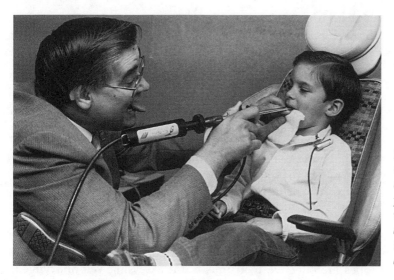

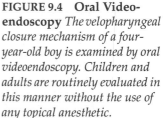

FIGURE 9.4   Oral Video-endoscopy *The velopharyngeal closure mechanism of a four-year-old boy is examined by oral videoendoscopy. Children and adults are routinely evaluated in this manner without the use of any topical anesthetic.*

For many of us who work in the area of cleft palate or who work with those who have velopharyngeal inadequacy due to structural defects (such as postcancer surgery) or neurological defect (such as one of the dysarthrias, discussed in Chapter 4) the use of nasovideoendoscopy of the VP mechanism has become the "gold standard." With nasal endoscopy one can assess the complex function of the VP mechanism during the dynamic speech act. Watterson and McFarlane (1990) discuss in detail the use of transnasal videoendoscopy of the velopharyngeal port mechanism. They discuss the use of sustained vowels, sustained consonants, single words and sentences, and phrases as speech stimuli in speech testing for VP competency. The use of high vowels such as /i/ and /u/ as well as stops (/p/ /t/), fricatives, and affricates allows for the examiner to make important statements about the ability of the VP mechanism to successfully manage complex speech tasks. The information gained by using such stimuli will guide therapy and management decisions. For example, it is important to know if the patient is always having nasal air escape on a particular phoneme, such as /s/, or if there is only a breakdown of the VP function at the phrase level or when the /s/ is in the context of a blend.

In the September 1998 ASHA Supplement No. 18, a joint statement by the American Academy of Otolaryngology Voice and Swallow Committee and by ASHA indicated that,

> Strobovideolaryngoscopy (including rigid and flexible endoscopy) is a laryngeal imaging procedure that may be used by otolaryngologists and other voice professionals as a diagnostic procedure.... Speech–language pathologists with expertise in voice disorders and with specialized training in strobovideolaryngoscopy are professionals qualified to use this procedure for the purpose of assessing voice production and vocal function.

As McFarlane (1990) and Boone and McFarlane (1994) have indicated, even children can be examined with naso- or orovideoendoscopy without the use of any topical anesthetics. Figure 9.4 shows a child being examined with nasoendoscopy

(Figure 5.7) without the aid of topical anesthesia. Indeed, in a recent prospective, double-blind study, Leder, Ross, Briskin, and Sasaki (1997) concluded that "speech–language pathologists can perform independent and comfortable transnasal endoscopy without administration of any substance to the nasal mucosa" (p. 1352).

Distinct variations in patterns of velopharyngeal closure have been demonstrated by Zwitman, Sonderman, and Ward (1974) and Zwitman (1990). Some subjects have only velar movement without associated pharyngeal wall movement, some subjects primarily have lateral and posterior pharyngeal wall constriction, and some subjects achieve closure by a combination of velar and pharyngeal movements. With a nasal fiberoptic endoscope, which places a small flexible scope through the nose and down into the pharynx, the clinician can see velopharyngeal closure from above the closure site (Miyazaki, Matsuya, and Yamaoka, 1975; Watterson and McFarlane, 1990) and the dynamics of VP function can been studied. The primary advantage of the flexible endoscope is that it is not invasive to the oral cavity and consequently does not impede tongue, lip, or jaw movements during dynamic articulation (a limitation of the oral endoscope). The oral and nasal endoscopic probes are effective instruments for assessing velopharyngeal competence in patients with nasal resonance problems, because they offer direct observation of velar length and movement, degree of lateral and posterior pharyngeal wall movement, and the kind of velopharyngeal closure the patient is using. Perhaps, most importantly, this examination allows the clinician and the patient to see the various types and degrees of velopharyngeal closure during a variety of phonetic contexts. As mentioned earlier, Watterson and McFarlane (1990) have described five useful classes of VP function and provide a basis for making recommendations for clinical treatment.

Treatment of Nasal Resonance Disorders

Hypernasality.   The presence of excessive nasal resonance (hypernasality) is relatively dependent on the judgment of the listener. That is, some languages and regional dialects require heavy nasal resonance and therefore consider pronounced nasalization of vowels to be normal. Others, however, such as general U.S. English, tolerate little nasal resonance beyond the three nasal consonants. Thus, a native New Englander with a nasal "twang" exhibits normal voice resonance in Portland, Maine, but when he or she travels to New Knoxville, Ohio, the people there perceive his or her voice as excessively nasal. Variations do exist in the degree of nasality among the voices of the people in Ohio, of course, but a certain amount of resonance variability can exist among any particular population without anyone being bothered by it. If, however, a particular voice in Ohio (or any other place) stands out as "excessively nasal," then that voice will be considered to have a resonance disorder. The judgment of hypernasality, then, is as dependent on the speech–language milieu of the speaker and his or her listeners as it is on the actual performance of the speaker.

The speaker who is judged to be hypernasal increases the nasalization of his or her vowels by failing to close his or her velopharyngeal port. This failure to close the velopharyngeal opening may be related to structural–organic defects, or it may have a functional etiology. Hypernasality frequently accompanies unrepaired cleft palate or a short palate. Among other organic causes of the disorder are surgical trauma (e.g., postadenoidectomy), accidental injury to the soft palate, and impaired innervation of the soft palate as a result of poliomyelitis or some other form of bulbar disease. Sometimes temporary hypernasality may follow surgical removal of the adenoids and tonsils as the patient attempts to minimize the pain by not moving his or her velopharyngeal mechanism. But when hypernasality persists for two or three months or more following adenoidectomy or tonsillectomy, the adequacy of the velopharyngeal mechanism must be suspected and evaluated. Some people speak with hypernasal resonance for purely functional reasons, perhaps to maintain a lingering internal model of a previously acceptable form of resonance, or perhaps to imitate the voice of someone they consider particularly attractive (such as a famous political figure or performer). Although the majority of people with hypernasal voices probably have some structural basis for their lack of velopharyngeal competence, the ease of imitating a hypernasal voice tells us that it could be relatively easy to become hypernasal with perfectly adequate and normal velopharyngeal equipment. Hypernasality is one voice problem in which the distinction must be made between organic and functional causes, as the treatment recommended is quite specific to the diagnosis.

If there are any indications of physical inadequacy of velopharyngeal closure, the primary role of the speech pathologist is to refer the patient to a specialist who can provide the needed physical correction, a plastic surgeon, say, or a prosthodontist. The speech–language pathologist will make the determination of the mechanism's adequacy for speech purposes and together the patient and other professionals will determine the best corrective approach. If surgery is selected, the speech pathologist will share the results of the speech–voice evaluation to aid with the selection of an appropriate surgical procedure. Postsurgically, the speech–language pathologist will evaluate the repaired VP mechanism to determine its adequacy for speech–language production. If dental appliances are to be selected, the speech–language pathologist will suggest the type of appliance, lift or prosthesis with a bulb, and the SLP will assist with the design and fitting of the appliance. If a prosthetic form of management is used, then the speech pathologist will be involved in the initial fabrication and fitting of the velar lift or obturator. Subsequent modifications of these devices will be directed by the speech pathologist, based on the results of his or her speech testing and the patient's response to clinical speech stimulation. There is very little evidence that voice therapy to improve resonance has any positive effect in the presence of physical inadequacy. In fact, there is some indication that voice therapy to improve the oral resonance of patients with palatal insufficiency (those who lack the physical equipment to produce closure) will usually not only fail, but will also be interpreted by the patient as his or her own fault—as a defeat indicating low personal worth—and thus will take an obvious toll on the patient's self-image. An example of the uselessness of speech therapy in the presence of a severe inadequacy of velopharyngeal closure is provided by this case of a teenage girl who had received speech therapy for both articulation and resonance for a period of seven years:

> Barbara, aged fourteen, had received seven years of group and individual speech therapy in the public schools and in a community speech and hearing clinic for "a

severe articulation defect characterized by sibilant distortion, and for a severely nasal voice." Barbara's mother became upset because of Barbara's continued lack of progress and her tendency to withdraw from social contact with her peers, which, the mother felt, was related to her embarrassment over her continued poor speech. Barbara was evaluated by a comprehensive cleft-palate team, which, after reviewing her history, found that her nasality dated from a severe bout of influenza when she was six years old. The influenza had been followed immediately by a deterioration of speech. Subsequent speech therapy records were incomplete, although the mother reported that the therapy had included extensive blowing drills, tongue–palate exercises, and articulation work. Physical examination of the velar mechanism found that Barbara had good tongue and pharyngeal movements, but bilateral paralysis of the soft palate; even on gag reflex stimulation, only a "flicker" of palatal movement was observed. Lateral cinefluorographic films confirmed the relatively complete absence of velar movement. The examining speech pathologist found that Barbara had normal articulation placement of the tongue for all speech sounds, despite severe nasal emission of airflow for fricative and affricate phonemes. Low back vowels were relatively oral in resonance, whereas middle and high vowels became increasingly nasal. It was the consensus of the evaluation team that, with her structural inadequacy, Barbara was (and had been) a poor candidate for speech therapy. It was recommended that she receive a pharyngeal flap and be evaluated again several weeks after the operation. The surgery was successful and had an amazingly positive effect on Barbara's speech. Although hypernasality disappeared, some slight nasal emission remained. Barbara was subsequently enrolled in individual speech therapy, where she experienced total success in developing normal fricative–affricate production.

Such a case dramatically shows the futility of continued speech therapy when real structural inadequacy exists. Without the operation, Barbara could have received speech therapy for the rest of her life, with no effect whatsoever on her speech. If velopharyngeal insufficiency is found, there are two primary alternatives for treatment, surgical or dental. When structural adequacy is achieved, remediation services of the speech–language pathologist can produce further changes in the patient's speech and resonance.

Surgical Treatment for Hypernasality.   The evaluation may reveal the existence of such structural inadequacies as open fistulas, open bony and soft tissue clefts, submucosal clefts, and short or relatively immobile soft palates. The plastic surgeon is usually the medical specialist most experienced in making decisions about when and if surgical closure of palatal openings is required, based on the recommendation of the speech–language pathologist. The speech pathologist is best able to assess the adequacy of the velopharyngeal port mechanism during speech. Usually, the major reason (often the only reason) for surgical or prosthetic treatment in these patients is to improve speech.

A plastic surgeon wrote, "The surgeon requires the involvement of the speech pathologist in diagnosis as well as therapy" (Grace, 1984, p. 152). This includes preoperative testing, pressure and flow measurements, and mutual evaluation of cineradiographic studies. Paralleling the widespread use of direct endoscopic visual observation in medicine, the development of oral and nasoendoscopy has become an indispensable tool for diagnosing many speech disorders. Although nasoendoscopy is used by some plastic surgeons, it is also often used by speech–language pathologists. It should be routinely available in centers managing organically based resonance disorders.

When the diagnostic tests have been completed, the speech pathologist and surgeon must arrive at the plan for management. The speech pathologist should be familiar with available options for anatomic correction and should participate in the decision for surgery. "The surgeon must know the alternative treatments and anticipated results of his operations. The timing of surgery can be a mutual decision" (Grace, 1984, p. 152). For those individuals who have cleft palate, the primary surgical procedure usually involves closing the cleft and still maintaining adequate palatal length. Most patients with cleft palate, however, require multiple secondary surgical procedures at later times, such as rebuilding structures or eliminating earlier surgical scars. Many patients with hypernasality have velums that are too short for closure or velums that do not move adequately for closure. Such patients often profit from a surgically constructed pharyngeal flap.

In this procedure, the surgeon takes a small piece of mucosal tissue from the pharynx and uses it to bridge the excessive velopharyngeal opening, attaching the tissue to the soft palate. This tissue acts as a substitute structure for an inadequate velum by deflecting both airflow and sound waves into the oral cavity and allowing the walls of the pharynx to close adequately onto the lateral margins of the pharyngeal flap. Bzoch (1989), discussing the physiological and speech results for forty patients who had received pharyngeal flap surgery, reported that the procedure was most effective in reducing both hypernasality and nasal emission (if present) in most of the subjects. Although pharyngeal flap surgery, or any other form of palatal surgery, must not be considered a panacea for all resonance problems, it often helps align oral–nasal structures in such a way that (allowing open or closed coupling of the nasal and oral cavity), for the first time, speech and voice therapy can be effective.

Regarding the use of surgical methods to correct speech problems, Grace observed:

> Postoperative speech testing is mandatory to objectively evaluate the results of surgery and reassess speech goals. The surgeon may profit from observing a postoperative evaluation, much as the speech pathologist would profit from seeing surgery. All too often there is a tendency for the surgeon to divorce the patient when the surgery is completed, with the expectation that the battle will be won or lost by the speech pathologist (Grace, 1984, p. 154).

When speaking of surgery in cleft palate patients, Grace went on to say: "In truth, the success of surgery varies widely from patient to patient, and it cannot be assumed that anatomy is restored to normal upon completion of the operation" (p. 154).

Dental Treatment of Hypernasality. Both orthodontists and prosthodontists can play important roles in treating individuals with hypernasality, particularly those with cleft palate. The orthodontist may have to expand the dental arches so that the patient can experience more normal palatal growth and dentition. The prosthodontist, by constructing various prosthetic speech appliances and obturators, may be able to help the patient preserve his or her facial contour and, by filling in various maxillary defects with prostheses, may cover open palatal defects such as fistulas and clefts. The prosthodontist may also be able to build speech-training appliances to provide posterior velopharyngeal closure. In evaluating twenty-one adults with acquired or congenital palate problems, Arndt, Shelton, and Bradford (1965) found that both groups made significant "articulation and voice gains with obturation." Many cleft-palate subjects are fitted by prosthodontists with acrylic bulbs at the ends of their appliances; if the bulbs are well positioned near the posterior and lateral pharyngeal walls, often a noticeable reduction of both nasality and air escape results. Articulation, which is dependent on adequate intraoral air pressure and normal resonance, may be achieved with speech–voice therapy in conjunction with a properly fitted speech appliance such as an obturator or palatal lift device. Two lateral views of obturators are shown in Figure 9.5. Figure 9.6 shows a palatal lift device designed for an adult male with a paralyzed palate following traumatic brain injury in an accident.

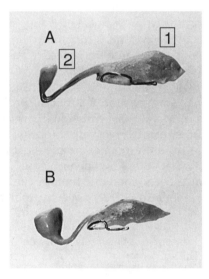

FIGURE 9.5   Two Views of Speech Appliances (Obturators) *(A) is from an adult with a neurogenic (dysarthria) problem of hypernasality; (B) is from a five-year-old girl with structural (cleft palate) hypernasality with an extremely short velum following surgical repair. (1) is the palatal part, and (2) is the pharyngeal part. Note that the size of the pharyngeal part of the adult appliance is smaller than the corresponding part of the child's prosthesis.*

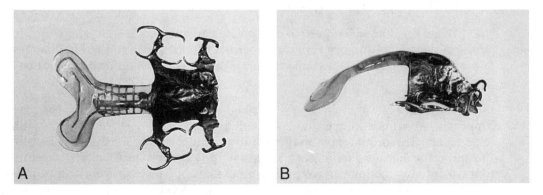

FIGURE 9.6   A Palatal Lift Device *(A) is a superior or top view; (B) is a lateral or side view.*

When commenting on the role of the speech pathologist in the prosthodontic management of patients with velopharyngeal inadequacy, Ahlstrom (1984), a prosthodontist, stated, "One of the primary diagnostic services that a speech pathologist can offer is the determination of velopharyngeal competence in patients. This helps the prosthodontist in determination of what type of appliance or procedure may be necessary" (p. 150). Many patients with dysarthria, which may include a hypernasality component, have immobile velums and thus lack sufficient velar movement to achieve closure. Such patients, who experience weakened or paralyzed soft palates, might well profit from consulting a prosthodontist about being fitted with a lift appliance to hold the immobile palate in a higher position so that some pharyngeal contact will be possible (Mazaheri, 1979). The palatal lift in Figure 9.6 was made for just such a patient who now has normal resonance with the device. For nasality problems related to velopharyngeal inadequacy, speech pathologists should freely consult both orthodontists and prosthodontists for their ideas on how to achieve adequate functioning of the oral structures.

Track 5

Voice Therapy for Hypernasality.   Any attempts at voice therapy for hypernasality should be deferred until both the evaluation of the problem and attempts at physical correction (surgical or prosthodontic) have been completed. The primary requirement for developing good oral voice quality is the structural adequacy of the velopharyngeal closing mechanism. Without adequate closure, voice therapy will be futile. However, for individuals who speak with hypernasality for functional reasons, voice therapy can help develop more oral resonance. Added to this group are occasional patients who have had surgical or dental treatment that has left them with only a marginal velopharyngeal closing mechanism; in voice therapy, this mechanism may be trained to work more optimally. Watterson, York, and McFarlane (1994) studied nasalance in the speech of thirty normal young adults and found that, while there was no statistical difference in nasalance scores under three different loudness levels, there was a strong systematic trend for the lowest nasalance scores to occur in the loudest conditions, while the highest nasalance scores occurred under the softest conditions. The implication is to experiment with increased loudness levels in cases of minimal or borderline VPI.

The Nasometer, mentioned earlier, is a less expensive and more practical adaptation or outgrowth of the Tonar II. The computer display gives the patient instant feedback information about the peak nasalance level, the target level of oral–nasal ratio, and the moment-to-moment level of nasalance. If the patient is capable of developing greater oral resonance, he or she works incrementally, using the Nasometer feedback system, toward goals of acceptable oral resonance. Various facilitating techniques (described in Chapter 6) may be used successfully with the Nasometer or with a tape recorder, nasal listening tube, U-tube manometer, Facilitator loop feedback, See Scape, nasal mirror, or stethoscope. They can even be used with the unaided ear. In a proposed new use of instrumentation, Kuehn (1997) has experimented with the use of continuous positive airway pressure (with sleep apnea equipment) as a possible means to reduce hypernasality. To date, studies of the approach seem to indicate that the levator veli palatini muscle works harder and contracts with more force when presented with positive airway pressure. This seems to be true for both normal people and those with repaired cleft palates.

Some techniques that have been helpful clinically are:

1. Altering Tongue Position. A high, forward carriage of the tongue sometimes contributes to nasal resonance. Efforts to develop a lower, more posterior carriage may decrease the perceived nasality.

2. Change of Loudness. A voice that has been perceived as hypernasal will sometimes be perceived as more normal if some other change in vocalization is made. One change that often accomplishes this is an increase in loudness; by speaking in a louder voice, the patient frequently sounds less hypernasal. (Watterson, York, and McFarlane, 1994). One should try both **increased and decreased** loudness levels with each patient to determine which condition best reduces nasality.

3. Auditory Feedback. If the patient is motivated to reduce his or her hypernasality, a great deal of therapy time should be spent learning to hear the differences between his or her nasal and oral resonances.

4. Establishing New Pitch. Some patients with hypernasality speak at inappropriately high pitch levels, which contribute to the listener's perception of nasality. Speaking at the lower end of one's pitch range seems to contribute to greater oral resonance.

5. Counseling. No voice therapy should ever be started without first explaining to the patient what the problem seems to be and the general course of therapy that is being planned.

6. Feedback. Developing an aural awareness of hypernasality with some oral–pharyngeal awareness of what hypernasality "feels" like is a most helpful therapeutic device.

7. Open-Mouth. Hypernasality is sometimes produced by an overall restriction of the oral opening. In such cases, efforts to develop greater oral openness may reduce the listener's perception of excessive nasality.

8. Focus. Although, for some patients, focusing on the facial mask area seems to increase nasality, for other patients, particularly those whose hypernasality is of functional origin, doing so noticeably improves resonance.

9. Respiration Training. Increased loudness is often achieved by respiration training.

These techniques achieve their results by altering the speech production, for example, by pitch modification, increased or decreased airflow, reduced air pressure on the velopharyngeal port, or enhanced feedback to the patient by using mirror fogging, acoustic changes, or changes in the location of vibratory patterns. We find these methods very successful with patients who have resonance disorders or whose velopharyngeal ports are "borderline adequate" or better. When the velopharyngeal mechanism is less adequate, surgical or prosthetic management is in order prior to initiating voice therapy techniques. When the degree of velopharyngeal mechanism adequacy is seriously in question, a period of intensive trial voice and articulation therapy may determine the need for other management approaches. This trial therapy should be intensive (three sessions per week minimum) but of short duration (six weeks), and it should be conducted with the understanding that it is a trial to determine if further therapy is indicated or if some other management approach is required. Under no circumstances should voice therapy for resonance disorders be continued when success is not forthcoming. Long periods of time without any progress are poor for motivation and the patient's self-image.

Denasality. Except for the nasal resonance required for /m/, /n/, and /ng/, vowels in U.S. English require only slight nasal resonance. In severe cases lack of nasal resonance produces actual articulatory substitutions for the three nasal phonemes as well as slight alterations of vowels. Denasality (hyponasality) is characterized by the diversion of sound waves and airflow out through the oral cavity, which permits little or no nasal resonance. More often than not, this problem is related to some kind of nasal or nasopharyngeal obstruction, such as excessive adenoidal growth, severe nasopharyngeal infection, as in head colds, large polyps in the nasal cavity, and so on. Some patients who are hypernasal before surgical or dental treatment emerge from such treatment with complete or highly excessive velopharyngeal obstruction. Perhaps the pharyngeal flap is too broad and permits little or no ventilation of the nasopharynx, or perhaps an obturator bulb fits too tightly (which can be easily reduced) and results in no nasal airflow or nasal resonance. Some kind of obstruction is the usual reason for a denasality problem, and the search for it must precede any attempt at voice therapy. We have seen a few cases, however, whose denasality was caused by psychological or other functional factors.

Nasal airflow competence can be tested simply as part of an overall resonance evaluation: Ask the patient to take a big breath, close his or her mouth, and exhale through the nose. Then test the airflow through each nostril separately, compressing the nares of one nostril at a time with a finger. If there is any observable decrement in airflow, the nasal passage should be investigated medically. Appropriate medical therapy (medications, reduction of turbinates surgically, septal repair, etc.) should precede any voice therapy for denasality. Only rarely do patients have markedly denasal voices for wholly functional reasons. Even though their denasal resonance may originally have had a physical cause, that cause may be no longer present, and the denasality may remain as a habit, a "set." One TV newsman with whom we worked had a denasal voice quality after many years of suffering from allergies. After moving to a new area of the country where the allergies were no longer a problem, he maintained his denasal voice by strength of habit until voice therapy produced a normal voice quality. Occasionally a patient has chosen a denasal voice as a model, for whatever reason, and has learned to match its denasality with some consistency. We once had a patient who would use a marked denasal voice quality when he was challenged at work. Voice therapy was helpful in both these cases.

Voice therapy for increasing nasal resonance might include:

1. Auditory Feedback. Considerable effort must be expended in contrasting for the patient the difference between the nasal and oral production of /m/, /n/,

and /ng/. Oral and nasal resonance of vowels can also be presented for listening contrast. The Facilitator mentioned in Chapter 6 can be helpful with this technique.

2. Counseling. The resonance requirements for normal English must be explained to the patient, and his or her own lack of nasal resonance, particularly for /m/, /n/, and /ng/, pointed out. If the patient's problem is wholly functional, this explanation is of primary importance.

3. Feedback. Emphasis must be given to contrasting what it sounds like and "feels" like to produce oral and nasal resonance. The patient should be encouraged to make exaggerated humming sounds both orally and nasally, concentrating on the "feel" of the two types of productions.

4. Nasal/Glide stimulation. This technique is one of the most powerful for denasality treatment. The phrases listed under this technique in Chapter 6 are very helpful ("Momma made lemon jam," etc.).

5. Focus. Direction of the tone into the facial mask is usually successful.

Assimilative Nasality.   The nasalization of vowels immediately before and after nasal consonants is known as *assimilative nasality.* Performance on stimulability testing will provide a good clue whether such nasal resonance is related to poor velar functioning or is functionally induced. A few neurological disorders, such as bulbar palsy or multiple sclerosis, prevent the patient from moving the velum quickly enough to facilitate the movements required for normal resonance. The velar openings begin too soon and are maintained too long, lagging behind the rapid requirements of normal speech and nasalizing vowels that occur next to nasal phonemes. Any patient who presents with sudden onset of hypernasality or assimilative nasality should be suspect for a neurological disorder or disease until proven otherwise and referral to a neurologist is in order. Most cases of assimilative nasality, however, are of functional origin, and the patient shows good oral resonance under special conditions of stimulability. Remember that in connected speech, all sounds are interdependent; as one sound is being produced, articulators are positioning for the next sound. This phonemic interdependence allows for a certain amount of assimilation, even in normal speech. Assimilative nasality, therefore, is another perceptual problem: Whether the speaker's nasalization of vowels adjacent to nasal phonemes is excessive or not depends on the perception of the listener. The perception of assimilative nasality is, of course, related to the perception of excessive nasality; a normal, minor amount of nasality in the vowels following nasal phonemes would not be perceived, and increased amounts of nasal resonance would be judged quite differently by different listeners, according to their individual standards and experience. Therapy for assimilative nasality is likewise highly variable. It is, in fact, largely related to the locale (in some areas such resonance is a normal voice pattern), the standards of the speaker or clinician, their motivations, and so on.

The Nasometer is a useful therapy instrument for the patient who wants to reduce his or her assimilative nasality. The clinician should be aware of the limitations of such instrumentation (Hardin et al., 1992; Watterson et al., 1993). The clinician and the patient can set oral–nasal ratio goals that favor orality and then work incrementally toward eliminating the assimilative nasal resonance. Voice therapy for assimilative nasality is best attempted only by those patients who are strongly motivated to develop more oral resonance. Facilitating approaches (see Chapter 6) might include:

1. Auditory Feedback. Ear training should help patients discriminate between their nasalized vowels and their oral vowels. Patients should listen to recordings of their own oral/consonant/vowel/oral/consonant words as contrasted with their nasal consonant/vowel/nasal consonant words, such as these pairs: *bad–man, bed–men, bead–mean, bub–mum,* and so on. Voice and diction books often contain word pairs matching monosyllabic words using /b/, /d/, and /g/ with those using /m/, /n/, and /ng/. Once the patient can hear the differences between oral and nasal cognates, determine whether he or she can produce them.

2. Counseling. Because nasal assimilations are difficult to explain verbally, any attempt at explanation should be accompanied by demonstration. The best demonstration is to present the contrast between oral and nasal resonance of vowels that follow or precede the three nasal phonemes.

Therapy for Oral–Pharyngeal Resonance Problems

Although during speech both the oral and pharyngeal cavities are constantly changing in size and shape, the oral cavity is the most changeable resonance cavity. Speech is possible only because of the capability for variation of such oral structures as the lips, mandible, tongue, and velum. The most dramatic oral movements in speech are those of the tongue, which makes various constrictive–restrictive contacts at different sites within the oral cavity to produce consonant articulation. Vowel and diphthong production are possible only because of size–shape adjustments of the oral cavity that require a delicate blend of muscle adjustment of all oral muscle structures. Although many individuals display faulty positioning of oral structures for articulation, and thus articulate "badly," fewer individuals are recognized to have problems positioning their oral structures for resonance. Slight departures in articulatory proficiency are much more easily recognized than are minor problems in voice resonance. Even though an articulation error may be viewed consistently as a problem, faulty oral–pharyngeal resonance is usually accepted as "the way he or she talks," or as a regional dialect. Nasality problems are more likely to be recognized by lay and professional listeners as requiring correction than are oral–pharyngeal resonance departures. Any judgment of resonance is heavily influenced by the appropriateness of pitch, the degree of glottal competence, as heard in the periodic quality of phonation, and the degree of accuracy of articulation. Because quality of resonance, then, appears basically to be a subjective experience, the goal in resonance therapy must be to achieve whatever voice "sounds best."

Singing teachers have long been aware of the vital role the tongue plays in influencing the quality of the voice, and they devote considerable instructional and practice time to helping singing students develop optimum carriage of the tongue (Coffin, 1981). Although the postures needed to produce various phonemes will attract the tongue to different anatomic sites within the oral cavity, with noticeable changes of oral resonance, more objective evidence of the role of the tongue in oral resonance may be obtained through spectrographic and video-fluorographic analysis. In the spectral analyses afforded by the spectrograph, we can study the effects of tongue positioning and the distribution of spectral formants. The second formant seems to "travel" the most, changing position up and down the spectrum for various vowel productions. Boone and McFarlane (1993) demonstrate this in their study of the "Yawn–Sigh Technique" (Chapter 6). The primary oral shaper for production of vowels appears to be the tongue. Decisions about quality of resonance (for example, is the voice hypernasal or denasal) are, however, almost impossible to render from the visual inspection of spectrograms. It is most difficult to quantify formant variations and relate them to variations in voice quality.

In describing the difficulty of spectrographic analysis, Moll (1968) has written that "this presumably more 'objective' measure involves overall judgments which probably are more difficult than those made in judging nasality from actual speech" (p. 99). Visual inspection of the spectrogram is a difficult task, particularly when one attempts to relate formant positioning to judgments of voice quality. As for the videofluorograph, its use for studying tongue, velar, mandibular, and pharyngeal movements, when such movements apply to voice quality, becomes far more effective when a voice track is added. The addition of the speaker's voice not only enables the viewer to match the sound of the voice with the analysis of the speaker's movements, but, more important, provides the viewer with the primary vehicle for determining whether a problem of quality exists. Quality judgments cannot be made from the visual study of oral movements alone, but depend primarily on hearing the sound of the voice. By using both the pitch and intensity readings at the same time on the Visi-Pitch, we have found that the stored tracings on the Visi-Pitch scope give useful information specific to better resonance. Often the resonance that sounds better to the ear is represented on the scope as less aperiodic (the frequency write-out has less scatter) and more intense (greater amplitude of the intensity curve). The "better-sounding" voice often comes quite unexpectedly as the clinician and the patient use various facilitating approaches in their search for good oral resonance. Once the "good" voice is achieved, the Visi-Pitch offers useful feedback for the patient, often confirming by improvement in the scope tracings the subjective judgments the clinician and patient have made.

Reducing the Strident Voice.   One of the most annoying oral–pharyngeal resonance problems is the strident voice. We use the term *stridency,* which means the unpleasant, shrill, metallic-sounding voice that appears to be related to hypertonicity of the pharyngeal constrictors (walls of the pharynx). Fisher (1975) described the strident voice as having brilliance of high overtones sounding "brassy, tinny, blatant." Physiologically, stridency may be produced by the elevation of the larynx and hypertonicity of the pharyngeal constrictors, which decrease both the length and the width of the pharynx. The surface of the pharynx becomes taut because of the tight pharyngeal constriction. The smaller pharyngeal cavity, coupled with its tighter, reflective mucosal surface, produces the ideal resonating structure for accentuating high frequency resonance. Stridency may be developed deliberately–for example, by a carnival barker or a store demonstrator for its obvious attention-getting effects—or it may emerge when a person becomes overly tense and constricts the pharynx as part of his or her overall response to stress. A person who has this sort of strident voice—and who wants to correct it—can, in voice therapy, often develop some relaxed oral–pharyngeal behaviors that decrease pharyngeal constriction (increasing the size of the pharynx) and lessen the amount of stridency. Anything that an individual can do to lower the larynx, decrease pharyngeal constriction, and promote general throat relaxation will usually reduce stridency. The following facilitating techniques (described in Chapter 6) are most helpful in greatly reducing stridency:

1. Inhalation Phonation. This tends to increase the size of the pharynx, relax the walls of the pharynx and open the laryngeal aditus.

2. Auditory Feedback. Explore various vocal productions with the patient, with the goal of producing a nonstrident voice. When the patient is able to produce good oral resonance, contrast this production with recorded strident vocalizations using loop tape feedback devices and following the various ear-training procedures. The Facilitator can be helpful here.

3. Establishing New Pitch. The strident voice is frequently accompanied by an inappropriately high voice pitch. Efforts to lower the pitch level often produce a voice that sounds less strident. We have found that a piano keyboard or an inexpensive electric keyboard or the CSL and even the Facilitator are valuable tools in helping patients find and establish a new pitch level or range that produces a much less strident-sounding voice.

4. Counseling. Although it is difficult to explain problems of resonance to someone else, sometimes such an explanation is essential if the patient is ever to develop any kind of self-awareness about the problem.

5. Glottal Fry. The glottal fry produces two beneficial effects. First, the fundamental frequency is somewhat lower following production of the glottal fry; second, the resonating cavity of the laryngeal aditus is enlarged following the production of the glottal fry (especially on ingressive glottal fry). The relaxation of the folds and the opening of the laryngeal aditus effectively reduce strident vocal quality.

6. Hierarchy Analysis. For the individual whose voice becomes strident whenever he or she is tense, it is important to try to isolate those situations in which his or her nonstridency is maintained.

7. Open-Mouth. Because stridency is generally the product of over constriction, oral openness is an excellent way to counteract these tight, constrictive tendencies.

8. Relaxation. It is difficult to produce strident resonance under conditions of relaxation and freedom from tension. Either general relaxation or a more specific relaxation of the vocal tract is helpful in reducing oral–pharyngeal tightness.

9. Tongue Protrusion /i/. This increases the length and width of the pharynx (the whole throat cavity).

10. Yawn–Sigh. Because the yawn–sigh approach produces an openness and relaxation that is completely the opposite of the tightness of pharyngeal constriction, it is perhaps the most effective approach in this list for reducing stridency.

Improving Oral Resonance.   Two problems of oral resonance are related to faulty tongue position, a **thin type** of resonance produced by excessively anterior tongue carriage and a **cul-de-sac-type** produced by backward retraction of the tongue. The thin voice lacks adequate oral resonance, and its user sounds immature and unsure of himself or herself. This problem, which is somewhat common among both men and women, is characterized by a generalized oral constriction with high, anterior carriage of the tongue and only minimal lip–mandibular opening. The user of such a voice appears to be holding back psychologically, either withdrawing from interpersonal contact by demonstrating all the symptoms of withdrawal, or retreating psychologically to a more infantile level of behavior by demonstrating a "baby–like" vocal quality. The first type, who withdraws from interpersonal contact, employs his or her thin resonance situationally, particularly when he or she feels most insecure; the second type uses the thin voice, the "baby resonance," more intentionally, in situations in which he or she wants to appear cute, to "get his or her own way," and so on. The following facilitating approaches (described in Chapter 6) have been useful in promoting a more natural adult oral resonance:

1. Change of Loudness. When the resonance problem is part of a general picture of psychological withdrawal in particular situations, efforts to increase voice loudness are appropriate for overall improvement of resonance.

2. Digital Manipulation. This is especially helpful when the pitch of the voice is too high or the quality is breathy.

3. Establishing New Pitch. The thin voice is perceived by listeners to be drastically lacking in authority. Frequently, the pitch is too high. Efforts to lower the voice pitch often have a positive effect on resonance.

4. Focus. In Chapter 6, we looked at tongue position and its influence on voice quality. The "babylike" voice may disappear with greater posterior tongue carriage.

5. Glottal Fry. The larger pharyngeal adjustment produced by glottal fry is generally helpful to produce improved resonance.

6. Hierarchy Analysis. Symptomatic voice therapy is based on the premise that it is often possible to isolate particular situations in which we function poorly, with maladaptive behavior, and other situations in which we function comparatively well. By isolating the various situations and their modes of behavior, we can often introduce more effective behavior into "bad" situations in place of the maladaptive behavior. For those individuals who use a thin voice in specific situations, particularly during moments of tension, hierarchy analysis may be a necessary preliminary step to eliminate the aberrant vocal quality.

7. Open-Mouth. The restrictive oral tendencies of a thin-voiced speaker may be effectively reduced by developing greater oral openness.

8. Relaxation. If the thin vocal quality is highly situational and the obvious result of tension, relaxation approaches may be helpful, particularly when used in combination with hierarchy analysis.

9. Respiration Training. Sometimes direct work on increasing voice loudness requires some work increasing control of the airflow during expiration.

10. Visual Feedback. Those patients whose anterior resonance focus is related to situational tensions may use feedback apparatuses to become aware of their varying states of tension. Feedback is best used with relaxation and hierarchy analysis.

11. Yawn–Sigh. The yawn–sigh approach is an excellent way of developing a more relaxed, posterior tongue carriage.

Patients with a thin voice are often judged by listeners to be immature, young, or lacking in authority. We have provided successful voice therapy to several attorneys, managers, and executives who suffered from thin voice quality, which was ineffective in their work. We helped one attorney improve his voice and his performance in the courtroom and during client conferences by using the open-mouth and glottal fry techniques.

The cul-de-sac voice is found in individuals from various etiologic groups: patients with oral apraxia; cerebral palsied children, particularly the athetoid type, who have a posterior focus to their resonance added to their dysarthria; some patients with bulbar or pseudobulbar-type lesions, who have a pharyngeal focus to their vocal resonance; and deaf children. The cul-de-sac voice, regardless of its initial physical cause, is produced by the deep retraction of the tongue into the oral cavity and hypopharynx, sometimes touching the pharyngeal wall and sometimes not. The body of the tongue literally obstructs the escaping airflow and the periodic sound waves generated from the larynx below. Although such a voice is often found in individuals with neural lesions who cannot control their muscles, and among deaf children and adults, it is also produced situationally by certain individuals for wholly functional reasons. Such posterior resonance is very difficult to correct in patients who have muscle disorders related to various problems of innervation, particularly dysarthric patients. Resonance deviations in the deaf may be changed somewhat in voice therapy, as described in Chapter 7, by dealing with special problems. For individuals who produce cul-de-sac resonance for purely functional reasons (whatever they are), the following facilitating approaches from Chapter 6 are useful:

1. Auditory Feedback. If, in the search for a better voice, the patient is able to produce a more forward, oral-sounding one, this should be contrasted with his or her cul-de-sac voice by listening to auditory feedback.

2. Focus. The forward focus in resonance required to place the voice in the facial mask makes the approach a useful one for patients with a cul-de-sac focus. High front vowels and front-of-the-mouth consonants are particularly good practice sounds to use with the place-the-voice approach.

3. Glottal Fry. The production of the glottal fry opens the pharynx and the laryngeal aditus, thus enlarging the resonance cavity and adding to the openness of the whole vocal tract. The whole pharynx is relaxed, eliminating the cul-de-sac resonance.

4. Hierarchy Analysis. If cul-de-sac resonance occurs only in particular situations, perhaps at those times when the individual is tense and under stress, the hierarchy approach may be useful. If the individual can produce good oral resonance in low-stress situations, he or she should practice using the same resonance at levels of increasing stress, on up the hierarchy.

5. Nasal–Glide Stimulation. This helps to get a forward placement of the tongue and the sound and can be used in conjunction with focus.

6. Relaxation. Posterior tongue retraction during moments of stress is often a learned response to tension. The patient who can learn a more relaxed positioning of the overall vocal tract may be able to reduce excessive tongue retraction.

7. Tongue Protrusion /i/. Because the tongue is extended outside of the mouth and the pitch is elevated, the base of the tongue is pulled forward and out of the oral pharynx and this is emphasized with the /i/ vowel. This eliminates the retracted tongue position that produces the back quality.

8. Visual Feedback. Posterior focus of voice resonance may for some patients be situationally related to tension. Feedback is often useful for helping these patients monitor their varying tension states.

Summary

Resonance deviations of the voice are often produced by physical problems of structure or function at various sites within the upper airway. Primary efforts must be given to identifying any structural abnormalities and correcting these problems by dental, medical, or surgical intervention. Speech–language pathologists play an important role in the early evaluation and diagnosis of a resonance problem, as well as in providing needed voice therapy to correct the problem. For both organic and functional resonance problems, specific facilitating approaches are listed to help patients develop better nasal and oral resonance.

REFERENCES

*Aerophone II. Model 6800. (1995). Lincoln Park, NJ: Kay Elemetrics.

*B & K Real-Time Frequency Analyzer. Naerum, Denmark: Bruel & Kjaer.

*Computerized Speech Lab. (1997). Lincoln Park, NJ: Kay Elemetrics.

*Dr. Speech. (1997). Richmond, VA: Kelleher Medical Instruments.

*Facilitator. Model 3500. (1998). Lincoln Park, NJ: Kay Elemetrics.

*Hearit. (1995). 8346 N. Mammoth Dr., Tucson, AZ 85743.

*Language Master. 7100 N. McCormick Road, Chicago, IL: Bell and Howell.

*Nasometer. Lincoln Park, NJ: Kay Elemetrics.

*Nasometer. (1994). Lincoln Park, NJ: Kay Elemetrics.

*Phonatory Function Analyzer, FS-77. Nagashima Medical Instruments. Richmond, VA: Kelleher Medical Instruments.

*Phonic Ear Vois. 250 Camino Alto, Mill Valley, CA 94941. H. C. Electronics.

*PM 100 Pitch Analyzer. Lincoln Park, NJ: Kay Elemetrics.

*Tonar II. This instrument, developed by S. G. Fletcher in 1970, is no longer commercially available.

*Tunemaster III. Berkshire Instruments, 170 Chestnut Street, Ridgewood, NJ 07450.

*Visi-Pitch, Model 6087. Lincoln Park, NJ: Kay Elemetrics.

*Vocaid. Texas Instruments, Communication Builders, PO Box 42030, Tucson, AZ 85733.

*Vocal Loudness Indicator. Suite 806, 1630 Fifth Avenue, Moline, IL 61265. LinguiSystems.

*Voice Instrumentation. 1022 Nicollet Avenue, Minneapolis, MN 55043. Artic Arion Products.

*Voice Monitor. Hollins College, Hollins, VA. Communication Research Unit.

Abitbol, J. (1998). Laser voice surgery. Third International Workshop on Laser Voice Surgery and Voice Care. Paris.

Abitbol, J. (1994). Atlas of Laser Surgery. San Diego, CA: Singular.

ADVANCE for Speech–Language Pathologists & Audiologists. (1998). Voice improvement patterns following botulinum toxin injection. Advance, 7, 25.

Ahlstrom, R. H. (1984). Speech pathology: Views from medicine and dentistry. In S. C. McFarlane (Ed.), Coping with Communicative Handicaps. San Diego: College Hill Press.

Ainsworth, S. (1980). Disorders of voice. In G. M. English (Ed.), Otolaryngology (Vol. 4, Chap. 13). Philadelphia: Harper & Row.

American Cancer Society. (1980). Cancer facts and figures, 1980. New York: Author. American Journal of Respiratory and Critical Care Medicine, 155, 2.

Aminoff, M. T., Dedo, H. H., & Izdebski, L. (1978). Clinical aspects of spasmodic dysphonia. Journal of Neurology, Neurosurgery and Psychiatry, 41, 361–365.

Andrews, M. L. (1995). Manual of Voice Treatment: Pediatrics through Geriatrics. San Diego, CA: Singular.

Andrews, M. L. (1991). Voice Therapy for Children. New York: Longman.

Arndt, W. B., Shelton, R. L., & Bradford, L. J. (1965). Articulation, voice, and obturation in persons with acquired and congenital palate defects. Cleft Palate Journal, 2, 377–383.

Arnold, G. E. (1962). Vocal rehabilitation of paralytic dysphonia. Arch Otolaryngol, 76, 358–368.

Aronson, A. E. (1990). Clinical Voice Disorders: An Interdisciplinary Approach (3rd ed.). New York: Thieme-Stratton.

Aronson, A. E. (1985). Clinical Voice Disorders (2nd ed.). New York: Thieme-Stratton.

Aronson, A. E., Peterson, H. W., & Litin, E. M. (1966). Psychiatric symptomatology in hypernasality in cleft palate children. Cleft Palate Journal, 1, 329–335.

Aronson, A. E., & DeSanto, L. W. (1983). Adductor spastic dysphonia: Three years after recurrent laryngeal nerve resection. Annals of Otolaryngology, Rhinology, and Laryngology, 93, 1–8.

ASHA. (1998). The role of otolaryngologist and speech–language pathologist in the performance and interpretation of strobovideolaryngoscopy. ASHA Supplement No. 18, 40, 32.

ASHA. (1992A). ASHA's special interest divisions. Asha, 34, 17.

ASHA. (1992B). Vocal tract visualization and imaging. ASHA Supplement No. 7, 34, 37–40.

ASHA. (1991). Amplification as a remediation technique for children with normal peripheral hearing. Asha, 33, 22–24.

Baken, R. J. (1987). Clinical Measurement of Speech and Voice. Boston, MA: College-Hill.

Baken, R. J. & Daniloff, R. G. (1991). Readings in Clinical Spectrography of Speech. San Diego, CA: Singular Publishing Group.

Baken, R. J., & Orlikoff, R. F. (1988). Changes in vocal fundamental frequency at the segmental level. *Journal of Speech and Hearing Research, 31,* 207–211.

Balestrieri, F., & Watson, C. B. (1982). Intubation granuloma. *Otolaryngol Clin No America, 15,* 567–579.

Barry, H. C., & Eathorne, S. W. (1994). Exercise and aging: Issues for the practitioner. *Medical Clinics of North America, 78,* 357–377.

Behrman, A., & Orlikoff, R. F. (1997). Instrumentation in voice assessment and treatment: What's the use? *American Journal of Speech–Language Pathology, 6,* 9–16.

Benninger, M., & Jacobson, B. (1995). Vocal nodules, microwebs, and surgery. *Journal of Voice, 9:3,* 326–331.

Berkow, R., Beers, M. H., & Fletcher, A. J. (1997). *Merck Manual.* West Point, PA: Merck & Co.

Bickley, C. A., & Stevens, K. N. (1987). Effects of vocal tract constriction of the glottal source: Data from voiced consonants. In T. Baer, C. Sasaki, & K. Harris (Eds.), *Laryngeal Functioning Phonation and Respiration.* Boston: Little, Brown.

Blager, F. B. (1995). Treatment of paradoxical vocal cord dysfunction. *Voice and Voice Disorders, 5,* 8–11.

Blakeley, R. W. (1991). Voice assessment without instrumentation. *Seminars in Speech and Language, 12,* 142–53.

Blakiston, J. (1985). *Blakiston's Gould Medical Dictionary.* NY: McGraw-Hill.

Blaugrund, S. M., Isshiki, N., & Taira, T. (1992). Phonosurgery. In A. Blitzer, M. F. Brin, C. T. Sasaki, S. Fahu, & K. S. Harris (Eds.) *Neurologic Disorders of the Larynx.* NY: Thieme Medical.

Bless, D. M., & Swift, E. (1996). Paradoxical vocal fold dysfunction. Paper presented at American Speech and Hearing Convention.

Bless, D., & Saxman, J. H. (1970). Maximum phonation time, flow rate, and volume change during phonation: Normative information on third-grade children. Paper presented at American Speech and Hearing Convention.

Blitzer, A., & Brin, M. F. (1991). Laryngeal dystonia: A series with botulinum toxin therapy. *Annals of Otolaryngology, Rhinology, and Laryngology, 100,* 85–90.

Blitzer, A., Brin, M. F., Fahn, S., & Lovelace, R. E. (1988). Localized injections of botulinum toxin for the treatment of vocal laryngeal dystonia (spastic dysphonia). *Laryngoscope, 98,* 195–197.

Blom, E. D. (1995). Tracheoesophageal speech. *Seminars in Speech & Language, 12,* 191–204.

Blonigen, J. (1994). *Remediation of Vocal Hoarseness.* Austin, TX: Pro-Ed.

Blood, G. W., Luther, A. R., & Stemple, J. C. (1992). Coping and adjustment in alaryngeal speakers. *American Journal of Speech–Language Pathology, 1,* 63–69.

Boone, D. R. (1998). *Facilitator Application Manual.* Lincoln Park, NJ: Kay Elemetrics.

Boone, D. R. (1997). *Is Your Voice Telling on You?* (2nd ed.). San Diego: Singular.

Boone, D. R. (1996). Clinical relevance of controlling chaos and complexity: Implications for the speech pathologist. *Vocal Fold Physiology.* San Diego: Singular.

Boone, D. R. (1993). *The Boone Voice Program for Children* (2nd ed.). Austin, TX: Pro-Ed.

Boone, D. R. (1983). *The Voice and Voice Therapy* (3rd ed.). Englewood Cliffs, NJ: Prentice-Hall.

Boone, D. R. (1982). *The Boone Voice Program for Adults.* Austin, TX: Pro-Ed.

Boone, D. R. (1977). Voice disorders: Communicative disorders. *An Audio Journal for Continuing Education.* New York: Grune & Stratton.

Boone, D. R. (1973). Voice therapy for children. *Journal of Human Communication, 1,* 30–43.

Boone, D. R. (1971). *The Voice and Voice Therapy.* Englewood Cliffs, NJ: Prentice-Hall.

Boone, D. R. (1966a). Modification of the voices of deaf children. *Volta Review, 68,* 686–692.

Boone, D. R. (1966b). Treatment of functional aphonia in a child and an adult. *Journal of Speech and Hearing Disorders, 31,* 69–74.

Boone, D. R., & McFarlane, S. C. (1994). *The Voice and Voice Therapy* (5th ed.). Englewood Cliffs, NJ: Prentice-Hall.

Boone, D. R., & McFarlane, S. C. (1993). A critical study of the yawn–sigh technique. *Journal of Voice, 7,* 75–80.

Boone, D. R., & Plante, E. (1993). *Human Communications and Its Disorders* (2nd ed.). Englewood Cliffs, NJ: Prentice-Hall.

Borden, G. J., Harris, K. S., & Raphael, L. J. (1994). *Speech Science Primer: Physiology, Acoustics, and Perception of Speech* (4th ed.). Baltimore, MD: Williams & Wilkins.

Bouhuys, A., Proctor, D. F., & Mead, T. (1966). Kinetic aspects of singing. *Applied Physiology, 21,* 483–496.

Bowman, S. A., & Shanks, J. C. (1978). Velopharyngeal relationships of /i/ and /s/ as seen cephalometrically. *Journal of Speech and Hearing Disorders, 43,* 185–191.

Bradford, L. I., Brooks, A. R., & Shelton, R. L. (1964). Clinical judgment of hypernasality in cleft palate children. *Cleft Palate Journal, 1,* 329–335.

Brodnitz, F. S. (1971). *Vocal Rehabilitation.* Rochester, MN: Whiting Press.

Brodnitz, F. S., & Froeschels, E. (1954). Treatment of nodules of vocal cords by the chewing method. *Archives of Otolarngology, 59,* 560–566.

Brown, O. L. (1996). *Discover Your Voice.* San Diego, CA: Singular.

Bouchayer, M., & Cornut, G. (1988). Microsurgery for benign lesions of the vocal folds. *Ear, Nose, and Throat Journal, 67,* 446–466.

Buller, A. (1942). Nasality: Cause and remedy of our American blight. *Quarterly Journal of Speech, 28,* 83–84.

Bzoch, K. R. (1989). *Communicative Disorders Related to Cleft Lip and Palate* (3rd ed.). Austin, TX: Pro-Ed.

Case, J. (1996). *Clinical Management of Voice Disorders* (3rd ed.). Austin, TX: Pro-Ed.

Case, J. L. (1991). *Clinical Management of Voice Disorders* (2nd ed.). Rockville, MD: Aspen Systems.

Casper, J., Colton, R., & Brewer, D. (1986). Selected therapy techniques and laryngeal physiological changes in patients with vocal fold immobility. *Folia Phoniatricia, 38,* 288–289.

Cherry, I., & Margulies, S. (1968). Contact ulcer of the larynx. *Laryngoscope, 78,* 1937–1940.

Christopher, K. L., Wood, R. P., Eckert, R. C., Blager, F. B., Raney, R. A., & Soutrada, D. F. (1983). Vocal cord dysfunction presenting as asthma. *New England Journal of Medicine, 308,* 1566–1570.

Coffin, B. (1981). *Overtones of bel canto.* New Jersey: Scarecrow.

Colton, R. H., & Casper, J. K. (1996). *Understanding Voice Problems: A Physiological Perspective for Diagnosis and Treatment* (2nd ed.). Baltimore, MD: Williams & Wilkins.

Colton, R. H., & Casper, T. K. (1990). *Understanding Voice Problems: A Physiological Perspective for Diagnosis and Treatment.* Baltimore: Williams & Wilkins.

Colton, R. H., Woo, P., Brewer, D. W., Griffin, B., & Casper, J. (1995). Stroboscopic signs associated with benign lesions of the vocal folds. *Journal of Voice, 9:3,* 312–325.

Cooper, M. (1990). *Winning with Your Voice.* Hollywood, FL: Fell.

Courey, M. S., Shohet, J. A., Scott, M. A., & Ossoff, R. H. (1996). Immunohistochemical characterization of benign laryngeal lesions. *Annals of Otology, Rhinology, and Laryngology, 105,* 525–531.

Crumley, R. L., & Izdebski, K. (1986). Voice quality following laryngeal reinnervation by ansa hypoglossi transfer. *Laryngoscope, 96,* 611–616.

Curry, E. T. (1949). Hoarseness and voice change in male adolescents. *Journal of Speech and Hearing Disorders, 16,* 23–24.

D'Antonio, L. L., Wigley, T. L., & Zimmerman, G. J. (1995). Quantitative measures of laryngeal function following Teflon ® injection or thyroplasty type 1. *Laryngoscope, 105,* 256–262.

Daniloff, R. G. (1973). Normal articulation process. In F. D. Minifie, T. J. Hixon, & F. Williams (Eds.), *Normal Aspects of Speech, Hearing, and Language.* Englewood Cliffs, NJ: Prentice-Hall.

Daniloff, R. G., (1985). *Speech Science.* San Diego: College Hill.

Darley, F. L., Aronson, A. E., & Brown, J. R. (1975). *Motor-Speech Disosrders.* Philadelphia, PA: Saunders.

Davis, P. J., Boone, D. R., Carroll, R. L., Darveniza, F., & Harrison, G. A. (1988). Adductor spastic dysphonia: Heterogeneity of physiological and phonatory characteristics. *Archives of Otolaryngology, 97,* 179–185.

Davis, P. J., Zhang, S. P., Winkworth, A., & Bandler, R. (1996). Neural control of vocalization: Respiratory and emotional influences. *Journal of Voice, 10:1,* 23–38.

Dedo, H. H. (1997). *Comments at Tenth Annual Pacific Voice Conference.* San Francisco.

Dedo, H. H. (1976). Recurrent laryngeal nerve section for spastic dysphonia. *Annals of Otology, Rhinology, and Laryngology, 85,* 451–459.

Dedo, H. H., & Carlsöö, B. (1982). Histologic evaluation of Teflon granulomas of human vocal cords: A light and electron microscopic study. *Acta Otolaryngology, 93,* 475–484.

Dedo, H. H., & Izdebski, K. (1983). Intermediate results of 306 recurrent laryngeal nerve sections for spastic dysphonia. *Laryngoscope, 93,* 9–16.

Dedo, H. H., & Jackler, R. K. (1982). Laryngeal papilloma: Results of treatment with the C02 laser and podophyllum. *Annals of Otolaryngology, Rhinology, and Laryngology, 91,* 425–430.

Delahunty, J., & Cherry, J. (1968). Experimentally produced vocal cord granulomas. *Laryngoscope, 78,* 1941–1947.

Dickson, D. R. (1962). Acoustic study of nasality. *Journal of Speech and Hearing Research, 5,* 103–111.

Diedrich, W. M., & Youngstrom, K. A. (1966). *Alaryngeal Speech.* Springfield, IL: Charles C. Thomas.

Djukanovíc, R., Homeyard, S., Gratziou, C., Madden, J., Walls, A., Montefort, S., Peroni, D., Polosa, R., Holgate, S., & Howarth, P. (1997). The effect of treatment with oral corticosteroids on asthma symptoms and airway inflammation. *American Journal of Respiratory Critical Care Medicine, 155,* 826–832.

Dursan, G., Sataloff, R. T., Spiegel, J. R., Mandel, S., Heurer, R. J., & Rosen, D. C. (1996). Superior laryngeal nerve paresis and paralysis. *Journal of Voice, 10:2,* 206–211.

Eckel, F. C., & Boone, D. R. (1981). The s/z ratio as an indicator of laryngeal pathology. *Journal of Speech and Hearing Disorders, 46,* 147–150.

Eliot, R. S. (1994). *From Stress to Strength: How to Lighten Your Load.* New York, NY: Chelsea House.

Ellis, P. D. M., & Bennett, J. (1977). Laryngeal trauma after prolonged endotracheal intubation. *Journal of Laryngology, 91,* 69–76.

Élö, J., Hídvégi, J., & Bajtai, A. (1995). Papova viruses and recurrent laryngeal papillomatosis. *Acta Otolaryngology, 115,* 322–325.

Eysenck, H. (Ed.). (1961). *Handbook of Abnormal Psychology.* New York: Basic Books.

Fairbanks, G. (1960). *Voice and Articulation Drillbook.* New York: Harper Brothers.

Fant, G. (1960). *Acoustic Theory of Speech Production.* The Hague: Mouton.

Farmakides, M. N., & Boone, D. R. (1960). Speech problems of patients with multiple sclerosis. *Journal of Speech and Hearing Disorders, 25,* 385–390.

Feldman, R. S. (1992). *Understanding Stress.* New York, NY: *Venture.*

Filter, M. D., & Urioste, K. (1981). Pitch imitation abilities of college women with normal voices. *Journal of Speech Hearing Association, 22,* 20–26.

Finitzo, T., & Freeman, F. (1989). Spasmodic dysphonia, whether and where: results of seven years of research. *Journal of Speech and Hearing Research, 32,* 541–555.

Fisher, H. B. (1975). *Improving voice and articulation* (2nd ed.). New York: Houghton Mifflin.

Fletcher, S. G. (1972). Contingencies for bioelectronic modification of nasality. *Journal of Speech and Hearing Disorders, 37,* 329–346.

Fletcher, S. G., & Daly, D. A. (1976). Nasalance in utterances of hearing impaired speakers. *Journal of Communication Disorders, 9,* 63–73.

Flower, W. M. (1991). Communication problems in patients with AIDS. In J. Mukand (Ed.), *Rehabilitation for Patients with HIV Disease.* New York, NY: McGraw-Hill.

Flower, W. M., & Sooy, D. C. (1987). AIDS: An introduction for speech-language pathologists and audiologists. *Asha, 30,* 25–30.

Ford, C. N., Bless, D. M., & Loftus, J. M. (1992). Role of injectable collagen in the treatment of glottic insufficiency: A study of 119 patients. *Ann Otol Rhinol Laryngol, 101,* 237–247.

Ford, C. N., Inagi, K., Bless, D. M., Khidr, A., & Gilchrist, K. W. (1996). Sulcus vocalis: A rational analytical approach to diagnosis and management. *Ann Otol Rhinol Laryngol, 105,* 189–200.

Froeschels, E. (1952). Chewing method as therapy. *Archives of Otolaryngology, 56,* 427–434.

Froeschels, E., Kastein, S., & Weiss, D. A. (1955). A method of therapy for paralytic conditions of the mechanisms of phonation, respiration, and glutination. *Journal of Speech and Hearing Disorders, 20,* 365–370.

Fujimoto, F. A., Madison, C. L., & Larrigan, L. B. (1991). The effects of a tracheostoma valve on the intelligibility and quality of tracheoesophageal speech. *Journal of Speech and Hearing Research, 34,* 33–36.

Gallivan, G. J., Hoffman, L., & Gallivan, K. H. (1996). Episodic paroxysmal laryngospasm: Voice and pulmonary function assessment and management. *Journal of Voice, 10:1,* 93–105.

Garfield, T. J., & Kimmelman, C. P. (1982). Neurological disorders: Amyotrophic lateral sclerosis, myasthenia gravis, multiple sclerosis, and poliomyelitis. *American Journal of Otolaryngology, 3,* 204–212.

Gerberding, J. L. (1988). Occupational health issues for providers of care to patients with HIV infection. *The Medical Management of AIDS.* Philadelphia: Saunders.

Gilbert, H. R., & Campbell, M. I. (1980). Speaking fundamental frequency in three groups of hearing-impaired individuals. *Journal of Communication Disorders, 13,* 195–205.

Gordon, M. T., Morton, F. M., & Simpson, I. C. (1978). Airflow measurements in diagnosis assessment and treatment of mechanical dysphonia. *Folia Phoniatrica, 30,* 372–379.

Gould, W. J. (1975). Quantitative assessment of voice function in microlaryngology. *Folia Phoniatrica, 27,* 190–200.

Grace, S. G. (1984). Speech pathology: Views from medicine and dentistry. In S. C. McFarlane (Ed.), *Coping with Communicative Handicaps.* San Diego: College-Hill.

Green, G. (1989). Psycho-behavioral characteristics of children with vocal nodules: WPBIC ratings. *Journal of Speech and Hearing Disorders, 54,* 306–312.

Greene, M. C. L., & Mathieson, L. (1991). *The Voice and Its Disorders* (5th ed.). London: Whurr.

Gumpert, L., Kalach, N., Dupont, C., & Contencin, P. (1998). Hoarseness and gastroesophageal reflux in children. *Journal of Laryngology and Otology, 112,* 49–54.

Hall, K. D. (1995). Variations across time in acoustic and electroglottographic measures of phonatory function in women with and without vocal nodules. *Journal of Speech and Hearing Research, 38,* 783–793.

Hall, S. W., & Merricort, R. D. (1995). Chemotherapy and radiation therapy for laryngeal cancer. *Seminars in Speech & Language, 12,* 233–239.

Hamaker, R. C., & Hamaker, R. A. (1995). Surgical treatment of laryngeal cancer. *Seminars in Speech & Language, 12,* 221–232.

Hardin, M. A., Van DeMark, D. R., Morris, H. L., & Payne, M. M. (1992). Correspondence between nasalance scores and listener judgments of hypernasality and hyponasality. *Cleft Palate-Craniofacial Journal, 29,* 346–351.

Harrison, G. A., Davis, P. J., Troughear, R. H., & Winkworth, A. L. (1992). Inspiratory speech as a management option for spastic dysphonia. *Annals of Otology, Rhinology, and Laryngology, 101,* 375–382.

Hartman, D. E., & Vishwanat, B. (1984). Spastic dysphonia and essential (voice) tremor treated with primadone. *Archives of Otolaryngology, 110,* 394–397.

Hirano, M. (1989). Surgical alteration of voice quality. In C. W. Cummings, J. M. Frederickson, L. A. Harker, C. J. Krause, & D. E. Schuller (Eds.), *Otolaryngology: Head and Neck Surgery.* Philadelphia: J. B. Lippincott.

Hirano, M. (1981). Clinical examination of the voice. New York: Springer-Verlag.

Hirano, M., Yoshida, T., Tanaka, S., & Hibi, S. (1990). Sulcus vocalis: Functional aspects. *Annals of Otology, Rhinology, and Laryngology, 99,* 679–683.

Hixon, T. J., & Abbs, J. H. (1980). Normal speech production. In T. J. Hixon, L. D. Shriberg, & J. H. Saxman (Eds.), *Introduction to Communication Disorders.* Englewood Cliffs, NJ: Prentice-Hall.

Hixon, T. J., Goldman, M. D., & Mead, J. (1973). Kinematics of the chest wall during speech production: Volume displacements of the rib cage, abdomen, and lung. *Journal of Speech and Hearing Research, 19,* 297–356.

Hoit, J. D. (1995). Influence of body position on breathing and its implications for the evaluation and treatment of speech and voice disorders. *Journal of Voice, 9,* 341–347.

Hoit, J. D., & Hixon, T. J. (1992). Age and laryngeal airway resistance during vowel production in women. *Journal of Speech and Hearing Research, 35,* 309–313.

Hollien, H. (1962). Vocal fold thickness and fundamental frequency of phonation. *Journal of Speech and Hearing Research, 5,* 237–243.

Hopkins, L. C. (1994). Clinical features of myasthenia gravis. *Neurologic Clinics, 12,* 243–261.

Hoshiko, M. S. (1962). Electromyographic investigation of the intercostal muscles during speech. *Archives of Physical Medicine & Rehabilitation, 43,* 115–119.

Inagi, K., Ford, C. N., Bless, D. M., & Heisey, D. (1996). Analysis of factors affecting botulinum toxin results in spasmodic dysphonia. *Journal of Voice, 10,* 306–313.

Iskowitz, M. (1998). In pursuit of natural sound. *Advance,* April 20, 7–9.

Isshiki, N. (1989). Medical displacement of the vocal cord. *Phonosurgery: Theory and Practice.* Tokyo: Springer-Verlag.

Isshiki, N., & von Leden, H. (1964). Hoarseness: Aerodynamic studies. *Archives of Otolaryngology, 80,* 206–213.

Izdebski, K., Dedo, H. H., & Boles, L. (1984). Spastic dysphonia: A patient profile of 200 cases. *American Journal of Otolaryngology, 5,* 7–14.

Jackson, C., & Jackson, C. L. (1942). Motor neuroses of the larynx. In *Diseases and Injuries of the Larynx* (pp. 287–294). New York: Macmillan.

Johnson, T. S. (1996). *Vocal Abuse Reduction Program,* Austin, TX: Pro-Ed.

Kantner, C. E. (1947). The rationale of blowing exercises for patients with repaired cleft palates. *Journal of Speech Disorders, 12,* 281–286.

Karnell, M. F. (1992). Adductor and abductor spasmodic dysphonia: Related until proven otherwise. *American Journal of Speech-Language Pathology, 1,* 17–18.

Kent, R. D., Kim, H., Weismer, G., & Kent, J. (1994). Laryngeal dysfunction in neurological disease: Amyotrophic lateral sclerosis, Parkinson Disease, and stroke. *Journal of Medical Speech-Language Pathology, 2:3,* 157–175.

Kingdom, T. T., & Lee, K. C. (1996). Invasive aspergillosis of the larynx in AIDS. *Otolaryngology Head and Neck Surgery, 115,* 135–137.

Kleinsasser, O. (1979). *Microlaryngoscopy and Endolaryngeal Microsurgery: Technique and Typical Findings.* Baltimore: University Park.

Koschkee, D. L., & Rammage, L. (1997). *Voice Care in the Medical Setting.* San Diego, CA: Singular.

Kotby, M. N. (1995). *The Accent Method of Voice Therapy.* San Diego, CA: Singular.

Koufman, J. A. (1991). The otolaryngologic manifestations of gastroesophageal reflux disease (GERD). *Laryngoscope, 101,* 1–78.

Koufman, J. A. (1986). Laryngoplasty for vocal cord medialization: An alternative to Teflon. *Laryngoscope, 96,* 726–731.

Koufman, J. A., & Blalock, P. D. (1991). Functional voice disorders. In J. A. Kougman & G. Isaacson (Eds.), *Voice Disorders: Otolaryngology Clinics in North America.* W.B. Saunders.

Koufman, J. A., Radomski, T. A., Joharji, G. M., Russell, G. B., & Pillsbury, D. C. (1996). Laryngeal biomechanics of the singing voice. *Otolaryngology Head and Neck Surgery, 115,* 527–537.

Koufman, J., Sataloff, R. T., & Toohill, R. (1996). Laryngopharyngeal reflux: Consensus conference report. *Journal of Voice, 10,* 215–216.

Kuehn, D. P. (1997). The development of a new technique for treating hypernasality. CPAP. *American Journal of Speech–Language Pathology, 6,* 5–8.

Larson, C. R. (1988). Brain mechanisms involved in the control of vocalization. *Journal of Voice, 2,* 301–311.

Laver, J. (1980). *The Phonetic Description of Voice Quality.* Cambridge, England: Cambridge University Press.

Lavorato, A. S. (1991). Evaluation and treatment of the professional voice with minimal instrumentation. *Seminars in Speech and Language, 12,* 154–167.

Lavorato, A. S., & McFarlane, S. C. (1983). Treatment of the professional voice. In W. H. Perkins (Ed.), *Current Therapy of Communication Disorders: Voice Disorders.* New York: Thieme-Stratton.

Lecoq, M., & Drape, F. (1996). Epidemiological survey of dysphonia in children at primary school. *Revue de Laryngologie Otologie Rhinologie, 117:4,* 323–325.

Leder, S. B., Ross, D. A., Briskin, K. B., & Sasaki, C. T. (1997). A prospective, double-blind, randomized study on the use of a topical anesthetic, vasoconstrictor, and placebo during transnasal flexible fiberoptic endoscopy. *Journal of Speech and Hearing Research, 40,* 1352–1357.

Leeper, H. A. (1976). Voice initiation characteristics of normal children and children with vocal nodules: A preliminary investigation. *Journal of Communication Disorders, 9,* 83–94.

Leeper, H. A., Millard, K. M., Bandur, D. L., & Hudson, A. J. (1996). An investigation of deterioration of vocal function in subgroups of individuals with ALS. *Journal of Medical Speech–Language Pathology, 4:3,* 163–181.

Lehmann, Q. H. (1965). Reverse phonation: A new maneuver for eliminating the larynx. *Radiology, 84,* 215–222.

Lewy, R. B. (1983). Teflon injection of the vocal cord: Complications, errors, and precautions. *Annals of Otology, Rhinology, and Laryngology, 92,* 473–474.

Lieberman, A. (1992). An integrated approach to patient management in Parkinson's disease. *Parkinson's Disease, 10:2,* 553–565.

Lim, R. Y. (1985). Laser arytenaidectomy. *Archives of Otolaryngology, 111,* 262–263.

Linviile, S. E. (1987). Acoustic-perceptual studies of aging voice in women. *Journal of Voice, 1,* 44–48.

Lu, F., Casiano, R. R., Lundy, D. S., & Xue, J. (1996). Longitudinal evaluation of vocal function after thyroplasty type 1 in the treatment of unilateral vocal paralysis. *Laryngoscope, 106,* 573–577.

Luchsinger, R., & Amold, G. E. (1965). *Voice–Speech–Language Clinical Communiculogy: Its Physiology and Pathology.* Belmont, CA: Wadsworth.

Ludlow, C. L., Naunton, R. F., Fujita, M., & Sedory, S. E. (1990). Spasmodic dysphonia: Botulinum toxin injection after recurrent nerve surgery. *Otolaryngology Head and Neck Surgery, 102,* 122–131.

Lundquist, P. G., Haglund, S., Carlson, B., Strander, H., & Lundgren, E. (1984). Interferon therapy in juvenile laryngeal papillomatosis. *Otolaryngology Head and Neck Surgery, 92,* 386–391.

Martensson, A. (1968). The functional organization of the intrinsic laryngeal muscles. In M. Krauss (Ed.), *Sound Production in Man* (pp. 91–97). New York: New York Academy of Sciences.

Mason, R. M., & Warren, D. W. (1980). Adenoid involution and developing hypernasality in cleft palate. *Journal of Speech and Hearing Disorders, 45,* 469–480.

Mazaheri, M. (1979). Prosthodontic care. In H. K. Cooper, R. L. Harding, M. M. Krogman, M. Mazaheri, & R. T. Millard (Eds.), *Cleft Palate and Cleft Lip: A Team Approach.* Philadelphia: Saunders.

McFarlane, S. C. (1990). Videolaryngoendoscopy and voice disorders. *Seminars in Speech and Language, 11,* 162–171.

McFarlane, S. C. (1988). Treatment of benign laryngeal disorders with traditional methods and techniques of voice therapy. *Ear, Nose, and Throat 1, 67,* 425–435.

McFarlane, S. C., & Brophy, J. W. (1992). *Effects of drugs on voice. ASHA Special Interest Division 2: Voice, 2,* 9–10.

McFarlane, S. C., Fujiki, M., & Brinton, B. (1984). *Coping with Communicative Handicaps: Resources for the Practicing Clinician.* San Diego, CA: College Hill.

McFarlane, S. C., Holt, T. L., & Lavorato, A. S. (1985). Unilateral cord paralysis: Vocal characteristics following three methods of treatment. *Asha, 27,* 114.

McFarlane, S. C., Holt-Romeo, T. L., Lavorato, A. S., & Warner, L. (1991). Unilateral vocal fold paralysis: Perceived vocal quality following three methods of treatment. *American Journal of Speech–Language Pathology, 1,* 45–48.

McFarlane, S. C., & Lavorato, A. S. (1984). The use of videoendoscopy in the evaluation and treatment of dysphonia. *Communicative Disorders, 9,* 117–126.

McFarlane, S. C., & Lavorato, A. S. (1983). Treatment of psychogenic hyperfunctional voice disorders. In W. H. Perkins (Ed.), *Current Therapy of Communication Disorders: Voice disorders.* New York: Thieme-Stratton.

McFarlane, S. C., Nelson, W., & Watterson, T. L. (1998). Acoustic, physiologic and aerodynamic effects of tongue protrusion /i/ in dysphonia. *ASHA Leader*, August, *18*, 72.

McFarlane, S. C., & Shipley, K. G. (1979). Spastic dysphonia: Laryngeal stuttering? *Asha, 21*, 710.

McFarlane, S. C., & Von Berg, S. (1998). Facilitative techniques in intervention for dysphonia. *Current Opinion in Otolaryngology & Head and Neck Surgery, 6*, 161–165.

McFarlane, S. C., & Watterson, T. L. (1995A). General principles of working to develop alaryngeal speech. *Seminars in Speech & Language, 12*, 175–180.

McFarlane, S. C., & Watterson, T. L. (1995B). Laryngectomee rehabilitation. *Seminars in Speech & Language, 12*, 175–239.

McFarlane, S. C., & Watterson, T. L. (1990). Vocal nodules: Endoscopic study of their variations and treatment. *Seminars in Speech and Language, 11*, 47–59.

McFarlane, S. C., Watterson, T. L., & Brophy, J. (1990). *Transnasal videoendoscopy of the laryngeal mechanisms. Seminars in Speech and Language, 11*, 8–16.

McFarlane, S. C., Watterson, T. L., Lewis, K., and Boone, D. R. (1998). Effect of voice therapy facilitation techniques on airflow in unilateral paralysis patients. *Phonoscope, 1*, 187–191.

McFerran, D. J., Abdullah, V., Gallimore, A. P., Pringle, M. B., & Croft, C. B. (1994). Vocal process granulomata. *Journal of Laryngology and Otology, 108*, 216–220.

McKinney, J. C. (1994). *The Diagnosis and Correction of Vocal Faults*. San Diego, CA: Singular.

McWilliams, B. J., Lavorato, A. S., & Bluestone, C. D. (1973). Vocal cord abnormalities in children with velopharyngeal valving problems. *Laryngoscope, 83*, 1745–1753.

Michel, J. F., & Wendahl, R. (1971). Correlatives of voice production. In L. E. Travis (Ed.), *Handbook of Pathology and Audiology*. Englewood Cliffs, NJ: Prentice-Hall.

Milisen, R. (1957). Methods of evaluation and diagnosis of speech disorders. In L. E. Travis (Ed.), *Handbook of Speech Pathology*. New York: Appleton-Century-Crofts.

Miller, R. H., Woodson, G. E., & Jankovic, J. (1987). Botulinum toxin injection of the vocal fold for spasmodic dysphonia. *Archives of Otolaryngology & Head and Neck Surgery, 113*, 603–608.

Minckler, J. (1972). Functional organization and maintenance. *Introduction to Neuroscience*. St. Louis, MO: C. V. Mosby.

Minifie, F. D. (1994). *Introduction to Communication Sciences and Disorders*. San Diego, CA: Singular.

Minifie, F. D. (1973). Speech acoustics. In F. D. Minifie, T. J. Hixon, & F. Williams (Eds.), *Normal Aspects of Speech, Hearing, and Language*. Englewood Cliffs, NJ: Prentice Hall.

Miyazaki, T., Matsuya, T., & Yamaoka, M. (1975). Fiberscopic methods for assessment of velopharyngeal closure during various activities. *Cleft Palate Journal, 12*, 107–114.

Moll, K. L. (1968). Speech characteristics of individuals with cleft lip and palate. In D. C. Spriestersbach & D. Sherman (Eds.), *Cleft Palate and Communication*. New York: Harper & Row.

Monsen, R. B. (1976). Second formant transitions in speech of deaf and normal-hearing children. *Journal of Speech and Hearing Research, 19*, 279–289.

Monsen, R. B., Engebretson, A. M., & Vernula, N. R. (1979). Some effects of degrees on the generation of voice. *Journal of Acoust. Soc. Amer., 66*, 1680–1690.

Moolenaar-Bijl, A. (1953). The importance of certain consonants in esophageal voice after laryngectomy. *Annals of Otolaryngology, Rhinology, and Laryngology, 62*, 979–989.

Moore, G. P., & von Leden, H. (1958). Dynamic variations of the vibratory pattern in the normal larynx. *Folia Phoniatrica, 10*, 205–238.

Morris, H. L., & Smith, J. K. (1962). A multiple approach evaluating velopharyngeal competency. *Journal of Speech and Hearing Disorders, 27*, 218–226.

Morris, R. J., & Brown, W. S., Jr. (1994). Age-related differences in speech intensity among adult females. *Folio Phoniatrica et Logapedica, 46*, 64–69.

Morrison, M., & Rammage, L. (1994). *The Management of Voice Disorders*. San Diego, CA: Singular.

Murdoch, B. E., & Chenery, H. J. (1997). *Dysarthria*. San Diego, CA: Singular.

Murray, J. F., & Nadel, J. A. (1994). *Textbook of Respiratory Medicine*. Philadelphia: Saunders.

Murry, T. & Doherty, E. T. (1980). Selected acoustic characteristics of pathologic and normal speakers. *Journal of Speech and Hearing Research, 23*, 361–369.

Murry, T., & Woodson, G. E. (1995). Combined-modality treatment of adductor spasmodic dysphonia with botulinum toxin and voice therapy. *Journal of Voice, 9*, 460–465.

Nash, E. A., & Ludlow, C. L. (1996). Laryngeal muscle activity during speech breaks in adductor spasmodic dysphonia. *Laryngoscope, 106*, 484–489.

Negus, V. E. (1957). The mechanism of the larynx. *Laryngoscope, 67*, 961–986.

Netsell, R. (1973). Speech physiology. In F. D. Minifie, T. J. Hixon, & F. Williams (Eds.), *Normal Aspects of Speech, Hearing, and Language*. Englewood Cliffs, NJ: Prentice-Hall.

Netsell, R., & Hixon, T. J. (1978). A noninvasive method for clinically estimating subglottal air pressure. *Journal of Speech and Hearing Disorders, 43*, 326–330.

Newby, H. A. (1972). *Audiology.* New York: Appleton-Century-Crofts.

Offer, D. (1980). Normal adolescent development. In H. I. Kaplan, A. M. Freedman, & B. J. Sadock (Eds.), *Comprehensive Textbook of Psychiatry* (3rd ed.). Baltimore: Williams & Wilkins.

O'Hollaren, M. T. (1995). Dysphea and the larynx. *Annals of Allergy, Asthma, and Immunology, 75,* 1–4.

O'Hollaren, M. T., & Everts, E. C. (1991). Evaluating the patient with stridor. *Annals of Allergy, Asthma, and Immunology, 67,* 301–306.

Palmer, J. M. (1993). *Anatomy for Speech and Hearing* (4th ed.). Baltimore, MD: Williams & Wilkins.

Pauloski, B. R., Fisher, H. B., Kempster, G. B., & Blom, E. D. (1989). Statistical differentiation of tracheoesophageal speech produced under four prosthetic/occlusion speaking conditions. *Journal of Speech and Hearing Research, 32,* 591–599.

Pearl, N. B., & McCall, G. N. (1986). *Laryngeal function during two types of whisper: A fiberoptic study.* Paper presented at ASHA convention, Detroit.

Perkins, W. H. (1983). Optimal use of voice: Prevention of chronic vocal abuse. *Seminars in Speech and Language,* 4, 273–286.

Perkins, W. H. (1977). *Speech Pathology, an Applied Behavioral Science* (2nd ed.). St. Louis, MO: Mosby.

Perkins, W. H., & Kent, R. D. (1986). *Functional Anatomy of Speech, Language, and Hearing.* San Diego, CA: College Hill.

Pershall, K. E., & Boone, D. R. (1986). A videoendoscopic and computerized tomographic study of hypopharyngeal and supraglottic activity during assorted vocal tasks. In V. Lawrence (Ed.), *Transcripts of the Fourteenth Symposium: Care of the Professional Voice.* New York: Voice Foundation.

Peterson, G. E., & Barney, H. L. (1952). Control methods used in a study of the vowels. *Journal of the Acoustical Society, 24,* 175–184.

Pillsbury, H. C., & Sasaki, C. T. (1982). Granulomatous diseases of the larynx. *Otolaryngologic Clinics of America, 15,* 539–551.

Plassman, B. L., & Lansing, R. W. (1990). Preceptual cues used to reproduce an inspired lung volume. *Journal of Applied Physiology, 69,* 1123–1130.

Pontes, P., & Behlau, M. (1993). Treatment of sulcus vocalis: auditory perceptual and acoustic analysis of the slicing mucosa surgical technique. *Journal of Voice, 7,* 365–376.

Prasad, U. (1985). C02 surgical laser in the management of bilateral vocal cord paralysis. *Journal of Laryngology and Otology, 99,* 891–894.

Ptacek, F. H., & Sander, E. K. (1963). Maximum duration of phonation. *Journal of Speech and Hearing Disorders, 28,* 171–182.

Ramig, L. O., Bonitati, C. M., Lemke, J. H., & Horii, Y. (1994). Voice treatment for patients with Parkinson disease: Development of an approach and preliminary efficacy data. *Journal of Medical Speech–Language Pathology, 2:3,* 191–209.

Ramig, L. O., & Verdolini, K. (1998). Treatment efficacy: Voice disorders. *Journal of Speech and Hearing Research, 41,* 5101–5116.

Renner, M. J. (1995). Counseling laryngectomees and families. *Seminars in Speech & Language, 12,* 215–220.

Rogers, J. H., & Stell, P. M. (1978). Paradoxical movement of the vocal cords as a cause of stridor. *Laryngology otology, 92,* 157–158.

Rosen, C. A., Woodson, G. E., Thompson, J. W., Hengesteg, A. P., & Bradlow, H. L. (1998). Preliminary results of the use of indole-3-carginol for recurrent respiratory papillomatosis. *Current Opinion in Otolaryngology and Head and Neck Surgery, 118:6,* 810–815.

Roth, C. R., Glaze, L. E., Goding, G. S., & David, W. S. (1996). Spasmodic dysphonia symptoms as initial presentation of amyotrophic lateral sclerosis. *Journal of Voice, 10,* 362–367.

Roy, N., Bless, D. M., Heisey, D., Ford, C. N. (1997). Manual circumlaryngeal therapy for functional dysphonia: An evaluation of short- and long-term treatment outcomes. *Journal of Voice, 11:3,* 321–331.

Roy, N., Ford, C. N., & Bless, D. M. (1996). Muscle tension dysphonia and spasmodic dysphonia: The role of manual laryngeal tension reduction in diagnosis and management. *Annals of Otology, Rhinology, & Laryngology, 105,* 851–856.

Roy, N., & Leeper, H. A. (1993). Effects of the manual laryngeal musculoskeletal tension reduction technique as a treatment for functional voice disorders: Perceptual and acoustic measures. *Journal of Voice, 7,* 242–249.

Salmon, S. (1986). Adjusting to laryngectomy. *Seminars in Speech and Language, 7,* 67–93.

Sansone, F. E., & Emanuel, F. W. (1970). Spectral noise levels and roughness severity ratings for normal and simulated rough vowels produced by adult males. *Journal of Speech and Hearing Research, 13,* 489–502.

Sapir, S., Keidar, A., & Mathers-Schmidt, B. (1993). Vocal attrition in teachers: Survey findings. *European Journal of Disorders of Communication, 28,* 177–185.

Sataloff, R. T. (1997a). Common infections and in-
flammations and other conditions. In R. T. Sataloff (Ed.), *Professional Voice: The Science and Art
of Clinical Care* (2nd ed.). (pp. 429–436). San
Diego, CA: Singular.

Sataloff, R. T., Ed. (1997b). *Professional Voice: The Science and Art of Clinical Care* (2nd ed.). San
Diego, CA: Singular.

Sataloff, R. T. (1997c). Voice surgery. In R. T. Sataloff
(Ed.), *Professional Voice: The Science and Art of
Clinical Care* (2nd ed.). San Diego, CA: Singular.

Sataloff, R. T. (1981). Professional singers: The science and art of clinical care. *American Journal of
Otolaryngology, 2,* 251–266.

Shanks, J. C. (1995). Coping with laryngeal cancer.
Seminars in Speech & Language, 12, 180–190.

Shaw, G. Y., Searl, J. P., Young, J. L., & Miner, P. B.
(1996). Subjective, laryngoscopic, and acoustic
measurements of laryngeal reflux before and
after treatment with omeprazole. *Journal of
Voice, 10,* 410–418.

Shelton, R. L., & Trier, W. C. (1976). Issues involved
in the evaluation of velopharyngeal closure.
Cleft Palate Journal, 13, 127–137.

Shelton, R. L., Hahn, E., & Morris, H. L. (1968). Diagnosis and therapy. In D. C. Spriestersbach &
D. Sherman (Eds.), *Cleft Palate and Communication.* New York: Academic Press.

Sherman, D. (1954). The merits of backward playing
of connected speech in the scaling of voice
quality disorders. *Journal of Speech and Hearing
Disorders, 19,* 312–321.

Shindo, M., Zaretsky, L. S., & Rice, D. H. (1996). Autologous fat injection for unilateral vocal fold
paralysis. *Annals of Otology, Rhinology, and
Laryngology, 105,* 602–606.

Shipp, T., Mueller, P., & Zwitman, D. (1980). Letter:
Intermittent abductory dysphonia. *Journal of
Speech and Hearing Disorders, 45,* 283.

Shipp, T., Qi, Y., Huntley, R., & Hollien, H. (1992).
Acoustic and temporal correlates of perceived
age. *Journal of Voice, 6,* 211–216.

Shulman, S. (1991). Voice therapy for spasmodic
dysphonia. *Proceedings of the Fourth Annual Pacific Voice Conference.* San Francisco.

Silbergleit, A. K., Johnson, A. F., & Jacobson, B. H.
(1997). Acoustic analysis of voice in individuals
with amyotrophic lateral sclerosis and perceptually normal vocal quality. *Journal of Voice,
11:2,* 222–231.

Singer, M. I., & Blom, E. D. (1980). An endoscopic
technique for restoring voice after laryngectomy. *Annals of Otolaryngology, Rhinology, and
Laryngology, 89,* 529–533.

Skolnick, M. L., Glaser, E. R., & McWilliams, B. J.
(1980). The use and limitations of the barium
pharyngogram in detection of velopharyngeal
insufficiency. *Radiology, 135,* 301–304.

Smith, E., Gray, S., Dove, H., Kirchner, L., & Heras,
H. (1997). Frequency and effects of teacher's
voice problems. *Journal of Voice, 11:1,* 81–87.

Solomon, N. P., & Hixon, T. J. (1993). Speech breathing in Parkinson's disease. *Journal of Speech and
Hearing Research, 36,* 294–310.

Spriestersbach, D. C. (1955). Assessing nasal quality
in cleft palate speech of children. *Journal of
Speech and Hearing Disorders, 20,* 266–270.

Stacy, M., & Jankovic, J. (1992). Differential diagnosis of Parkinson's disease and the parkinsonism plus syndromes. *Neurology Clinical, 10,*
341–359.

Stemple, J., Gerdeman, B. K., & Glaze, L. E. (1994). *Clinical Voice Management.* San Diego, CA: Singular.

Stemple, J. C., & Holcomb, B. (1988). *Effective Voice
and Articulation.* Columbus, OH: Merrill.

Stetson, R. H. (1937). Can all laryngectomized patients be taught esophageal speech? *Transactions
of American Laryngological Association, 59,* 59–71.

Stewart, C. F., Allen, E. L., Tureen, P., Diamond, B. E.,
Blitzer, A., & Brin, M. F. (1997). Adductor spasmodic dysphonia: Standard evaluation of symptoms and severity. *Journal of Voice, 11,* 95–103.

Stone, R. E. (1982). Management of childhood dysphonia's organic bases. In M. D. Filter (Ed.),
Phonatory Voice Disorders in Children. Springfield, IL: Charles C. Thomas.

Strauss, L., Hejal, R., Galan, G., Dixon, L., & McFadden, E. R., Jr. (1997). Observations on the effects
of aerosolized albuterol in acute asthma. *American Journal of Respiratory Critical Care Medicine,
155,* 826–832.

Stroebel, C. (1983). *Quieting Reflex Training for
Adults.* York: BMA Audio Cassettes.

Strome, M. (1982). Common laryngeal disorders in
children. In M. D. Filter (Ed.), *Phonatory Voice
Disorders in Children.* Springfield, IL: Charles C.
Thomas.

Strong, M. S., & Jako, G. J. (1972). Laser surgery in
the larynx: Early clinical experience with continuous CO2 laser. *Annals of Otology, Rhinology,
and Laryngology, 81,* 791–798.

Subtelny, J., Whitehead, R., & Klueck, E. (1989). Therapy to improve pitch in young adults with profound hearing loss. *Volta Review, 91,* 261–268.

Tait, N. A., Michel, J. F., & Carpenter, M. A. (1980).
Maximum duration of sustained /s/ and /z/
in children. *Journal of Speech and Hearing Disorders, 45,* 239–246.

Takahashi, H., & Koike, Y. (1975). Some perceptual dimensions and acoustical correlates of pathologic voices. *Acta Oto-Laryngologica, 338*, 1–24.

Tanaka, S., Hirano, M., & Umeno, H. (1994). Laryngeal behavior in unilateral superior laryngeal nerve paralysis. *Annals of Otolaryngology, Rhinology, and Laryngology, 103*, 93–97.

Templin, M. C., & Darley, F. L. (1980). *The Templin-Darley Tests of Articulation*. Iowa City: Bureau of Education Research and Service.

Thompson, A. E. (1978). Nasal airflow during normal speech production. Unpublished Master's Thesis, University of Arizona, Tucson.

Thurman, W. L. (1958). Intensity relationships and optimum pitch level. *Journal of Speech and Hearing Research, 1*, 117–123.

Titze, I. R., Jiang, J. J., & Lin, E. (1997). Populations in the U.S. workforce who rely on voice as a primary tool of trade: A preliminary report. *Journal of Voice, 11:3*, 254–259.

Titze, I. R., Lemke, J., & Montequin, D. (1997). Populations in the U.S. Workforce Who Rely on Voice as a Primary Tool of Trade. *Journal of Voice, 11*, 254–259.

Toohill, R. J. (1975). The psychosomatic aspects of children with vocal nodules. *Archives of Otolaryngology, 101*, 591–595.

Trudeau, M. D. (1998). Paradoxical vocal cord dysfunction among juveniles. *Voice and Voice Disorders, 8*, 11–13.

Tucker, H. M., & Lavertu, P. (1992). Paralysis and paresis of the vocal folds. In A. Blitzer, M. F. Brin, C. T. Sasaki, & K. S. Harris (Eds.), *Neurologic Disorders of the Larynx*. New York, NY: Thieme Medical.

Tucker, H. M., Wood, B. G., Levine, H., & Katz, R. (1979). Glottic reconstruction after near total laryngectomy. *Laryngoscope, 89*, 609–618.

Tyler, A. A., & Watterson, T. L. (1991). VOT as an indirect measure of laryngeal function. *Seminars in Speech & Language, 12*, 131–141.

Van den Berg, J. W. (1968). Register problems. In M. Krauss (Ed.), *Sound Production in Man*. New York: New York Academy of Sciences.

Varvares, M. A., Montgomery, W. W., & Hillman, R. E. (1995). Teflon granuloma of the larynx: Etiology, pathophysiology, and management. *Annals of Otology, Rhinology, and Laryngology, 104:7*, 511–515.

Von Berg, S. (1996). The efficacy of visual feedback in reducing abnormal pitch and nasalance in the deaf. Unpublished Master's Thesis, University of Nevada, Reno.

Warren, D. W. (1979). PERCI: A method for rating palatal efficiency. *Cleft Palate Journal, 16*, 279–285.

Watterson, T. L. (1991). Current trends in voice evaluation. *Seminars in Speech and Language, 12*, 57–64.

Watterson, T. L., Cox, T. L., & McFarlane, S. C. (1998). Speech intelligibility using four different electric-neck larynges. *Phonoscope, 1*, 21–26.

Watterson, T. L., Gibbins, C., & McFarlane, S. C. (1998). Diagnosis of adductor spasmodic dysphonia: A survey. *Phonoscope, 1*, 193–202.

Watterson, T., Hansen-Magorian, H., & McFarlane, S. C. (1990). A demographic description of laryngeal contact ulcer patients. *Journal of Voice, 4*, 71–75.

Watterson, T. L., Hinton, J., & McFarlane, S. C. (1996). Novel stimuli for obtaining nasalance measures from young children. *Cleft Palate-Craniofacial Journal, 33*, 67–73.

Watterson, T. L., Lewis, K. E., & Deutsch, C. (1998). Nasalance and nasality in low pressure and high pressure speech. *Cleft Palate-Craniofacial Journal, 35*, 293–298.

Watterson, T. L., & McFarlane, S. C. (1995). The artificial larynx. *Seminars in Speech and Language, 12*, 205–215.

Watterson, T., & McFarlane, S. C. (1992). Adductor and abductor spasmodic dysphonia: Different disorders. *American Journal of Speech–Language Pathology, 1*, 19–20.

Watterson, T. L., & McFarlane, S. C. (1991). Transoral and transnasal laryngeal endoscopy. *Seminars in Speech and Language, 12*, 77–87.

Watterson, T. L., & McFarlane, S. C. (1990). Transnasal videoendoscopy of the velopharyngeal port mechanism. *Seminars in Speech and Language, 11*, 27–37.

Watterson, T. L., McFarlane, S. C., & Brophy, J. W. (1990). Some issues and ethics in oral and nasal videoendoscopy. *Seminars in Speech and Language, 11*, 1–7.

Watterson, T., McFarlane, S. C., & Diamond, K. L. (1993). Phoneme effects on vocal effort and vocal quality. *American Journal of Speech and Language Pathology, 2*, 74–78.

Watterson, T., McFarlane, S. C., & Menicucci, A. (1990). Vibratory characteristics of Teflon-injected and noninjected paralyzed vocal folds. *Journal of Speech and Hearing Disorders, 55*, 61–66.

Watterson, T., McFarlane, S. C., & Wright, D. (1993). Nasalance (nasometer), nasality and speech intelligibility. *Journal of Communication Disorders, 26*, 13–28.

Watterson, T. L., York, S. L., & McFarlane, S. C. (1994). Effect of vocal loudness on nasalance measures. *Journal of Communication Disorders, 27*, 257–262.

Weed, D. T., Jewett, B. S., Rainey, C., Zealear, D. L., Stone, R. E., Ossoff, R. H., & Netterville, J. L.

(1996). Long-term follow-up of recurrent laryn-geal nerve avulsion for the treatment of spastic dysphonia. *Annals of Otology, Rhinology, and Laryngology, 105,* 592–601.

Weiss, L., & McFarlane, S. C. (1998) Responses to clinical stimulation as prognostic indicators of vocal recovery. *Phonoscope, 1,* 165–177.

Wetmore, S. I., Key, J. M., & Suen, J. Y. (1985). Complications of laser surgery for laryngeal papillomatosis. *Laryngoscope, 95,* 798–801.

Whited, R. E. (1979). Laryngeal dysfunction following prolonged intubation. *Annals of Otolaryngology, Rhinology, and Laryngology, 89,* 474–478.

Williamson, A. B. (1945). Diagnosis and treatment of seventy-two cases of hoarse voice. *Quarterly Journal of Speech, 31,* 189–202.

Wilson, D. K. (1987). *Voice Problems of Children* (3rd ed.). Baltimore: Williams & Wilkins.

Wilson, F. B., Oldring, D. J., & Mueller, J. (1980). Recurrent laryngeal nerve dissection: A case report involving return of spastic dysphonia after initial surgery. *Journal of Speech and Hearing Disorders, 45,* 112–118.

Wolpe, J. (1987). *Essential Principles and Practices of Behavior Therapy.* Phoenix: Milton H. Erickson Foundation.

Woo, P., Casper, J., Colton, R., & Brewer, D. (1992). Dysphonia in the aging: Physiology versus disease. *Laryngoscope, 102,* 139–144.

Yamaguchi, H., Yotsukura, Y., Kondo, R., Hanyuu, Y., Horiguchi, S., Imaizumi, S., & Hirose, H. (1986). Nonsurgical therapy for vocal nodules. *Folia Phoniatrica, 38,* 372–373.

Yanagihara, N. Y., & von Leden, H. (1967). Respiration and phonation. *Folia Phoniatrica, 19,* 153–166.

Yates, A., & Dedo, H. H. (1984). Carbon dioxide laser enucleation of polypoid vocal cords. *Laryngoscope, 94,* 731–736.

Yorkston, K. M., Beukelman, D. R., & Bell, K. R. (1988). *Clinical Management of Dysarthric Speakers.* Austin, TX: Pro-Ed.

Yorkston, K. M., Miller, R. M., & Strand, E. A. (1994). *Management of Speech and Swallowing in Degenerative Diseases.* Tuscon, AZ: Communication Skill Builders.

Yorkston, K. M., Strand, E., Miller, R., Hillel, A., & Smith, K. (1993). Speech deterioration in amyotrophic lateral sclerosis: Implications for the timing of intervention. *Journal of Medical Speech–Language Pathology, 1:1,* 35–46.

Zemlin, W. R. (1998). *Speech and Hearing Science: Anatomy and Physiology* (4th ed.). Englewood Cliffs, NJ: Prentice-Hall.

Zemlin, W. R. (1988). *Speech and Hearing Science: Anatomy and Physiology.* (3rd ed.). Englewood Cliffs, NJ: Prentice-Hall.

Zwitman, D. H. (1990). Utilization of transoral endoscopy to assess velopharyngeal closure. *Seminars in Speech and Language, 11,* 38–46.

Zwitman, D. H., Gyepes, M. T., & Ward, P. H. (1976). Assessment of velar and lateral wall movement by oral telescope and radiographic examination in patients with velopharyngeal inadequacy and in normal subjects. *Journal of Speech and Hearing Disorders, 41,* 381–389.

Zwitman, D. H., Sonderman, J. C., & Ward, P. H. (1974). Variations in velopharyngeal closure assessed by endoscopy. *Journal of Speech and Hearing Disorders, 39,* 366–372.

Zwitman, D. G., & Calcaterra, T. C. (1973). The "silent cough" method for vocal hyperfunction. *Journal of Speech and Hearing Disorders, 38,* 119–125.

INDEX